McGraw-Hill Education

TEAS
Review

McGraw-Hill Education

McGraw-Hill Education

TEAS Review

CARA CANTARELLA

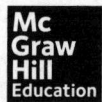

New York Chicago San Francisco Athens London Madrid
Mexico City Milan New Delhi Singapore Sydney Toronto

1 2 3 4 5 6 7 8 9 10   RHR/RHR   1 2 1 0 9 8 7 6 5

ISBN   978-0-07-184120-7
MHID   0-07-184120-2

e-ISBN   978-0-07-184121-4
e-MHID   0-07-184121-0

TEAS® is a trademark of Assessment Technologies Institute™ LLC, which was not involved in the production of, and does not endorse, this product.

McGraw-Hill Education products are available at special quantity discounts to use as premiums and sales promotions or for use in corporate training programs. To contact a representative, please visit the Contact Us pages at www.mhprofessional.com.

Contents

CHAPTER 47   Active vs. Passive Voice   439

Introduction

If you're applying to nursing school and you've picked up a copy of this book, chances are you're already familiar with the Test of Essential Academic Skills (TEAS) and have decided you'd like help with reviewing what's on the test before taking the exam. This book focuses on just that: content review and review questions. Inside, you'll see content review regarding the major topics on all four subjects tested on the TEAS, and you'll also have 600 review questions to help reinforce your skills.

Before we begin, let's take a look at the subjects you'll encounter on the TEAS. We'll also make some recommendations regarding how to use this book for optimal results.

TEAS Overview

The Test of Essential Academic Skills is a test administered to nursing candidates to test exactly what the name implies: essential academic skills. These are fundamental skills that are considered to be required for success in nursing school. The skills tested fall into four subject categories: Reading, Mathematics, Science, and English and Language Usage. You will see them on the TEAS in that order. The TEAS V test has four sections, as described in the table below:

Subject	Number of Questions	Time Allowed
Reading	48	58 minutes
Mathematics	34	51 minutes
Science	54	66 minutes
English and Language Usage	34	34 minutes
Total	170	209 minutes

The Reading section of the test covers two main areas: paragraph and passage comprehension and informational source comprehension. Paragraph and passage comprehension questions test your understanding of what you read when reviewing academic passages, articles, advertisements, e-mails, and other forms of written correspondence. Informational source comprehension questions test your ability to gather information from maps, labels, diagrams, and other resources.

The Mathematics section of the test covers four subjects: numbers and operations, algebraic applications, data interpretation, and measurement.

Numbers and operations questions test your ability to perform basic math and to solve problems involving fractions, ratios, proportions, and percentages. Algebraic applications questions test your ability to solve problems involving an unknown quantity, and data interpretation questions require you to answer questions based on information obtained from graphs and charts. Measurement questions require you to measure various dimensions of an object and to convert measurements from one form to another.

The Science section of the test also covers four main areas. These are scientific reasoning, human body science, life science, and earth and physical science. Scientific reasoning questions test your understanding of the scientific method and principles underlying scientific inquiry. Human body science questions test your knowledge of the anatomy and physiology of specific body systems. Life science questions are largely concerned with cell biology, evolutionary biology, taxonomy, and genetics. Earth and physical science questions focus mainly on chemistry and Newtonian physics.

Finally, the English and Language Usage section of the test covers three subcategories. The first tests your understanding of grammar and the meanings of words based on their context. The second subcategory assesses your knowledge of the rules of spelling, capitalization, and punctuation. The third English subcategory, structure, tests your ability to recognize sentences that are well written, not just in terms of grammar but also in terms of style. This subcategory also tests your understanding of correct paragraph organization.

How to Use this Book

The content review presented in this book does not include every possible topic that might be tested on the TEAS V. Instead it presents a review of important topics you are likely to see on the test, and it explains different question types you may encounter.

Sometimes understanding what a question is asking for can be key to identifying the correct answer. In the Reading sections, for instance, you'll see some questions that ask about details from the passage, and other questions that ask you to draw conclusions based on information given in the passage. The answer to a detail question will *always* be given right in the passage, and the answer to a conclusions question will *never* be stated directly. Just knowing what to expect on these different question types can help you choose the correct answer.

While understanding the question types is important, there's no substitute for learning the content actually covered on the exam. This book is chock-full of relevant content, but how you choose to learn that content will depend on where the gaps in your knowledge lie—and the time you have to prepare.

If you feel fairly confident about certain sections of the test, you can focus your study on just those topics or sections that you feel are your weak areas. This approach works best if you have limited time to study as well. However, if you'd like to brush up on the content of the test as a whole, you can review each chapter of the book in its entirety. This "whole book" approach requires time and will work best if you have ample time in your study schedule to prepare for the test. It also has another distinct advantage: in addition to helping you improve your weak areas, it can help you strengthen the areas that are your strong suits. This way, you can pick up more points in the areas that you're already successful in to help boost your score.

Test Information and Registration

The TEAS is administered by ATI Nursing Education. To register for the test or to obtain more information, contact ATI at:

ATI Nursing Education

11161 Overbrook Road

Leawood, KS 66211

(800) 667-7531

(913) 685-2381

www.atitesting.com

For further practice on this exam we recommend *McGraw-Hill Education: 5 TEAS Practice Tests*.

PART 1

Reading

TEAS Reading questions test two different types of comprehension: paragraph and passage comprehension, and informational source comprehension. Paragraph and passage comprehension questions are accompanied by a single paragraph or an entire passage. These questions test your ability to understand the text that you have read. Informational source comprehension questions often include figures, such as maps or graphs, and excerpts from other resources, such as outlines, directions, or ingredient lists.

The questions that you'll see on the TEAS can be grouped into different question types, depending on the issues they address. They range in scope from overarching, big-picture questions to questions that test more in-depth detail.

CHAPTER 1
Main Idea

Main Idea questions test understanding of the overall content of a passage or selection. They ask about the general point or "big picture" idea. They are commonly phrased "What is the passage mainly about?" or "Which of the following best reflects the main idea of the passage?"

When answering Main Idea questions, keep in mind the following:

> The answer to a Main Idea question must not be too broad or too specific. It must be just right to capture the "big picture" of the passage.

Consider this example:

Public highways are used constantly with little thought of how important they are to the everyday life of a community. It is understandable that most people think about their local public highway only when it affects their own activities. People usually don't focus on highway improvements unless the subject is brought to their attention by increased taxes or advertising.

Highway improvements are an important issue, however. It is important for the economies of most communities to keep highways in good repair. Products purchased in one location are often manufactured in other locations, and safe highways are required to transport the products to their final destination. Good transportation facilities contribute greatly to community prosperity.

The type and amount of the highway improvement needed in any area depend on the traffic in that area. In low-population areas, the amount of traffic on local roads is likely to be small, and highways will not require as much work. But as an area develops, the use of public highways increases, and maintenance demands increase. In small towns, residents are also more able to adapt to the condition of the roads. A road shutdown does not have the same impact on business as it would in busy areas. In large districts with many activities, however, roads must be usable year-round in order for business progress to continue.

In planning improvements of highway systems, several different types of traffic may be encountered. These range from business traffic to agricultural shipping to residential transportation. Improvement activities must meet the requirements of all classes of traffic, the most important being provided for first. Those improvements of lesser importance can be performed as soon as finances permit.

Which title best conveys the main idea of the passage?

A. America's Rural Highways: How They Contribute to Economic Growth
B. America's Rural Highways: Their History and Development
C. America's Rural Highways: What Can Be Done About Traffic
D. America's Rural Highways: Why Improvement Is Important

The correct answer is **D**. Most of the article focuses on why improvement is an important issue for those who use rural highways. Therefore, choice D best captures the main idea of the passage. The passage mentions the economic role of the highways, but that is not the main idea, so choice A can be eliminated. There is little attention to history in the passage, nor does the passage focus on traffic control as an issue in itself, so choices B and D are also incorrect.

Some Main Idea questions ask you to identify what a passage is "mainly about," as in the example below. This passage concerns the town of Stratford-upon-Avon, where Shakespeare was born.

The English town of Stratford-upon-Avon is visited yearly by tourists wanting to view the birthplace of William Shakespeare. William's father, John Shakespeare, bought the family home on Henley Street, and it is here that William is believed to have been born in 1564. Shakespeare's birth home remained in his family until the early 1800s, and it is now a public museum.

Shakespeare attended school at the King Edward VI Grammar School, which occupied the first floor of a building known as the Guildhall. It was in this Guildhall that Shakespeare first experienced theater, when he saw a theatrical performance given by a group of traveling actors. The Royal Shakespeare Company still performs in the town at the Royal Shakespeare and Swan Theaters.

Close to the Guildhall is the site of a house known as New Place, which was bought by Shakespeare himself. Here Shakespeare lived during the later part of his life, until his death in 1616. Although he spent most of his career in London, with trips back to Stratford, he moved permanently to New Place in the last years of his life and is believed to have written some of his later works there. Only the foundations of the New Place house now remain.

In the town of Shottery, one mile from Stratford, is the cottage where Shakespeare's wife, Anne Hathaway, was born. The Hathaway cottage, now also a museum, is actually a large, thatch-roofed farmhouse with sprawling gardens where Shakespeare is believed to have developed his relationship with Anne. They married in 1582 and had three children.

What is this passage mainly about?

A. The importance of Stratford-upon-Avon for theatrical performances
B. The importance of Stratford-upon-Avon in Shakespeare's plays
C. The importance of Stratford-upon-Avon in Shakespeare's life
D. The importance of Stratford-upon-Avon in English history

The correct answer is **C**. This passage focuses on Shakespeare's relationship to Stratford-upon-Avon throughout his life. It does not mention whether the town appeared in his plays, although there is a short statement that he wrote some of his plays there. The passage does deal with theatrical performances and history, but those are broad topics and not the main idea.

Main Idea questions may sometimes ask you to identify which statement from the passage best reflects the "big picture" of the passage. Here, we are looking for the sentence that comes closest to describing the main idea, without being too broad or too specific.

One of the most important gymnastic exercises in the original Montessori school approach is that of the "line." For this exercise, a line is drawn in chalk or paint on the floor. Instead of one line, there may also be two lines drawn. The children are taught to walk on these lines like tightrope walkers, placing their feet one in front of the other.

To keep their balance, the children must make efforts similar to those of real tightrope walkers, except that they have no danger of falling, since the lines are drawn only on the floor. The teacher herself performs the exercise first, showing clearly how she places her feet, and the children imitate her without her even needing to speak. At first it is only certain children who follow her, and when she has shown them how to walk the line, she leaves, letting the exercise develop on its own.

The children for the most part continue to walk, following with great care the movement they have seen, and making efforts to keep their balance so they don't fall. Gradually the other children come closer and watch and try the exercise. In a short time, the entire line is covered with children balancing themselves and continuing to walk around, watching their feet attentively.

Music may be used at this point. It should be a very simple march, without an obvious rhythm. It should simply accompany and support the efforts of the children.

When children learn to master their balance in this way, Dr. Montessori believed, they can bring the act of walking to a remarkable standard of perfection.

Which of the following sentences best reflects the main idea of the entire passage?

A. Instead of one line, there may also be two lines drawn.
B. Music may be used at this point.
C. One of the most important gymnastic exercises in the original Montessori school approach is that of the "line."
D. The children for the most part continue to walk, following with great care the movement they have seen, and making efforts to keep their balance so they don't fall.

The correct answer is **C**. Choice C best reflects the main idea of the entire passage, because it introduces the "big picture" concept developed in the passage. The entire passage talks about the Montessori exercise of the "line." Choices A, B, and D reflect details from the passage; they are too narrow to be the main idea.

Let's look at two more examples:

Percy Bysshe Shelley was one of the second-generation Romantic poets. Along with John Keats and Lord Byron, Shelley was considered one of the most masterful poets of his generation.

Shelley was born in England in 1792, as a member of the aristocracy. He was educated at two prestigious English schools, Eton College and Oxford University. Shelley believed that poets were visionaries who could serve as societal leaders because of the creative power of their imaginations. The second generation of Romantic poets, in particular, believed that poets were going to help change the world. Shelley's generation believed that, through the imagination, anything was possible. They believed that they could use the creative power of the mind to change the government and even change the world. Shelley's poems reflect this belief. He was a truly idealistic thinker, and he claimed that poets were the "unacknowledged legislators of the world." The poet's creative vision could let him or her see things that other people could not.

Shelley's ideas were heavily influenced by the politics of his time. He grew up at a time when governments were under transformation. In fact, he came of age in the shadow of the French Revolution. This period was very violent, and since France was so close to England, Shelley was acutely aware of the violence that was occurring there. That may have led him to concentrate even more on his belief that artists were able to change the world and improve living conditions.

Shelley's poem "Mont Blanc" focuses on the Romantic notion of the sublime. The Romantic poets believed that when people interacted with Nature, it sometimes caused them to be in a state of wonder—or it caused them to be awestruck. For example, when a person gazed at a mountain, the huge size of the mountain could cause the person to become speechless with wonder. This was the effect that the sublime quality of Nature could have on a viewer.

In "Mont Blanc," Shelley describes the mountain in a way that attempts to explain its effects on the viewer's mind. According to Shelley, the mountain itself causes the viewer's thoughts to enter a kind of strange trance, and to be affected in a way that resembles how a poet or an artist feels whenever he or she is caught in the midst of a creative inspiration. In the poem, Shelley draws a comparison between the effect of the mountain on the viewer and the power that the imagination has over the artist's mind.

What is the passage mainly about?

A. It focuses on the history of the French Revolution.
B. It discusses English poetry that addresses Nature.
C. It covers Shelley's ideas about the imagination.
D. It deals generally with the artist's role in society.

The correct answer is **C**. The passage is mainly about how Shelley explores the role of the creative imagination and what it means for a poet. Choice A is incorrect because the discussion about the French Revolution is only a reference to the historical background in which Shelley lived; choice A is therefore too narrow to reflect the main idea. Although the passage does discuss English poetry that addresses Nature, the main focus of the passage concerns Shelley's views on how poets could use the power of imagination to help change the world. The passage describes what Shelley thought about the imagination specifically, so choice D can be eliminated, as it is too broad to capture the main idea.

Now try this passage:

CPR, an acronym that stands for cardiopulmonary resuscitation, is a widely utilized method of attempting to save someone's life. It is especially applicable to scenarios in which a patient's heart has stopped beating. Frequently, it is also used in cases where a person is in danger of drowning.

Almost all approaches to CPR suggest that a person begin resuscitation efforts with chest compressions. To perform a chest compression, the individual places both hands flat on the patient's chest and then begins pushing down carefully but firmly, most likely at equal intervals. The compressions should be counted, so that the individual can keep track of how many compressions have been administered. The unofficial recommendation of how many chest compressions to provide is around 100 per minute.

There are many resources through which potential lifesavers can acquire training and even certification so that they can more effectively administer this life-saving technique to a potential patient. However, the American Heart Association stresses that even if someone has not received any type of formal training, attempting to help a person who needs to be resuscitated is far better than offering no help. This is why 911 operators sometimes request that bystanders at the scene of an emergency administer CPR. The operators may even coach the bystanders verbally, over the phone. These approaches have been shown to be effective in many cases.

If a bystander at an emergency scene has received CPR training—even if the training occurred a long time ago—the bystander should attempt further techniques in addition to chest compressions, especially if the patient has been underwater. The lifesaver should start first by checking the patient's airway. He or she might also administer mouth-to-mouth rescue breathing. However, lifesavers should only perform these additional techniques if they are confident of their skills and remember their training. Otherwise, any potential lifesaver should just administer chest compressions.

Some important items to remember in administering CPR are as follows. First, the lifesaver should always check whether the patient is conscious or not. Verbal interaction or communication can be a key way of determining if a person is conscious. If the emergency is related to drowning, the lifesaver should start chest compressions. These should be conducted for about a minute or so before the lifesaver calls 911. However, if one person can perform the compressions, and there is another person available who can call 911, then these steps should happen simultaneously.

For persons who are trained in CPR, one of the best ways to remember the order in which steps should be administered is to recall the memory cue CAB. This cue stands for Circulation, Airway, Breathing. The goal of CPR is to help an unresponsive person to start breathing on his or her own. First, use chest compressions to restore circulation. This is the C of CAB. Second, check the patient's airway for possible blockages. The A in CAB stands for airway. Finally, administer rescue breathing. This is, of course, the B of CAB.

What is the passage mainly about?

A. It focuses on how to administer CPR techniques.
B. It focuses on several ways to save people in danger.
C. It covers various ways that people can learn about CPR.
D. It presents a review of how people can use CPR daily.

The correct answer is **A**. The passage is mainly about how to administer CPR techniques. Choice B is incorrect because the passage focuses more on CPR than on lifesaving approaches in general. The passage discusses how to use CPR and not how to learn about it, per se, so choice C can be eliminated.

Review Questions

1. Literary scholars have frequently compared the characteristics of poetry written by the first and second generation of Romantic poets. Poets such as William Wordsworth established the foundations of the exaltation of the imagination that later influenced writers such as John Keats and Percy Bysshe Shelley. The first generation of poets was attempting to advocate for the importance of artistry and creativity. The second generation of poets built on this foundation and went even further in their speculations about what creativity could achieve, especially perhaps in a political sense. However, the second generation was also negatively impacted by their observation of the French Revolution, and this experience tempered their idealism.

    Which of the following best states the main idea of the passage?

    A. To describe the distinctions between the first and second generation Romantic poets
    B. To explain the influence of William Wordsworth as a poet
    C. To illustrate the importance of Percy Bysshe Shelley as a poet
    D. To discuss the political viewpoints of the British Romantic poets

2. The acoustics of various performance venues emerge as the result of careful planning and extensive decision making. Sound travels differently when it moves through air, and the objects it encounters in a particular environment strongly impact the way that listeners hear the sound. Venues that are designed primarily to house symphony orchestra performances require vastly different acoustic designs than do venues that

cater to more intimate performances. Engineers must take into account a wide variety of variables during the design process, including vibration, sound, ultrasound, and infrasound.

A sound wave consists of a fundamental, followed by a series of sequential overtones. The way that listeners perceive these sound waves is impacted by the material used in the listening environment, the physical layout of the environment, the position of the stage relative to the audience's seating, and even the height of the ceiling. Many acoustic engineers also must take into consideration the manner in which transducers impact listening. Transducers include loudspeakers, microphones, and sonar projectors. The addition of these tools to an acoustic environment can strongly influence and transform how audience members in different locations in the room perceive any sound being transmitted.

Which of the following best states the main idea of the passage?

A. Sound is a multifaceted and complex phenomenon impacted by numerous factors.
B. Acoustic engineers need to acquire an advanced degree to become qualified.
C. Acoustic engineering is a sophisticated science that requires complex decision making.
D. Multiple acoustic engineers should work on a single project to combine their expertise.

3. Michelangelo was arguably the most talented and prolific artist to emerge from the Italian Renaissance. Not only did he spend three years on his back lying on a scaffold to create the famous paintings adorning the Sistine Chapel, but he also created a sculpture of the Biblical hero David that has been emulated for centuries. Michelangelo himself reflected that he simply took a block of marble and removed all the pieces that did not belong to the David statue. Michelangelo is considered a consummate artist because he created works in so many different media, including painting and sculpture.

The passage is primarily concerned with which of the following?

A. Justifying the value of Michelangelo's art
B. Explaining why Michelangelo could create in multiple media
C. Analyzing the humility of great artists from the Renaissance
D. Arguing that Michelangelo's accomplishments are some of the greatest of his time

4. The current tests for measuring IQ, or an individual's intelligence quotient, were developed during the early and mid-twentieth century. Their use was popularized by Terman, who designed specific tests for use in the U.S. Army. Some psychologists today assert that the traditional system of measuring IQ should remain the sole method of assessing intelligence. Historically, the test has been constructed based on the assumption that there exists one general intelligence factor that impacts an individual's intellectual capacity.

The validity of this assumption has been challenged by other psychologists. In particular, Howard Gardner has emphasized that a unified conception of intelligence based on a single factor remains highly limited and unnecessarily constraining. Gardner has postulated an alternative theory concerning the existence of multiple intelligences. He posits that individuals can possess intelligence in particular areas, including linguistic intelligence, spiritual intelligence, spatial intelligence, intrapersonal intelligence, interpersonal intelligence, musical intelligence, mathematical intelligence, and kinesthetic intelligence, among others. Gardner asserts that individuals can be extremely intelligent and exhibit talent in one area, while failing to demonstrate the same level of prowess in another area. His theory has been discussed widely, although efforts to obtain empirical evidence to support his ideas remain in process.

Which of the following best states the main idea of the passage?

A. Traditional IQ tests are faulty and should be eliminated.
B. Howard Gardner's theory of IQ measurement focuses on multiple intelligences.
C. Both traditional IQ tests and Gardner's assessments should be used to measure intelligence.
D. Gardner's IQ test focuses predominantly on linguistic intelligence.

5. To All Department Supervisors:

The Acme Records Retrieval System will be undergoing scheduled maintenance this Friday, from 4:00 p.m. until midnight. Please inform all department personnel of the system outage, so that researchers can make alternative arrangements to access necessary data.

An archived copy of the Core Business Records Database will be accessible in the Web Services department office from 4:00 p.m. until 8:00 p.m. on Friday. However, this database contains only core records data and is limited in its scope.

Please direct any questions to Marcus Sampson, Web Services Maintenance Officer, at (617) 555-0004.

What is the memo mainly about?

A. It notifies employees of maintenance on the Records Retrieval System.
B. It notifies employees regarding who to contact in the Web Services office.
C. It describes the scope of the company's Core Business Records Database.
D. It explains the public availability of the Core Business Records Database.

6. The Beatles influenced the genre of rock and roll just as Beethoven expanded the genre of the symphony. John Lennon, Paul McCartney, George Harrison, and Ringo Starr expanded the public's understanding of their musical genre and reclassified it as an anthem for rebellion. Their music transformed into the hippies' theme songs of the sixties. Beethoven similarly altered the public's understanding of the symphony. His addition of a chorus in the last movement of the Ninth Symphony attests to this feat.

What is the passage mainly about?

A. It compares the effects that the Beatles and Beethoven had on their genres.
B. It explains how the Beatles helped reclassify rock and roll as a genre.
C. It contrasts the music styles of the Beatles with those of Beethoven.
D. It describes how the music of the Beatles became the hippies' theme songs.

7. In the animal kingdom, many symbiotic relationships exist between two species that take actions known to be mutually beneficial for both parties. In the water, clownfish have such a relationship with sea anemones. The fish are one of the only species that can swim unharmed in the anemone's waving tentacles, as typically the tentacles would sting any animal that swam near it. However, the clownfish is immune to the sting of the tentacles and is therefore protected by them; in return, its presence helps the anemone stay clean, avoid attack by parasites, and remain free from infection.

Which of the following best states the main idea of the passage?

A. Clownfish are one of the only species that can swim unharmed near sea anemones.
B. Clownfish and sea anemones have a mutually beneficial symbiotic relationship.
C. Sea anemones are able to protect clownfish and offer them a safe place to reside.
D. Clownfish typically help sea anemones to stay clean and avoid being attacked.

8. To Whom It May Concern,

I am writing to request a refund of the charge made to my credit card for the purchase of a water filter on Friday, September 18. The filter was the wrong type for my filtration system, so I had to return it. I returned the filter to the store on Saturday, September 19, and the customer service clerk had me complete the paperwork to refund my charges for the purchase. However, the credit never appeared on my credit card account. Please reverse the charges in the amount shown on the credit receipt attached to this e-mail.

Thank you for your assistance.

Claire Glendheim

The e-mail is primarily concerned with which of the following?

A. Explaining the reason for a return
B. Reporting a product failure
C. Complaining about poor service
D. Requesting a refund

9. Historically, the study of creativity has concentrated on persons known for their innovation. Early creativity studies focused on creative "geniuses," such as Einstein, Mozart, or Shakespeare. This type of creativity is known as "Big C" creativity. However, as research on creativity progressed, a corresponding interest in how people could be creative in smaller ways—on an everyday basis—emerged in the discipline. Scholars began to investigate how ordinary tasks, such as cleaning, driving particular familiar routes, and completing work and schoolwork, could be conducted in innovative ways. This focus of creativity research has been labeled "little c" creativity.

Which sentence best describes the main idea of this passage?

A. Creativity occurs not just in large ways, but through small, everyday actions.
B. The study of creativity has historically concentrated on innovative persons.
C. The study of creativity addresses both "Big C" and "little c" types of creativity.
D. Driving familiar routes to a destination can be considered an example of creativity.

10. Laurel Hill Botanic Gardens is pleased to announce the installation of the sculpture series by Laurel Hill artist-in-residence, Darryl C. Grant. The installation features mixed-media sculptures emphasizing the floral designs prominent in Mr. Grant's paintings, many of which are also on exhibit in the Michael and Frieda Sachs Viewing Room.

The sculpture exhibit will open at 10:00 a.m. on Thursday, June 5. The Botanic Gardens' art curator, Jessalyn Jones, will present an overview of the sculptures and lead a guided tour of the installation. The opening ceremony will end with refreshments served in the Nature Observatory from 2:00–3:00 p.m.

This is a members-only event. All Botanic Gardens members and their guests are invited to attend. Tickets are $50.00 per person and can be purchased at the registration desk beginning Monday, May 5.

What is the memo mainly about?

A. It invites Botanic Gardens members to a sculpture installation.
B. It explains the history of floral sculptures at the Botanic Gardens.
C. It describes details regarding the work of sculptor Darryl C. Grant.
D. It explains the role of the art curator in presenting the exhibit.

Answer Key

1. A	**6.** A
2. C	**7.** B
3. D	**8.** D
4. B	**9.** C
5. A	**10.** A

Answers and Explanations

1. (A) The passage describes the distinctions between the first and second generations of British Romantic poets. Choice D is incorrect because the poets' political sensibilities are included as an example of a factor that impacted their perspectives.

2. (C) The passage emphasizes the fact that performance venues have excellent acoustics as the result of extensive planning and careful decision making. Choice A is incorrect because this statement is too broad.

3. (D) The first sentence emphasizes Michelangelo's status as a master artist, and the passage describes his most well-known art works. Choice A is incorrect because the passage is more of an advocacy for Michelangelo rather than a defense of the value of his art.

4. (B) The passage describes Gardner's theory and indicates that it focuses on the idea of multiple intelligences. Choice C is incorrect because the passage does not address this topic directly.

5. (A) This memo is designed mainly to notify Acme employees of maintenance on the Records Retrieval System. Choices B, C, and D are mentioned in the memo, but they are details of the memo as opposed to the main idea.

6. (A) The focus of the passage is conveyed in the first sentence, which states that "the Beatles influenced the genre of rock and roll just as Beethoven expanded the genre of the symphony." The passage mainly compares the effects that the Beatles and Beethoven had on their respective genres. Choice B is a detail mentioned in the passage, and choice C can be eliminated because the passage does not contrast the styles of the artists, but instead compares their impact.

7. (B) The main idea of the passage is that clownfish and sea anemones have a mutually beneficial symbiotic relationship. Choices A, C, and D all represent supporting details of the passage, not the main idea.

8. (D) The e-mail is primarily concerned with requesting a refund. The first sentence of the e-mail clarifies the reason for the author's message. The author does explain why she returned the product, as choice A indicates, but this is a supporting detail of the e-mail, not its main focus.

9. (C) The main idea of the passage is that the study of creativity addresses both "Big C" and "little c" types of creativity. The passage focuses mainly on the study of creativity, not on defining what creativity is, so choice A can be eliminated. Choice B presents a supporting detail of the passage.

10. (A) The memo mainly invites Botanic Gardens members to a sculpture installation. Choice B is incorrect, because the memo does not discuss the history of floral sculptures. Choices C and D convey details mentioned in the passage, not the main idea.

CHAPTER 2

Identifying Details

Identifying Details questions ask about specific facts from the passage. They often start with the phrase "According to the author." They typically ask "how" and "what" questions. In a sense, Detail questions are the opposite of Main Idea questions. They ask about smaller issues raised in the passage rather than "big picture" ideas. When answering Detail questions, keep in mind the following:

> The answer to a Detail question is always given directly in the passage.

Some Detail questions may ask you to identify the correct order of events given in the passage, as in this example.

Imagine living in the year 1800. The railroads then were very scarce. Gas lights were not yet invented, and electric lights were not even dreamed of. Even kerosene wasn't used at that point. This was the world into which Samuel Morse, the inventor of the telegraph, was born.

Samuel Morse was born in Charlestown, Massachusetts, shortly before the turn of the century, in 1791. When he was seven years old, he was sent to boarding school at Phillips Academy, Andover. While he was there, his father wrote him letters, giving him good advice. He told him about George Washington and about a British statesman named Lord Chesterfield, who was able to achieve many of his goals. Lord Chesterfield was asked once how he managed to find time for all of his pursuits, and he replied that he only ever did one thing at a time, and that he "never put off anything until tomorrow that could be done today."

Morse worked hard at school and began to think and act for himself at quite a young age. His biggest accomplishment was in painting, and he established himself as a successful painter after graduating from college at Yale. But he also had an interest in science and inventions. He was passionate about the idea of discovering a way for people to send messages to each other in short periods of time.

In the early 1800s, it took a long time to receive news of any sort, even important news. Whole countries had to wait weeks to hear word of the outcomes of faraway wars. The mail was carried by stagecoach. In emergency situations, such as when ships were lost at sea, there was no way to send requests for help. Electricity had been discovered, but little application had been made of it up until that point. This was about to change when Morse set his mind to his invention.

On October 1, 1832, Morse was sailing to America from a trip overseas on a ship called the *Sully*. He became preoccupied with the thought of inventing a machine that would later become the telegraph. Morse thought about the telegraph night and day. As he sat upon the deck of the ship after dinner one night, he took out a little notebook and began to create a plan.

If a message could be sent ten miles without dropping, he wrote, "I could make it go around the globe." He said this over and over again during the years after his trip.

One morning at the breakfast table, Morse showed his plan to some of the other *Sully* passengers. Five years later, when the model of the telegraph was built, it was exactly like the one shown that morning to the passengers on the *Sully*.

Once he arrived in America, Morse worked for twelve long years to get people to notice his invention. Though some supported the idea of the telegraph, many people scoffed at it. Morse persisted, and eventually a bill was passed by Congress in 1842. It authorized the funds needed to build the first trial telegraph line.

After two years, the telegraph line was complete. Morse and his colleagues tested it in May 1844. The device worked, and the telegraph became a huge success. Morse's persistence had finally paid off.

According to the passage, which order of events below is correct?

A. Morse returns to America aboard the *Sully*, receives good advice from his father, and begins to draw a model for the telegraph.
B. Morse begins to draw a model for the telegraph, attends Yale, and receives funding from Congress.
C. Morse attends Yale, becomes a painter, and returns to America aboard the *Sully*.
D. Morse discovers electricity, draws a model for the telegraph, and returns to America aboard the *Sully*.

The correct answer is **C**. Only in choice C are the events placed in the correct order. Paragraph three states that Morse became a painter after graduating from Yale, and paragraph five describes Morse as sailing to America aboard the *Sully* after that. The passage states that Morse was returning to America from a trip overseas.

As the question in the following example shows, some Detail questions may ask you to identify a statement that paraphrases, or restates, information given in the passage.

Literary scholars have often speculated as to the personal characteristics of William Shakespeare. The Bard is known to many as the greatest writer the English language has ever known, but we have very few examples of his handwriting or even his own name written out in his hand. Some academics have gone so far as to speculate that Shakespeare was a pseudonym for an aristocrat. However, the majority of scholars have dismissed this proposal, and they concentrate instead on Shakespeare's thoughtful insights and dexterous construction of language.

Which sentence below best restates, or paraphrases, the third sentence of the passage?

A. Some scholars are convinced that Shakespeare was the name of an aristocratic family that fell from grace.
B. Some scholars think that Shakespeare got most of his insights from disguising himself as an aristocrat and infiltrating wealthy circles.
C. Some scholars have speculated that aristocrats did not like Shakespeare's plays and considered his insights pseudo-intellectual.
D. Some scholars have a theory that Shakespeare's works were really written by an aristocrat who used that name as an alias.

The correct answer is **D**. The third sentence states that some scholars speculate, or have the theory, that Shakespeare was a pseudonym, or alias, used by an aristocrat who wrote his works. Choice D therefore best restates the information given in the third sentence.

In the following example the question asks about a specific detail mentioned in one part of the passage.

Austrian-born Sigmund Freud, a psychoanalytic psychologist, lived from the mid-nineteenth to the mid-twentieth century. The psychoanalytic approach refers to the school of thought that unconscious memories or desires guide our emotions and actions. In personality theory, this equates to events from childhood shaping the individual self without a person's conscious awareness. These specific childhood events continue to exert a strong influence over our lives and dominate our emotions. If you are a life-of-the-party, extroverted personality, perhaps you had a healthy upbringing; however, quiet, deep-thinker types can be just as functional. How your caregivers responded to your natural urges will determine your level of mental health, according to the psychoanalytic approach.

Freud believed that as a child, an individual's actions are driven by hidden impulses—and that repression or denial of those impulses by parents or society can lead to fixations or personality disorders. Alternatively, if the child's impulses are accepted as normative to his or her development, then a functional adult behavioral pattern should take root. Now, by no means should parents allow every impulse to dictate behavior; each of us has a "censor," which Freud referred to as the "superego." This element of the psyche is largely helpful and acts as a conscience. However, if we let the superego dominate our personality, Freud believed, it could lead to repression and inauthentic behavior.

Freud often worked with highly distressed female clients, repressed in their natural modes of expression; this is how he developed many of his theories, which some people believe are not very scientific. By today's standards, they are not, but Freud's idea that unconscious urges drive our behavior was revolutionary for his time.

According to the passage, which of the following statements best describes Freud's theory of personality?

A. Individuals are shaped by childhood experiences.
B. Individuals are shaped by a superego, or censor.
C. Healthy individuals become outgoing, while unhealthy ones become introverted.
D. Women are more likely to repress their emotions than men.

The correct answer is A. To answer this question, it may be helpful to reread the first paragraph of the passage. The first paragraph states that Freud's personality theory is based on how childhood events shape individuals, choice A. The paragraph also states that extroverted and introverted individuals can be equally functional, making choice B incorrect. The superego is part of Freud's theory, but not the whole definition. The third paragraph states that Freud developed his theories by working with female patients who repressed their emotions, but the passage does not say whether women are more repressed than men.

The next two examples contain further explanations of Detail questions that ask about specific information from each passage.

CPR, an acronym that stands for cardiopulmonary resuscitation, is a widely utilized method of attempting to save someone's life. It is especially applicable to scenarios in which a patient's heart has stopped beating. Frequently, it is also used in cases where a person is in danger of drowning.

Almost all approaches to CPR suggest that a person begin resuscitation efforts with chest compressions. To perform a chest compression, the individual places both hands flat on the patient's chest and then begins pushing down carefully but firmly, most likely at equal intervals. The compressions should be counted, so that the individual can keep track of how many compressions have been administered. The unofficial recommendation of how many chest compressions to provide is around 100 per minute.

There are many resources through which potential lifesavers can acquire training and even certification so that they can more effectively administer this lifesaving technique to a potential patient. However, the American Heart Association stresses that even if someone has not received any type of formal training, attempting to help a person who needs to be resuscitated is far better than offering no help. This is why 911 operators sometimes request that bystanders at the scene of an emergency administer CPR. The operators may even coach the bystanders verbally, over the phone. These approaches have been shown to be effective in many cases.

If a bystander at an emergency scene has received CPR training—even if the training occurred a long time ago—the bystander should attempt further techniques in addition to chest compressions, especially if the patient has been underwater. The lifesaver should start first by checking the patient's airway. He or she might also administer mouth-to-mouth rescue breathing. However, lifesavers should only perform these additional techniques if they are confident of their skills and remember their training. Otherwise, any potential lifesaver should just administer chest compressions.

Some important items to remember in administering CPR are as follows. First, the lifesaver should always check whether the patient is conscious or not. Verbal interaction or communication can be a key way of determining if a person is conscious. If the emergency is related to drowning, the lifesaver should start chest compressions. These should be conducted for about a minute or so, before the lifesaver calls 911. However, if one person can perform the compressions and there is another person available who can call 911, then these steps should happen simultaneously.

For persons who are trained in CPR, one of the best ways to remember the order in which steps should be administered is to recall the memory cue CAB. This cue stands for Circulation, Airway, Breathing. The goal of CPR is to help an unresponsive person to start breathing on his or her own. First, use chest compressions to restore circulation. This is the C of CAB. Second, check the patient's airway for possible blockages. The A in CAB stands for airway. Finally, administer rescue breathing. This is, of course, the B of CAB.

According to the passage, what is the goal of CPR?

A. To prevent a person who has lost consciousness from drowning
B. To help an unconscious person regain consciousness
C. To help an unresponsive person start breathing again
D. To help an unresponsive person become mobile again

The correct answer is **C**. This Detail question asks you to identify the goal of CPR, according to the passage. Paragraph six states that the goal of CPR is to help an unresponsive person start breathing on his or her own. The correct answer is stated directly in the passage, as choice C reflects.

Now consider this passage:

The English town of Stratford-upon-Avon is visited yearly by tourists wanting to view the birthplace of William Shakespeare. William's father, John Shakespeare, bought the family home on Henley Street, and it is here that William is believed to have been born in 1564. Shakespeare's birth home remained in his family until the early 1800s, and it is now a public museum.

Shakespeare attended school at the King Edward VI Grammar School, which occupied the first floor of a building known as the Guildhall. It was in this Guildhall that Shakespeare first experienced theater, when he saw a theatrical performance given by a group of traveling actors. The Royal Shakespeare Company still performs in the town at the Royal Shakespeare and Swan Theaters.

Close to the Guildhall is the site of a house known as New Place, which was bought by Shakespeare himself. Here Shakespeare lived during the later part of his life, until his death in 1616. Although he spent most of his career in London, with trips back to Stratford, he moved permanently to New Place in the last years of his life and is believed to have written some of his later works there. Only the foundations of the New Place house now remain.

In the town of Shottery, one mile from Stratford, is the cottage where Shakespeare's wife, Anne Hathaway, was born. The Hathaway cottage, now also a museum, is actually a large, thatch-roofed farmhouse with sprawling gardens where Shakespeare is believed to have developed his relationship with Anne. They married in 1582 and had three children.

What does the passage state about the importance of the Guildhall to Shakespeare?

A. Shakespeare wrote some of his most important works there.
B. The Guildhall became the first home for the Royal Shakespeare Company.
C. Shakespeare's father bought the Guildhall, and Shakespeare was born there.
D. Shakespeare first saw theater at the Guildhall when he was a student there.

The correct answer is **D**. The second paragraph tells us that Shakespeare attended school at the Guildhall and that he saw his first theater production there. The passage does not mention that the Royal Shakespeare Company found its first home at the Guildhall, so choice B is incorrect. Although Shakespeare bought a home near the Guildhall, he did not actually live there, nor did his family own the building, based on information given in the passage, so C is incorrect.

Review Questions

1. Christopher Columbus was particularly influenced by the maps of the ancient geographer Ptolemy. Ptolemy argued that the world was round, which went against the belief of the day that the world was flat. Columbus sided with Ptolemy on this question and set out to prove that it was so.

At the time it was widely held that sailing west from Europe would lead to certain death. Believing that the world was round, Columbus thought that one who sailed west would wind up in the east. Other scientists of the day rejected this idea, so Columbus wrote to a respected Italian scholar, Paolo Toscanelli, to ask for his opinion on the matter.

Toscanelli supported the idea of Columbus's trip and sent word back to Columbus in 1474. After receiving Toscanelli's encouragement, Columbus focused all of his thoughts and plans on traveling westward. To make the journey, he would require the help of a generous financial backer, so he went to seek the aid of the king of Portugal. Columbus asked the king for ships and sailors to make the journey. In return, he promised to bring back wealth and to help to convert natives living on the lands to the Church. Portugal refused, and Columbus approached Italy unsuccessfully as well. He went to Spain next.

Queen Isabella of Spain agreed to support the journey. It took some time for Columbus to convince her, but he did succeed, and she paid for the trip. Part of what led the queen to believe in Columbus was the way that he focused on his goal for such a long time with great intent. He spent the best years of his life working toward his dream, remaining persistent and determined. Legend has it that even during his first voyage, members of his crew became frightened and uncertain, wanting to return home, but Columbus pressed on. The eventual discovery of the Americas was the reward for his commitment.

More than 500 years later, the geography of the world is often taken for granted, but Columbus was an early visionary whose results proved at least some of his theories correct.

Which country was responsible for funding Columbus's voyage to the Americas?

A. Italy
B. Spain
C. Turkey
D. Portugal

2. The English town of Stratford-upon-Avon is visited yearly by tourists wanting to view the birthplace of William Shakespeare. William's father, John Shakespeare, bought the family home on Henley Street, and it is here that William is believed to have been born in 1564. Shakespeare's birth home remained in his family until the early 1800s, and it is now a public museum.

Shakespeare attended school at the King Edward VI Grammar School, which occupied the first floor of a building known as the Guildhall. It was in this Guildhall that Shakespeare first experienced theater, when he saw a theatrical performance given by a group of traveling actors. The Royal Shakespeare Company still performs in the town at the Royal Shakespeare and Swan Theaters.

Close to the Guildhall is the site of a house known as New Place, which was bought by Shakespeare himself. Here Shakespeare lived during the later part of his life, until his death in 1616. Although he spent most of his career in London, with trips back to Stratford, he moved permanently to New Place in the last years of his life and is believed to have written some of his later works there. Only the foundations of the New Place house now remain.

In the town of Shottery, one mile from Stratford, is the cottage where Shakespeare's wife, Anne Hathaway, was born. The Hathaway cottage, now also a museum, is actually a large, thatch-roofed farmhouse with sprawling gardens where Shakespeare is believed to have developed his relationship with Anne. They married in 1582 and had three children.

How was William Shakespeare first introduced to plays?

A. When he was a boy, the Royal Shakespeare Company visited his classroom.
B. He read many scripts at the Guildhall, where he attended school as a child.
C. He watched a traveling group of performers in the same building as the King Edward VI Grammar School.
D. His wife, Anne Hathaway, began taking him to New Place, where she performed as an actress.

3. One of the most important gymnastic exercises in the original Montessori school approach is that of the "line." For this exercise, a line is drawn in chalk or paint on the floor. Instead of one line, there may also be two lines drawn. The children are taught to walk on these lines like tightrope walkers, placing their feet one in front of the other.

   To keep their balance, the children must make efforts similar to those of real tightrope walkers, except that they have no danger of falling, since the lines are drawn only on the floor. The teacher herself performs the exercise first, showing clearly how she places her feet, and the children imitate her without her even needing to speak. At first it is only certain children who follow her, and when she has shown them how to walk the line, she leaves, letting the exercise develop on its own.

   The children for the most part continue to walk, following with great care the movement they have seen, and making efforts to keep their balance so they don't fall. Gradually the other children come closer and watch and try the exercise. In a short time, the entire line is covered with children balancing themselves and continuing to walk around, watching their feet attentively.

   Music may be used at this point. It should be a very simple march, without an obvious rhythm. It should simply accompany and support the efforts of the children.

   When children learn to master their balance in this way, Dr. Montessori believed, they can bring the act of walking to a remarkable standard of perfection.

   Before the children begin to walk the line, what must they do?

   A. Master their balance
   B. Watch their teacher
   C. Watch their feet attentively
   D. Draw a line on the floor

The Myers-Briggs personality test is based on the sixteen personality types conceptualized by Carl Jung and Isabel Briggs Myers. The Myers-Briggs test was developed based on the presumption that most individuals would fall somewhere on a spectrum of the following binaries: introvert–extrovert, sensor–intuitor, thinker–feeler, and judger–perceiver. Although other personality tests measure different personality traits, the Myers-Briggs test notably bases its foundation on philosophical suppositions from Jung that are rooted in his discussion of archetypes. The test is distinctive due to its reliance on a nonempirical theoretical foundation.

The next two questions are based on this passage.

4. Which of the following statements summarizes why the Myers-Briggs test is unique?

    A. The Myers-Briggs test uses a total of 16 personality types.
    B. The Myers-Briggs test is based on the use of a set of binary traits.
    C. The Myers-Briggs test is based on empirical data rather than theory.
    D. The Myers-Briggs test is based on theory rather than empirical data.

5. Which of the following statements is true, based on the passage?

    A. Conclusions drawn from the test have no basis in reality.
    B. Conclusions drawn from the test are based on the archetypes of Carl Jung.
    C. Conclusions drawn from the test are based on neither fact nor opinion.
    D. Conclusions drawn from the test are based on historical evidence.

6. Austrian-born Sigmund Freud, a psychoanalytic psychologist, lived from the mid-nineteenth to the mid-twentieth century. The psychoanalytic approach refers to the school of thought that unconscious memories or desires guide our emotions and actions. In personality theory, this equates to events from childhood shaping the individual self without a person's conscious awareness. These specific childhood events continue to exert a strong influence over our lives and dominate our emotions. If you are a life-of-the-party, extroverted personality, perhaps you had a healthy upbringing; however, quiet, deep-thinker types can be just as functional. How your caregivers responded to your natural urges will determine your level of mental health, according to the psychoanalytic approach.

    Freud believed that as a child, an individual's actions are driven by hidden impulses—and that repression or denial of those impulses by parents or society can lead to fixations or personality disorders. Alternatively, if the child's impulses are accepted as normative to his or her development, then a functional adult behavioral pattern should take root. Now, by no means should parents allow every impulse to dictate behavior; each of us has a "censor," which Freud referred to as the "superego." This element of the psyche is largely helpful and acts as a conscience. However, if we let the superego dominate our personality, Freud believed, it could lead to repression and inauthentic behavior.

    Freud often worked with highly distressed female clients, repressed in their natural modes of expression; this is how he developed many of his theories, which some people believe are not very scientific. By today's standards, they are not, but Freud's idea that unconscious urges drive our behavior was revolutionary for his time.

Which of the following is a belief held by Sigmund Freud, according to the passage?

A. No scientific support exists for the idea that unconscious urges drive our behavior.
B. The superego serves as a censor that primarily causes repression and inauthenticity.
C. Parents should allow every impulse that a child has to dictate the child's behavior.
D. Functional adult behavior should result from accepting a child's impulses as normal.

7. The current tests for measuring IQ, or an individual's intelligence quotient, were developed during the early and mid-twentieth century. Their use was popularized by Terman, who designed specific tests for use in the U.S. Army. Some psychologists today assert that the traditional system of measuring IQ should remain the sole method of assessing intelligence. Historically, the test has been constructed based on the assumption that there exists one general intelligence factor that impacts an individual's intellectual capacity.

The validity of this assumption has been challenged by other psychologists. In particular, Howard Gardner has emphasized that a unified conception of intelligence based on a single factor remains highly limited and unnecessarily constraining. Gardner has postulated an alternative theory concerning the existence of multiple intelligences. He posits that individuals can possess intelligence in particular areas, including linguistic intelligence, spiritual intelligence, spatial intelligence, intrapersonal intelligence, interpersonal intelligence, musical intelligence, mathematical intelligence, and kinesthetic intelligence, among others. Gardner asserts that individuals can be extremely intelligent and exhibit talent in one area, while failing to demonstrate the same level of prowess in another area. His theory has been discussed widely, although efforts to obtain empirical evidence to support his ideas remain in process.

Which of the following statements is true, based on the passage?

A. Individuals who are extremely intelligent typically demonstrate equally high levels of skills in all areas.
B. The work of Howard Gardner emphasizes a unified conception of intelligence based on a single factor.
C. The use of IQ tests was made popular by Terman, who designed specific tests for use in the U.S. Army.
D. The traditional system of measuring IQ has remained the sole method of assessing intelligence.

Percy Bysshe Shelley was one of the second-generation Romantic poets. Along with John Keats and Lord Byron, Shelley was considered one of the most masterful poets of his generation.

Shelley was born in England in 1792, as a member of the aristocracy. He was educated at two prestigious English schools, Eton College and Oxford

University. Shelley believed that poets were visionaries who could serve as societal leaders because of the creative power of their imaginations. The second generation of Romantic poets, in particular, believed that poets were going to help change the world. Shelley's generation believed that, through the imagination, anything was possible. They believed that they could use the creative power of the mind to change the government and even change the world. Shelley's poems reflect this belief. He was a truly idealistic thinker, and he claimed that poets were the "unacknowledged legislators of the world." The poet's creative vision could let him or her see things that other people could not.

Shelley's ideas were heavily influenced by the politics of his time. He grew up at a time when governments were under transformation. In fact, he came of age in the shadow of the French Revolution. This war was very violent, and since France was so close to England, Shelley was acutely aware of the violence that was occurring there. That may have led him to concentrate even more on his belief that artists were able to change the world and improve living conditions.

Shelley's poem "Mont Blanc" focuses on the Romantic notion of the sublime. The Romantic poets believed that when people interacted with Nature, it sometimes caused them to be in a state of wonder—or it caused them to be awestruck. For example, when a person gazed at a mountain, the huge size of the mountain could cause the person to become speechless with wonder. This was the effect that the sublime quality of Nature could have on a viewer.

In "Mont Blanc," Shelley describes the mountain in a way that attempts to explain its effects on the viewer's mind. According to Shelley, the mountain itself causes the viewer's thoughts to enter a kind of strange trance, and to be affected in a way that resembles how a poet or an artist feels whenever he or she is caught in the midst of a creative inspiration. In the poem, Shelley draws a comparison between the effect of the mountain on the viewer and the power that the imagination has over the artist's mind.

The next two questions are based on this passage.

8. According to the passage, how did Shelley think poets could save the world?

    A. Through the creative power of the imagination
    B. By fighting in the French Revolution
    C. By writing more about Nature
    D. By speaking out against acts of violence

9. According to the passage, what effect can mountains have on a viewer?

    A. They can cause a viewer to become intimidated.
    B. They can frighten a viewer into being speechless.
    C. They can cause a viewer to become amused.
    D. They can cause a viewer to be filled with wonder.

10. CPR, an acronym that stands for cardiopulmonary resuscitation, is a widely utilized method of attempting to save someone's life. It is especially applicable to scenarios in which a patient's heart has stopped beating. Frequently, it is also used in cases where a person is in danger of drowning.

Almost all approaches to CPR suggest that a person begin resuscitation efforts with chest compressions. To perform a chest compression, the individual places both hands flat on the patient's chest and then begins pushing down carefully but firmly, most likely at equal intervals. The compressions should be counted, so that the individual can keep track of how many compressions have been administered. The unofficial recommendation of how many chest compressions to provide is around 100 per minute.

There are many resources through which potential lifesavers can acquire training and even certification so that they can more effectively administer this life-saving technique to a potential patient. However, the American Heart Association stresses that even if someone has not received any type of formal training, attempting to help a person who needs to be resuscitated is far better than offering no help. This is why 911 operators sometimes request that bystanders at the scene of an emergency administer CPR. The operators may even coach the bystanders verbally, over the phone. These approaches have been shown to be effective in many cases.

If a bystander at an emergency scene has received CPR training—even if the training occurred a long time ago—the bystander should attempt further techniques in addition to chest compressions, especially if the patient has been underwater. The lifesaver should start first by checking the patient's airway. He or she might also administer mouth-to-mouth rescue breathing. However, lifesavers should only perform these additional techniques if they are confident of their skills and remember their training. Otherwise, any potential lifesaver should just administer chest compressions.

Some important items to remember in administering CPR are as follows. First, the lifesaver should always check whether the patient is conscious or not. Verbal interaction or communication can be a key way of determining if a person is conscious. If the emergency is related to drowning, the lifesaver should start chest compressions. These should be conducted for about a minute or so, before the lifesaver calls 911. However, if one person can perform the compressions and there is another person available who can call 911, then these steps should happen simultaneously.

For persons who are trained in CPR, one of the best ways to remember the order in which steps should be administered is to recall the memory cue CAB. This cue stands for Circulation, Airway, Breathing. The goal of CPR is to help an unresponsive person to start breathing on his or her own. First, use chest compressions to restore circulation. This is the C of CAB. Second, check the patient's airway for possible blockages. The A in CAB stands for airway. Finally, administer rescue breathing. This is, of course, the B of CAB.

According to the passage, what is the best approach to using CPR for untrained lifesavers?

A. Untrained lifesavers should use chest compressions only.
B. Untrained lifesavers should refrain from using any form of CPR.
C. Untrained lifesavers should clear the patient's airway only.
D. Untrained lifesavers should administer rescue breathing.

11. Saltwater fish and freshwater fish are related, but their natural environments prove rather distinctive. In terms of being kept as pets, freshwater fish require less maintenance. They live in water that can be adapted from tap water, and they can be kept in many different types of containers in addition to aquariums. Saltwater fish, on the other hand, require a specific type of salt-infused water. Careful watch of the pH balance of the water must also be maintained.

According to the passage, what must people watch carefully when they have saltwater fish?

A. The type of food the fish ingest
B. The water temperature
C. The pH balance of the water
D. The type of light in the aquarium

12. Music can have a significant positive influence on individuals in many different circumstances. Persons who must spend time recuperating in the hospital are frequently soothed by the presence of soft music. Babies are trained to respond to auditory noises through the use of music. Persons going through emotional difficulties such as grief frequently listen to and create music as a means of dealing with the issues they are experiencing. Even people who simply need a short respite from the stresses of the day often use music as a calming and coping mechanism.

According to the passage, what can happen when a baby is exposed to music on a regular basis?

A. The baby can associate various sounds with different foods.
B. The baby can learn to distinguish between his or her parents' voices.
C. The baby can learn to respond to different noises.
D. The baby can learn to discriminate between the voices of siblings.

13. The acoustics of various performance venues emerge as the result of careful planning and extensive decision making. Sound travels differently when it moves through air, and the objects it encounters in a particular environment strongly impact the way that listeners hear the sound. Venues that are designed primarily to house symphony orchestra performances require vastly different acoustic designs than do venues that cater to more intimate performances. Engineers must take into account a wide variety of variables during the design process, including vibration, sound, ultrasound, and infrasound.

A sound wave consists of a fundamental, followed by a series of sequential overtones. The way that listeners perceive these sound waves is impacted by the material used in the listening environment, the physical layout of the environment, the position of the stage relative to the audience's seating, and even the height of the ceiling. Many acoustic engineers also must take into consideration the manner in which transducers impact listening. Transducers include loudspeakers, microphones, and sonar projectors. The addition of these tools to an acoustic environment can strongly influence and transform how audience members in different locations in the room perceive any sound being transmitted.

Which of the following is true regarding sound waves, according to the passage?

A. Sound waves impact the hard of hearing differently than other people.
B. Sound waves are distinctive for different musical genres.
C. Sound waves are unaffected by the physical layouts of performance venues.
D. A sound wave consists of a fundamental and a series of overtones.

14. Bees are a natural part of the pollination cycle of plants. Many plants require the assistance of bees in order to transfer their pollen so that flowers can be produced. Bees travel from flower to flower, and minuscule grains of pollen attach to the bees' legs. The pollen travels much more efficiently via bees than it might if it had to rely on the wind, for example. In this manner, bees assist in the natural pollination cycle through the action of gathering nectar from flowers. Bees are a critical component of this process; without them, plants would face much greater challenges in their reproduction.

The passage indicates which of the following about the migration of pollen via bees as opposed to migration by the wind?

A. Pollen travels much more efficiently via bees than it would by the wind.
B. Pollen can travel equally as effectively via bees or by the wind.
C. Pollen is too heavy to be transported by the wind, except during wind storms.
D. Bees are sometimes allergic to pollen, so it must be transported on the wind.

15. When artists achieve commercial successes, their emotional mindsets can be influenced by this experience. Claude Monet was one such example of this phenomenon. Monet's innovative style earned him considerable fame and public acclaim. In addition, he was extremely prolific as an artist because of his industrious work ethic. As a result, he was successful at his craft, and his paintings reflect a more contemplative and calm perspective than those of artists whose life experiences were fraught with poverty and struggle.

According to the passage, why did Monet's paintings reflect a contemplative perspective?

A. Because he did not achieve fame until after his death
B. Because he experienced artistic success during his lifetime
C. Because he became overly enthusiastic about painting
D. Because he was trying to cultivate an artistic persona

Answer Key

1.	B	**9.**	D
2.	C	**10.**	A
3.	B	**11.**	C
4.	D	**12.**	C
5.	B	**13.**	D
6.	D	**14.**	A
7.	C	**15.**	B
8.	A		

Answers and Explanations

1. **(B)** Choice A is incorrect because while Italy is the first county mentioned in the passage, and an Italian man named Toscanelli supported Columbus' travel idea, the passage never mentions Italy's *financial* support of Columbus. Choice D is incorrect because the passage specifically says that Portugal refused to financially support Columbus.

2. **(C)** Choice A is incorrect because the Royal Shakespeare Company was not yet established when William was a boy. Choice B offers information that was never stated in the passage, while choice D takes two elements of the passage, Anne Hathaway and New Place, and incorrectly links them. Choice C is, thus, correct.

3. **(B)** The children learn to master their balance by taking part in the activity, which requires practice; therefore, choice A is not a logical choice. Choice C occurs *after* the children have started walking the line, not before, and

choice D refers to an action the teacher must take, not the children. Choice B is the correct answer.

4. **(D)** The author states that the test is based upon a nonempirical theoretical foundation. *Empirical data* refers to data gained by observation. Choice C is incorrect because it is the opposite of the correct answer.

5. **(B)** The passage states that *the Myers-Briggs test notably bases its foundation on philosophical suppositions from Jung that are rooted in his discussion of archetypes*. Choice B is therefore correct.

6. **(D)** Choice D is the only offered statement that Freud himself believed. Choice B misrepresents information given in the passage, and choice C is the opposite of Freud's belief, according to paragraph two.

7. **(C)** The statement in choice C is mentioned in the first paragraph of the passage. Choice B is

the opposite of the correct answer, and choice A is incorrect as well, according to the work of Gardner described in paragraph three.

8. (A) In the beginning of the selection, the author explains that Shelley and his contemporaries believed very strongly in the power of the creative imagination. Shelley believed poets could see things that other people could not.

9. (D) The passage states that Shelley believed the size of a mountain could inspire a state of wonder in a viewer. This experience is similar to the same state of wonder a poet experiences through creative inspiration.

10. (A) In the beginning of the passage, the author explains that anyone can use chest compressions to try to save a patient. This is true even if the person has not been trained or certified in CPR in an official sense.

11. (C) The passage explains that saltwater aquariums require a fish owner to check the pH balance of the water carefully. Choice B is incorrect because the passage specifically describes pH balance.

12. (C) The passage suggests that babies who are exposed to music on a regular basis can learn to respond to noises. Choice A is incorrect because the passage explicitly mentions how music can foster auditory training in infants.

13. (D) The passage states that a sound wave consists of a fundamental followed by a series of sequential overtones. Choices A and B are incorrect because the passage does not mention these statements.

14. (A) The passage explains that pollen travels much more efficiently on bees' legs than it could by being blown on the wind. Choice C is incorrect because the passage never mentions the weight of pollen.

15. (B) The passage explains that when artists achieve commercial success, their emotional mindsets can be influenced by the experience. The passage mentions reasons Monet was successful and the effect this success had on his work.

CHAPTER 3

Topic and Theme

Topic and Theme questions may reflect one of two types. The first type asks the test taker to differentiate between the topic, theme, main idea, and supporting details in a Reading passage. The **topic** of a passage is the general subject matter addressed in the passage. A passage regarding key battles of the Civil War might address the topic of history (very general), military conflict (more specific), or Civil War battles (very specific). The **themes** of the passage are ideas or concepts that weave throughout a passage and frequently recur. A passage regarding key battles of the Civil War might contain themes of heroism, bravery, or strategic prowess, for instance.

This first question type is shown in the following three examples.

Imagine living in the year 1800. The railroads then were very scarce. Gas lights were not yet invented, and electric lights were not even dreamed of. Even kerosene wasn't used at that point. This was the world into which Samuel Morse, the inventor of the telegraph, was born.

Samuel Morse was born in Charlestown, Massachusetts, shortly before the turn of the century, in 1791. When he was seven years old, he was sent to boarding school at Phillips Academy, Andover. While he was there, his father wrote him letters, giving him good advice. He told him about George Washington and about a British statesman named Lord Chesterfield, who was able to achieve many of his goals. Lord Chesterfield was asked once how he managed to find time for all of his pursuits, and he replied that he only ever did one thing at a time, and that he "never put off anything until tomorrow that could be done today."

Morse worked hard at school and began to think and act for himself at quite a young age. His biggest accomplishment was in painting, and he established himself as a successful painter after graduating from college at Yale. But he also had an interest in science and inventions. He was passionate about the idea of discovering a way for people to send messages to each other in short periods of time.

In the early 1800s, it took a long time to receive news of any sort, even important news. Whole countries had to wait weeks to hear word of the outcomes of faraway wars. The mail was carried by stagecoach. In emergency situations, such as when ships were lost at sea, there was no way to send requests for help. Electricity had been discovered, but little application had been made of it up until that point. This was about to change when Morse set his mind to his invention.

On October 1, 1832, Morse was sailing to America from a trip overseas on a ship called the *Sully*. He became preoccupied with the thought of inventing a machine that would later become the telegraph. Morse thought about the telegraph night and day. As he sat upon the deck of the ship after dinner one night, he took out a little notebook and began to create a plan.

If a message could be sent ten miles without dropping, he wrote, "I could make it go around the globe." He said this over and over again during the years after his trip.

One morning at the breakfast table, Morse showed his plan to some of the other *Sully* passengers. Five years later, when the model of the telegraph was built, it was exactly like the one shown that morning to the passengers on the *Sully*.

Once he arrived in America, Morse worked for twelve long years to get people to notice his invention. Though some supported the idea of the telegraph, many people scoffed at it. Morse persisted, and eventually a bill was passed by Congress in 1842. It authorized the funds needed to build the first trial telegraph line.

After two years, the telegraph line was complete. Morse and his colleagues tested it in May 1844. The device worked, and the telegraph became a huge success. Morse's persistence had finally paid off.

Which of the following describes the word *telegraph* as it relates to the passage?

A. Main idea
B. Topic
C. Supporting detail
D. Theme

The correct answer is **B**. The word *telegraph* is the topic of the passage, because that is the passage's central focus.

Let's consider a second example:

Historically, the study of creativity has concentrated on persons known for their innovation. Early creativity studies focused on creative "geniuses," such as Einstein, Mozart, or Shakespeare. This type of creativity is known as "Big C" creativity. However, as research on creativity progressed, a corresponding interest in how people could be creative in smaller ways— on an everyday basis—emerged in the discipline. Scholars began to investigate how ordinary tasks, such as cleaning, driving particular familiar routes, and completing work and schoolwork, could be conducted in innovative ways. This focus of creativity research has been labeled "little c" creativity.

Is *creative geniuses* a topic, main idea, supporting detail, or theme of the above passage?

A. Topic
B. Main idea
C. Supporting detail
D. Theme

The correct answer is **C**. *Creative geniuses* are a supporting detail of this passage. The topic of the passage is the study of creativity, and the main idea is that the study of creativity addresses both "Big C" and "little c" types of creativity.

Now consider this passage:

> The current tests for measuring IQ, or an individual's intelligence quotient, were developed during the early and mid-twentieth century. Their use was popularized by Terman, who designed specific tests for use in the U.S. Army. Some psychologists today assert that the traditional system of measuring IQ should remain the sole method of assessing intelligence. Historically, the test has been constructed based on the assumption that there exists one general intelligence factor that impacts an individual's intellectual capacity.
>
> The validity of this assumption has been challenged by other psychologists. In particular, Howard Gardner has emphasized that a unified conception of intelligence based on a single factor remains highly limited and unnecessarily constraining. Gardner has postulated an alternative theory concerning the existence of multiple intelligences. He posits that individuals can possess intelligence in particular areas, including linguistic intelligence, spiritual intelligence, spatial intelligence, intrapersonal intelligence, interpersonal intelligence, musical intelligence, mathematical intelligence, and kinesthetic intelligence, among others. Gardner asserts that individuals can be extremely intelligent and exhibit talent in one area, while failing to demonstrate the same level of prowess in another area. His theory has been discussed widely, although efforts to obtain empirical evidence to support his ideas remain in process.
>
> Which of the following describes the phrase *IQ measurement* as it relates to the passage?
>
> A. Main idea
> B. Topic
> C. Supporting detail
> D. Theme

The correct answer is **B**. The phrase *IQ measurement* reflects the topic of this passage. This phrase is too broad to be a supporting detail of the passage.

The second type of Topic and Theme question asks the test taker to identify the topic sentence or summary sentence of a paragraph or passage. **Topic sentences** are introductory sentences that encapsulate the main idea to be developed in that paragraph or passage. **Summary sentences** are concluding sentences that restate the main idea of the paragraph or passage. They may also draw a conclusion based on information given in the paragraph or passage.

Normally we might think of topic sentences and summary sentences as applying only to text at the paragraph level. The topic sentence of a full passage would be referred to as its thesis statement, and the summary sentence of a full passage would be referred to as its conclusion. On the

TEAS, however, the term *topic sentence* is sometimes used to refer to a sentence at either the paragraph level or the level of the full passage. The term *summary sentence* is also used to refer to the concluding sentence for a single paragraph or the conclusion of a full passage.

CPR, an acronym that stands for cardiopulmonary resuscitation, is a widely utilized method of attempting to save someone's life. It is especially applicable to scenarios in which a patient's heart has stopped beating. Frequently, it is also used in cases where a person is in danger of drowning.

Almost all approaches to CPR suggest that a person begin resuscitation efforts with chest compressions. To perform a chest compression, the individual places both hands flat on the patient's chest and then begins pushing down carefully but firmly, most likely at equal intervals. The compressions should be counted, so that the individual can keep track of how many compressions have been administered. The unofficial recommendation of how many chest compressions to provide is around 100 per minute.

There are many resources through which potential lifesavers can acquire training and even certification so that they can more effectively administer this lifesaving technique to a potential patient. However, the American Heart Association stresses that even if someone has not received any type of formal training, attempting to help a person who needs to be resuscitated is far better than offering no help. This is why 911 operators sometimes request that bystanders at the scene of an emergency administer CPR. The operators may even coach the bystanders verbally, over the phone. These approaches have been shown to be effective in many cases.

If a bystander at an emergency scene has received CPR training—even if the training occurred a long time ago—the bystander should attempt further techniques in addition to chest compressions, especially if the patient has been underwater. The lifesaver should start first by checking the patient's airway. He or she might also administer mouth-to-mouth rescue breathing. However, lifesavers should only perform these additional techniques if they are confident of their skills and remember their training. Otherwise, any potential lifesaver should just administer chest compressions.

Some important items to remember in administering CPR are as follows. First, the lifesaver should always check whether the patient is conscious or not. Verbal interaction or communication can be a key way of determining if a person is conscious. If the emergency is related to drowning, the lifesaver should start chest compressions. These should be conducted for about a minute or so, before the lifesaver calls 911. However, if one person can perform the compressions and there is another person available who can call 911, then these steps should happen simultaneously.

For persons who are trained in CPR, one of the best ways to remember the order in which steps should be administered is to recall the memory cue CAB. This cue stands for Circulation, Airway, Breathing. The goal of CPR is to help an unresponsive person to start breathing on his or her own. First, use chest compressions to restore circulation. This is the C of CAB. Second, check the patient's airway for possible blockages. The A in CAB stands for airway. Finally, administer rescue breathing. This is, of course, the B of CAB.

Which of the following sentences is the topic sentence for paragraph two?

A. Almost all approaches to CPR suggest that a person begin resuscitation efforts with chest compressions.
B. The unofficial recommendation of how many chest compressions to provide is around 100 per minute.
C. The compressions should be counted, so that the individual can keep track of how many compressions have been administered.
D. To perform a chest compression, the individual places both hands flat on the patient's chest and then begins pushing down carefully but firmly, most likely at equal intervals.

The correct answer is **A**. Paragraph two focuses on how to give chest compressions. Choice A reflects the topic sentence, as this sentence comes first in the paragraph and describes the idea to be developed. Choices B, C, and D reflect supporting details of the paragraph.

Let's look at another example:

Christopher Columbus was particularly influenced by the maps of the ancient geographer Ptolemy. Ptolemy argued that the world was round, which went against the belief of the day that the world was flat. Columbus sided with Ptolemy on this question and set out to prove that it was so.

At the time it was widely held that sailing west from Europe would lead to certain death. Believing that the world was round, Columbus thought that one who sailed west would wind up in the east. Other scientists of the day rejected this idea, so Columbus wrote to a respected Italian scholar, Paolo Toscanelli, to ask for his opinion on the matter.

Toscanelli supported the idea of Columbus's trip and sent word back to Columbus in 1474. After receiving Toscanelli's encouragement, Columbus focused all of his thoughts and plans on traveling westward. To make the journey, he would require the help of a generous financial backer, so he went to seek the aid of the king of Portugal. Columbus asked the king for ships and sailors to make the journey. In return, he promised to bring back wealth and to help to convert natives living on the lands to the Church. Portugal refused, and Columbus approached Italy unsuccessfully as well. He went to Spain next.

Queen Isabella of Spain agreed to support the journey. It took some time for Columbus to convince her, but he did succeed, and she paid for the trip. Part of what led the queen to believe in Columbus was the way that he focused on his goal for such a long time with great intent. He spent the best years of his life working toward his dream, remaining persistent and determined. Legend has it that even during his first voyage, members of his crew became frightened and uncertain, wanting to return home, but Columbus pressed on. The eventual discovery of the Americas was the reward for his commitment.

More than 500 years later, the geography of the world is often taken for granted, but Columbus was an early visionary whose results proved at least some of his theories correct.

Which of the following sentences is the summary sentence for the entire passage?

A. Christopher Columbus was particularly influenced by the maps of the ancient geographer Ptolemy.
B. More than 500 years later, the geography of the world is often taken for granted, but Columbus was an early visionary whose results proved at least some of his theories correct.
C. Part of what led the queen to believe in Columbus was the way that he focused on his goal for such a long time with great intent.
D. Legend has it that even during his first voyage, members of his crew became frightened and uncertain, wanting to return home, but Columbus pressed on.

The correct answer is **B**. The passage continually emphasizes how Columbus worked to prove his belief that the world was round. His commitment to his vision enabled him to win the backing of Queen Isabella and eventually discover America. The statement in choice C summarizes how the persistence of Columbus impressed Queen Isabella. This statement highlights an important theme of the passage, *persistence*, rather than summarizing the entire passage.

Review Questions

Saltwater fish and freshwater fish are related, but their natural environments prove rather distinctive. In terms of being kept as pets, freshwater fish require less maintenance. They live in water that can be adapted from tap water, and they can be kept in many different types of containers in addition to aquariums. Saltwater fish, on the other hand, require a specific type of salt-infused water. Careful watch of the pH balance of the water must also be maintained.

The next two questions are based on this passage.

1. Which of the following describes the phrase *fresh versus saltwater fish* as it relates to the passage?

    A. Main idea
    B. Topic
    C. Supporting detail
    D. Theme

2. Is the phrase *maintenance requirements* a topic, main idea, supporting detail, or theme of the above passage?

    A. Main idea
    B. Topic
    C. Supporting detail
    D. Theme

Laurel Hill Botanic Gardens is pleased to announce the installation of the sculpture series by Laurel Hill artist-in-residence, Darryl C. Grant. The installation features mixed-media sculptures emphasizing the floral designs prominent in Mr. Grant's paintings, many of which are also on exhibit in the Michael and Frieda Sachs Viewing Room.

The sculpture exhibit will open at 10:00 a.m. on Thursday, June 5. The Botanic Gardens' art curator, Jessalyn Jones, will present an overview of the sculptures and lead a guided tour of the installation. The opening ceremony will end with refreshments served in the Nature Observatory from 2:00–3:00 p.m.

This is a members-only event. All Botanic Gardens members and their guests are invited to attend. Tickets are $50.00 per person and can be purchased at the registration desk beginning Monday, May 5.

The next two questions are based on this passage.

3. Is *floral designs* a topic, main idea, supporting detail, or theme of the above announcement?

A. Theme
B. Topic
C. Supporting detail
D. Main idea

4. Which of the following sentences is the topic sentence for the entire announcement?

A. The Botanic Gardens' art curator, Jessalyn Jones, will present an overview of the sculptures.
B. The installation features mixed-media sculptures emphasizing the floral designs prominent in Mr. Grant's paintings.
C. All Botanic Gardens members and their guests are invited to attend.
D. The opening ceremony will end with refreshments served in the Nature Observatory from 2:00–3:00 p.m.

To Whom It May Concern,

I am writing to request a refund of the charge made to my credit card for the purchase of a water filter on Friday, September 18. The filter was the wrong type for my filtration system, so I had to return it. I returned the filter to the store on Saturday, September 19, and the customer service clerk had me complete the paperwork to refund my charges for the purchase. However, the credit never appeared on my credit card account. Please reverse the charges in the amount shown on the credit receipt attached to this e-mail.

Thank you for your assistance.

Claire Glendheim

The next two questions are based on this passage.

5. Which of the following sentences is a summary sentence for the e-mail above?

   A. I am writing to request a refund of the charge made to my credit card for the purchase of a water filter on Friday, September 18.
   B. The filter was the wrong type for my filtration system, so I had to return it.
   C. However, the credit never appeared on my credit card account.
   D. Please reverse the charges in the amount shown on the credit receipt attached to this e-mail.

6. Which of the following describes the phrase *credit card refund request* as it relates to the above e-mail?

   A. Topic
   B. Theme
   C. Supporting detail
   D. Main idea

7. Jan,

Arthur from Human Resources let me know that you were requesting recommendations for interns who might fill the open position in the Graphics department. I would highly recommend Alex Hastings, who has worked with me this summer on several book designs. His work is consistently top quality. He has not only the experience we are looking for, but also the motivation and drive to excel. Alex will be graduating this fall and would be an ideal candidate to fill the position.

If I can provide you with any additional information, just let me know.

Henry

Is *intern recommendation* a topic, main idea, supporting detail, or theme of the above passage?

   A. Main idea
   B. Topic
   C. Supporting detail
   D. Theme

Historically, the study of creativity has concentrated on persons known for their innovation. Early creativity studies focused on creative "geniuses," such as Einstein, Mozart, or Shakespeare. This type of creativity is known as "Big C" creativity. However, as research on creativity progressed, a corresponding interest in how people could be creative in smaller ways—on an everyday basis—emerged in the discipline. Scholars began to investigate how ordinary tasks, such as cleaning, driving particular familiar routes, and completing work and schoolwork, could be conducted in innovative ways. This focus of creativity research has been labeled "little c" creativity.

The next two questions are based on this passage.

8. Is *types of creativity* a topic, main idea, supporting detail, or theme of the above passage?

 A. Supporting detail
 B. Theme
 C. Main idea
 D. Topic

9. Which of the following describes the phrase *driving particular familiar routes* as it relates to the above passage?

 A. Main idea
 B. Theme
 C. Topic
 D. Supporting detail

The way that scientists have envisioned the makeup of the universe has shifted and transformed as the centuries have passed. Prior to the work of Copernicus, people believed that the earth was at the center of the universe. The idea that the earth revolved around the sun was initially taken as heresy. The progression and gradual acceptance of these originally controversial ideas paved the way for the acceptance of later discoveries by Newton and Einstein. Their theories have revolutionized the ways in which science itself is conducted today.

The next two questions are based on this passage.

10. Which of the following sentences is the topic sentence for the entire passage?

 A. The way that scientists have envisioned the makeup of the universe has shifted and transformed as the centuries have passed.
 B. Prior to the work of Copernicus, people believed that the earth was at the center of the universe.
 C. The progression and gradual acceptance of these originally controversial ideas paved the way for the acceptance of later discoveries by Newton and Einstein.
 D. Their theories have revolutionized the ways in which science itself is conducted today.

11. Is *changing mindsets* a topic, main idea, supporting detail, or theme of the above passage?

 A. Supporting detail
 B. Topic
 C. Main idea
 D. Theme

The best method of treating individuals facing psychological difficulties is a blend of cognitive-behavioral therapy and medication. This approach not only serves to address the patient's potential chemical imbalances, but it also emancipates the patient by allowing him or her some autonomy in dealing with the issues associated with a possible malaise.

Cognitive-behavioral therapy requires the patient to examine his or her own behavior and to make moderations in a rational and well-thought-out manner. If a person's chemical makeup is preventing him or her from being able to carry out such a responsibility, then medication can help alleviate specific symptoms to allow the patient to deal with the underlying emotional and psychological issues in an effective manner. Nevertheless, psychologists have wide-ranging opinions on how to help these patients cope with challenges such as depression or anxiety.

Some trained professionals assert that medication alone can best serve psychological patients. Other psychologists believe that the utilization of Freud's psychoanalytic approach represents the best method for assisting persons with these emotional symptoms. Some counselors believe that each person's set of individual circumstances should be considered. Other counselors depend on the characteristics of behaviorism to modify the patients' behavior so that their behavioral patterns become more effective. Overall, however, many professionals agree that the combination of cognitive-behavioral therapy and medication will ultimately best serve the patient.

The next two questions are based on this passage.

12. Which of the following sentences is the summary sentence for the passage?

   A. The best method of treating individuals facing psychological difficulties is a blend of cognitive-behavioral therapy and medication.
   B. Some counselors believe that each person's set of individual circumstances should be considered.
   C. Overall, however, many professionals agree that the combination of cognitive-behavioral therapy and medication will ultimately best serve the patient.
   D. Nevertheless, psychologists have wide-ranging opinions on how to help these patients cope with challenges such as depression or anxiety.

13. Is *cognitive-behavioral therapy versus medication* a topic, main idea, supporting detail, or theme of the above passage?

   A. Main idea
   B. Topic
   C. Supporting detail
   D. Theme

14. One of the most important gymnastic exercises in the original Montessori school approach is that of the "line." For this exercise, a line is drawn in chalk or paint on the floor. Instead of one line, there may also be two

lines drawn. The children are taught to walk on these lines like tightrope walkers, placing their feet one in front of the other.

To keep their balance, the children must make efforts similar to those of real tightrope walkers, except that they have no danger of falling, since the lines are drawn only on the floor. The teacher herself performs the exercise first, showing clearly how she places her feet, and the children imitate her without her even needing to speak. At first it is only certain children who follow her, and when she has shown them how to walk the line, she leaves, letting the exercise develop on its own.

The children for the most part continue to walk, following with great care the movement they have seen, and making efforts to keep their balance so they don't fall. Gradually the other children come closer and watch and try the exercise. In a short time, the entire line is covered with children balancing themselves and continuing to walk around, watching their feet attentively.

Music may be used at this point. It should be a very simple march, without an obvious rhythm. It should simply accompany and support the efforts of the children.

When children learn to master their balance in this way, Dr. Montessori believed, they can bring the act of walking to a remarkable standard of perfection.

Is *the line* a topic, main idea, supporting detail, or theme of the above passage?

A. Supporting detail
B. Main idea
C. Topic
D. Theme

15. Imagine living in the year 1800. The railroads then were very scarce. Gas lights were not yet invented, and electric lights were not even dreamed of. Even kerosene wasn't used at that point. This was the world into which Samuel Morse, the inventor of the telegraph, was born.

Samuel Morse was born in Charlestown, Massachusetts, shortly before the turn of the century, in 1791. When he was seven years old, he was sent to boarding school at Phillips Academy, Andover. While he was there, his father wrote him letters, giving him good advice. He told him about George Washington and about a British statesman named Lord Chesterfield, who was able to achieve many of his goals. Lord Chesterfield was asked once how he managed to find time for all of his pursuits, and he replied that he only ever did one thing at a time, and that he "never put off anything until tomorrow that could be done today."

Morse worked hard at school and began to think and act for himself at quite a young age. His biggest accomplishment was in painting, and he established himself as a successful painter after graduating from college at Yale. But he also had an interest in science and inventions. He was passionate about the idea of discovering a way for people to send messages to each other in short periods of time.

In the early 1800s, it took a long time to receive news of any sort, even important news. Whole countries had to wait weeks to hear word of the outcomes of faraway wars. The mail was carried by stagecoach. In emergency situations, such as when ships were lost at sea, there was no way to send requests for help. Electricity had been discovered, but little application had been made of it up until that point. This was about to change when Morse set his mind to his invention.

On October 1, 1832, Morse was sailing to America from a trip overseas on a ship called the *Sully*. He became preoccupied with the thought of inventing a machine that would later become the telegraph. Morse thought about the telegraph night and day. As he sat upon the deck of the ship after dinner one night, he took out a little notebook and began to create a plan.

If a message could be sent ten miles without dropping, he wrote, "I could make it go around the globe." He said this over and over again during the years after his trip.

One morning at the breakfast table, Morse showed his plan to some of the other *Sully* passengers. Five years later, when the model of the telegraph was built, it was exactly like the one shown that morning to the passengers on the *Sully*.

Once he arrived in America, Morse worked for twelve long years to get people to notice his invention. Though some supported the idea of the telegraph, many people scoffed at it. Morse persisted, and eventually a bill was passed by Congress in 1842. It authorized the funds needed to build the first trial telegraph line.

After two years, the telegraph line was complete. Morse and his colleagues tested it in May of 1844. The device worked, and the telegraph became a huge success. Morse's persistence had finally paid off.

Which of the following describes the word *perseverance* as it relates to the passage?

A. Main idea
B. Topic
C. Supporting detail
D. Theme

Answer Key

1. B		**9.** D	
2. D		**10.** A	
3. C		**11.** D	
4. C		**12.** C	
5. D		**13.** B	
6. A		**14.** C	
7. B		**15.** D	
8. D			

Answers and Explanations

1. (B) *Fresh versus saltwater fish* is the general topic of this passage. Choice D is incorrect because the topic of a passage is its general subject matter, whereas a theme is a concept or idea that relates to the passage topic and recurs frequently throughout the passage.

2. (D) *Maintenance requirements* is a theme of this passage. The passage compares and contrasts saltwater and freshwater fish, with a focus on their respective maintenance requirements.

3. (C) *Floral designs* is a supporting detail of this announcement. The announcement mentions in the first paragraph that the installation features sculptures emphasizing the floral designs prominent in Mr. Grant's paintings.

4. (C) Choice C is the topic sentence of the entire announcement, because it introduces the main idea developed in the announcement. This announcement's purpose is to invite members of the Botanic Gardens to an event. The topic sentence is unusually positioned in that it appears in the middle of the announcement rather than at the beginning. The sentences in choices A, B, and D are incorrect because they offer supporting details.

5. (D) Choice D provides a summary sentence for the ideas addressed in the entire e-mail. Here, the author restates her main reason for the writing the e-mail: to have her credit card charges reversed. Choice A is the topic statement of the e-mail, while choices B and C are supporting details.

6. (A) The topic of this passage is a credit card refund request. The main idea of this e-mail might be stated as follows: "The author returned a water filtration system and is placing a second request for a credit card refund."

7. (B) The phrase *intern recommendation* is the specific topic of this passage. Two possible supporting details of the e-mail could be *motivation* and *extensive experience*, both of which describe the intern's qualifications.

8. (D) *Types of creativity* is the general topic of this passage, because it is what the passage is about.

9. (D) The phrase *driving particular familiar routes* is a supporting detail of the passage. This detail is mentioned as an example of an everyday task.

10. (A) Choice A is the topic sentence of the entire article, because it introduces the main idea developed in the article. Choice B is a supporting detail for the topic sentence. Choice C is another supporting detail.

11. (D) *Changing mindsets* is a theme of this passage, not the topic; the topic is not focused on changing mindsets but, more specifically, on scientific views of the universe.

12. (C) Choice C provides a summary sentence for the passage, while choice A is the topic sentence.

13. (B) *Cognitive-behavioral therapy versus medication* is the topic of this passage rather than the theme, because the topic is the general subject matter of the passage, while theme concerns reoccurring ideas related to the topic.

14. (C) *The line* is the general topic of this passage because it is what the passage is about; one theme throughout the passage is *mimicking behavior*.

15. (D) *Perseverance* is a theme of this passage. The passage discusses Morse's perseverance throughout, while the topic of the passage is the telegraph.

CHAPTER 4

Making Inferences and Drawing Conclusions

Inference questions ask about logical deductions or implications that can be drawn from what an author says. They usually contain the phrases "What does the author imply about X?" or "What can be inferred about X?" They also contain phrases such as "most likely" and "probably." A common Inference question is "Based on the passage, which of the following is most likely to be true?"

The correct answers to Inference questions must be logically deduced from the information presented. When answering Inference questions, therefore, it's important to remember that the correct answer will not be a detail found in the passage.

> The answer to an Inference question is never given directly in the passage.

Instead, you must use logical reasoning to determine the answer. Consider this example:

Aficionados of classical music frequently appreciate the characteristics of jazz, and some laypersons think the two genres are somewhat similar. However, jazz musicians are noted for their improvisational abilities, whereas classically trained musicians are often very reliant upon printed music. Although musicians in both genres must be very well versed in scales and various musical keys, jazz musicians must possess impeccable knowledge of this material in order to be able to perform and fulfill the requirements of their chosen genre.

Based on information given in the passage, which of the following statements is most likely to be true of jazz musicians?

A. Jazz musicians must rely on printed musical scores.
B. Jazz musicians can also play classical music if they wish.
C. Jazz musicians do not always need printed music.
D. Jazz musicians play better music than classical musicians.

The correct answer is **C**. The passage states that jazz musicians can improvise, whereas classical musicians rely on printed music, so we can therefore reason logically that jazz musicians do not always need printed scores. The passage does not suggest that jazz musicians can play classical music, although both types of musicians learn many of the same skills. The passage states that jazz musicians must develop excellent skills, but it does not imply that jazz is superior to classical music, so choice D is incorrect.

Here is another Inference question regarding the study of Shakespeare.

Literary scholars have often speculated as to the personal characteristics of William Shakespeare. The Bard is known to many as the greatest writer the English language has ever known, but we have very few examples of his handwriting or even his own name written out in his hand. Some academics have gone so far as to speculate that Shakespeare was a pseudonym for an aristocrat. However, the majority of scholars have dismissed this proposal, and they concentrate instead on Shakespeare's thoughtful insights and dexterous construction of language.

Based on information given in the passage, how do scholars most likely learn about Shakespeare?

A. Through speculation about his personality and his true identity
B. By studying diaries, letters, and other documents written in his hand
C. By studying his plays, his poetry, and other works attributed to him
D. By studying the architecture, construction, and other physical attributes of his historical era

The correct answer is **C**. The last sentence of the passage states that most scholars focus on Shakespeare's use of insights and language, which implies that scholars learn about him through what is expressed in his works. The passage makes clear that very few documents are actually written in his hand, so choice B is incorrect. Choice D is not mentioned anywhere in the passage, so we cannot make a logical inference about it.

In this next example, concerning Michelangelo, we are asked to draw an inference based on a specific sentence in the passage.

Michelangelo was arguably the most talented and prolific artist to emerge from the Italian Renaissance. Not only did he spend three years on his back lying on a scaffold to create the famous paintings adorning the Sistine Chapel, but he also created a sculpture of the Biblical hero David that has been emulated for centuries. Michelangelo himself reflected that he simply took a block of marble and removed all the pieces that did not belong to the David statue. Michelangelo is considered a consummate artist because he created works in so many different media, including painting and sculpture.

Which of the following is implied by the third sentence of the passage?

A. Michelangelo mused that the statue of David was inside the block of marble all along, and all he had to do was free it.
B. Michelangelo created his sculpture of David by using several pieces of marble, each of which had to be dug up or removed from the quarry separately.
C. Michelangelo created a reflection of his statue of David by removing all the marble that stood between the statue and a mirrored surface.
D. Michelangelo said that he worked by trial and error, removing pieces of marble to see what happened as he sculpted his statue of David.

The correct answer is **A**. The third sentence of the passage implies that by "removing" all the marble that did not belong to the statue of David,

Michelangelo was revealing something that he had envisioned within the marble all along. Choice A forms the best logical deduction that can be based on the third sentence. Choice B is outside the scope of the passage.

Drawing Conclusions questions require the same deductive logic as Inference questions, except they focus specifically on overall conclusions that can be drawn from a passage or paragraph. Conclusion questions ask about the "big ideas" implied in a selection, rather than the details. They may also ask about predictions that can be made, based on the information in a passage. The question that follows asks about the third paragraph of this example specifically.

> Public highways are used constantly with little thought of how important they are to the everyday life of a community. It is understandable that most people think about their local public highway only when it affects their own activities. People usually don't focus on highway improvements unless the subject is brought to their attention by increased taxes or advertising.
>
> Highway improvements are an important issue, however. It is important for the economies of most communities to keep highways in good repair. Products purchased in one location are often manufactured in other locations, and safe highways are required to transport the products to their final destination. Good transportation facilities contribute greatly to community prosperity.
>
> The type and amount of the highway improvement needed in any area depend on the traffic in that area. In low-population areas, the amount of traffic on local roads is likely to be small, and highways will not require as much work. But as an area develops, the use of public highways increases, and maintenance demands increase. In small towns, residents are also more able to adapt to the condition of the roads. A road shutdown does not have the same impact on business as it would in busy areas. In large districts with many activities, however, roads must be usable year-round in order for business progress to continue.
>
> In planning improvements of highway systems, several different types of traffic may be encountered. These range from business traffic to agricultural shipping to residential transportation. Improvement activities must meet the requirements of all classes of traffic, the most important being provided for first. Those improvements of lesser importance can be performed as soon as finances permit.

What conclusion can be drawn from the third paragraph of the passage?

A. People in small towns are more adaptable than those in more developed areas.
B. People move to small towns to avoid the traffic found in developed areas.
C. Good highway maintenance is more important in developed areas than in small towns.
D. Most people do not think about highway maintenance in rural or developed areas.

The correct answer is **C.** The last sentence of the paragraph states that roads in developed areas must be usable year-round, which indicates that maintenance in those areas is more important than in small towns. Choice A is incorrect because the author does not compare the adaptability of people in small towns versus developed areas. Choice B is not suggested in the passage. Finally, the first paragraph states that most people do not usually think about highway maintenance or improvements, but this is not a topic raised in the third paragraph, so choice D is incorrect as well.

The passage below is followed by another Drawing Conclusions question, this time concerning the passage's final paragraph.

Austrian-born Sigmund Freud, a psychoanalytic psychologist, lived from the mid-nineteenth to the mid-twentieth century. The psychoanalytic approach refers to the school of thought that unconscious memories or desires guide our emotions and actions. In personality theory, this equates to events from childhood shaping the individual self without a person's conscious awareness. These specific childhood events continue to exert a strong influence over our lives and dominate our emotions. If you are a life-of-the-party, extroverted personality, perhaps you had a healthy upbringing; however, quiet, deep-thinker types can be just as functional. How your caregivers responded to your natural urges will determine your level of mental health, according to the psychoanalytic approach.

Freud believed that as a child, an individual's actions are driven by hidden impulses—and that repression or denial of those impulses by parents or society can lead to fixations or personality disorders. Alternatively, if the child's impulses are accepted as normative to his or her development, then a functional adult behavioral pattern should take root. Now, by no means should parents allow every impulse to dictate behavior; each of us has a "censor," which Freud referred to as the "superego." This element of the psyche is largely helpful and acts as a conscience. However, if we let the superego dominate our personality, Freud believed, it could lead to repression and inauthentic behavior.

Freud often worked with highly distressed female clients, repressed in their natural modes of expression; this is how he developed many of his theories, which some people believe are not very scientific. By today's standards, they are not, but Freud's idea that unconscious urges drive our behavior was revolutionary for his time.

What conclusion can be drawn from the last paragraph of the passage?

A. Freud's theories of personality development are still considered revolutionary today.
B. Scientists are still trying to prove Freud's theories of the unconscious today.
C. Freud's views on the unconscious are not considered scientific fact today.
D. Women's emotions can be studied and analyzed scientifically today.

The correct answer is **C**. The last paragraph states that Freud's theories are not considered scientific today, and that would include his views on the unconscious, as the unconscious was part of his psychoanalytic theory. The paragraph does not provide information to suggest that women's emotions can be studied scientifically today, so choice D is incorrect.

Review Questions

1. The Beatles influenced the genre of rock and roll just as Beethoven expanded the genre of the symphony. John Lennon, Paul McCartney, George Harrison, and Ringo Starr expanded the public's understanding of their musical genre and reclassified it as an anthem for rebellion. Their music transformed into the hippies' theme songs of the sixties. Beethoven similarly altered the public's understanding of the symphony. His addition of a chorus in the last movement of the Ninth Symphony attests to this feat.

   What does the author imply about the influence that both the Beatles and Beethoven had on music?

   A. While different musically, both the Beatles and Beethoven invented radically new genres that the general public became skeptical about.
   B. The Beatles and Beethoven revolutionized the audience's perspective of their respective genres of music.
   C. Neither the Beatles nor Beethoven let societal concerns dictate the way they constructed music; as a result, their nonconformity gave birth to chaotic movements in music.
   D. Both inspired others to follow their lead to invent new genres of music.

2. Imagine living in the year 1800. The railroads then were very scarce. Gas lights were not yet invented, and electric lights were not even dreamed of. Even kerosene wasn't used at that point. This was the world into which Samuel Morse, the inventor of the telegraph, was born.

   Samuel Morse was born in Charlestown, Massachusetts, shortly before the turn of the century, in 1791. When he was seven years old, he was sent to boarding school at Phillips Academy, Andover. While he was there, his father wrote him letters, giving him good advice. He told him about George Washington and about a British statesman named Lord Chesterfield, who was able to achieve many of his goals. Lord Chesterfield was asked once how he managed to find time for all of his pursuits, and he replied that he only ever did one thing at a time, and that he "never put off anything until tomorrow that could be done today."

   Morse worked hard at school and began to think and act for himself at quite a young age. His biggest accomplishment was in painting, and he established himself as a successful painter after graduating from college at Yale. But he also had an interest in science and inventions. He was passionate about the idea of discovering a way for people to send messages to each other in short periods of time.

In the early 1800s, it took a long time to receive news of any sort, even important news. Whole countries had to wait weeks to hear word of the outcomes of faraway wars. The mail was carried by stagecoach. In emergency situations, such as when ships were lost at sea, there was no way to send requests for help. Electricity had been discovered, but little application had been made of it up until that point. This was about to change when Morse set his mind to his invention.

On October 1, 1832, Morse was sailing to America from a trip overseas on a ship called the *Sully*. He became preoccupied with the thought of inventing a machine that would later become the telegraph. Morse thought about the telegraph night and day. As he sat upon the deck of the ship after dinner one night, he took out a little notebook and began to create a plan.

If a message could be sent ten miles without dropping, he wrote, "I could make it go around the globe." He said this over and over again during the years after his trip.

One morning at the breakfast table, Morse showed his plan to some of the other *Sully* passengers. Five years later, when the model of the telegraph was built, it was exactly like the one shown that morning to the passengers on the *Sully*.

Once he arrived in America, Morse worked for twelve long years to get people to notice his invention. Though some supported the idea of the telegraph, many people scoffed at it. Morse persisted, and eventually a bill was passed by Congress in 1842. It authorized the funds needed to build the first trial telegraph line.

After two years, the telegraph line was complete. Morse and his colleagues tested it in May 1844. The device worked, and the telegraph became a huge success. Morse's persistence had finally paid off.

What does paragraph three imply about the character of Samuel Morse?

A. Morse was a solemn child who depended heavily on his family for support.
B. Morse had difficulty focusing on one project and so failed to find any real success early in life.
C. Morse was a well-rounded child with varied interests who exerted independence even at a young age.
D. Morse treasured independence above family; therefore, he threw himself into his projects for consolation.

One of the most important gymnastic exercises in the original Montessori school approach is that of the "line." For this exercise, a line is drawn in chalk or paint on the floor. Instead of one line, there may also be two lines drawn. The children are taught to walk on these lines like tightrope walkers, placing their feet one in front of the other.

To keep their balance, the children must make efforts similar to those of real tightrope walkers, except that they have no danger of falling, since the lines are drawn only on the floor. The teacher herself performs the exercise first, showing clearly how she places her feet, and the children imitate her without her even needing to speak. At first it is only certain children who follow her, and when she has shown them how to walk the line, she leaves, letting the exercise develop on its own.

The children for the most part continue to walk, following with great care the movement they have seen, and making efforts to keep their balance so they don't fall. Gradually the other children come closer and watch and try the exercise. In a short time, the entire line is covered with children balancing themselves and continuing to walk around, watching their feet attentively.

Music may be used at this point. It should be a very simple march, without an obvious rhythm. It should simply accompany and support the efforts of the children.

When children learn to master their balance in this way, Dr. Montessori believed, they can bring the act of walking to a remarkable standard of perfection.

The next two questions are based on this passage.

3. Based on the passage's tightrope walking example, what does the author imply about Montessori education?

   A. Dr. Montessori believed that children learned best through example and practice.
   B. Montessori schools provide unusual exercise regimens to keep children from getting bored.
   C. Dr. Montessori believed that children were incapable of learning to walk without strict instruction.
   D. Children in Montessori schools are subjected to rigorous exercise because it is believed to help children retain information.

4. Based on the passage, which of the following most likely reflects Dr. Montessori's belief about learning?

   A. Children cannot learn through experience.
   B. Not all children can learn through exercise.
   C. Children can learn only through demonstrations.
   D. Learning is less likely when fear is present.

5. Aficionados of classical music frequently appreciate the characteristics of jazz, and some laypersons think the two genres are somewhat similar. However, jazz musicians are noted for their improvisational abilities, whereas classically trained musicians are often very reliant upon printed music. Although musicians in both genres must be very well versed in scales and various musical keys, jazz musicians must possess impeccable knowledge of this material in order to be able to perform and fulfill the requirements of their chosen genre.

What does the author imply about the similarity between classical and jazz music?

A. It can be inferred that despite some opinions, classical and jazz music resemble each other quite remarkably.
B. Both genres have the same roots in folk music, so musicians from one genre can play in the other without too much trouble.
C. Despite some opinions that the classical and jazz genres are similar, musicians in the two genres have notably different skills.
D. Although the musical structures of the two are the same, jazz musicians are better at playing both kinds of music.

Christopher Columbus was particularly influenced by the maps of the ancient geographer Ptolemy. Ptolemy argued that the world was round, which went against the belief of the day that the world was flat. Columbus sided with Ptolemy on this question and set out to prove that it was so.

At the time it was widely held that sailing west from Europe would lead to certain death. Believing that the world was round, Columbus thought that one who sailed west would wind up in the east. Other scientists of the day rejected this idea, so Columbus wrote to a respected Italian scholar, Paolo Toscanelli, to ask for his opinion on the matter.

Toscanelli supported the idea of Columbus's trip and sent word back to Columbus in 1474. After receiving Toscanelli's encouragement, Columbus focused all of his thoughts and plans on traveling westward. To make the journey, he would require the help of a generous financial backer, so he went to seek the aid of the king of Portugal. Columbus asked the king for ships and sailors to make the journey. In return, he promised to bring back wealth and to help to convert natives living on the lands to the Church. Portugal refused, and Columbus approached Italy unsuccessfully as well. He went to Spain next.

Queen Isabella of Spain agreed to support the journey. It took some time for Columbus to convince her, but he did succeed, and she paid for the trip. Part of what led the queen to believe in Columbus was the way that he focused on his goal for such a long time with great intent. He spent the best years of his life working toward his dream, remaining persistent and determined. Legend has it that even during his first voyage, members of his crew became frightened and uncertain, wanting to return home, but Columbus pressed on. The eventual discovery of the Americas was the reward for his commitment.

More than 500 years later, the geography of the world is often taken for granted, but Columbus was an early visionary whose results proved at least some of his theories correct.

The next two questions are based on this passage.

6. Based on the passage, which of the following can be inferred about Queen Isabella?

   A. She wholeheartedly believed in Ptolemy's vision of the world.
   B. She was open to new ideas about the geography of the world.
   C. She was an enemy of Portugal and Italy.
   D. She believed Columbus's expedition would fail.

7. Based on the passage, what can be concluded about the king of Portugal?

   A. He lacked enough support for Columbus's vision to fund it.
   B. He agreed with Ptolemy's vision of the world.
   C. He had no financial resources to offer Columbus.
   D. He and Queen Isabella were enemies.

Public highways are used constantly with little thought of how important they are to the everyday life of a community. It is understandable that most people think about their local public highway only when it affects their own activities. People usually don't focus on highway improvements unless the subject is brought to their attention by increased taxes or advertising.

Highway improvements are an important issue, however. It is important for the economies of most communities to keep highways in good repair. Products purchased in one location are often manufactured in other locations, and safe highways are required to transport the products to their final destination. Good transportation facilities contribute greatly to community prosperity.

The type and amount of the highway improvement needed in any area depends on the traffic in that area. In low-population areas, the amount of traffic on local roads is likely to be small, and highways will not require as much work. But as an area develops, the use of public highways increases, and maintenance demands increase. In small towns, residents are also more able to adapt to the condition of the roads. A road shutdown does not have the same impact on business as it would in busy areas. In large districts with many activities, however, roads must be usable year-round in order for business progress to continue.

In planning improvements of highway systems, several different types of traffic may be encountered. These range from business traffic to agricultural shipping to residential transportation. Improvement activities must meet the requirements of all classes of traffic, the most important being provided for first. Those improvements of lesser importance can be performed as soon as finances permit.

The next two questions are based on this passage.

8. According to the passage, what can be inferred about the relationship between the lack of highway maintenance and local economies?

   A. Businesses do not consider highway systems when choosing their location.
   B. Consumers will frequent businesses despite the lack of highway maintenance.
   C. Businesses can thrive despite the lack of good highway systems.
   D. Poor roads decrease consumer traffic, which leads to a decline in business.

9. What conclusion can be drawn based on paragraph two of the passage?

   A. Public highways are important only as a means of bypassing rural areas.
   B. It costs much more to repair rural highways than city streets, so city streets are ultimately less important.
   C. Public highways play a vital role in transporting goods to and from different locations.
   D. People do not care about the upkeep of public highways because they do not understand their value.

10. Freud was the first psychologist to conceptualize the idea of the unconscious, or the proposal that people acted from motivations of which they were unaware. Freud believed that unconscious motivations were most effectively revealed through dreams, so he frequently had his patients review and analyze their dreams. Since Freud's initial proposal, psychologists have built upon his original conception.

    It can be inferred that Freud established what relationship between his theory of the unconscious and dreams?

    A. Dreams could reveal why people acted a certain way even if they were not conscious of the motives behind those actions.
    B. If people analyzed their dreams, they could learn how to motivate themselves and take action.
    C. Because dreams occurred while people were asleep, or unconscious, most people could not remember them until Freud developed his theories.
    D. Freud was the first serious scholar to study dreams and speculate on their meaning.

11. In the animal kingdom, many symbiotic relationships exist between two species that take actions known to be mutually beneficial for both parties. In the water, clownfish have such a relationship with sea anemones. The fish are one of the only species that can swim unharmed in the anemone's waving tentacles, as typically the tentacles would sting any animal that swam near it. However, the clownfish is immune to the sting of the tentacles and is therefore protected by them; in return, its presence helps the anemone stay clean, avoid attack by parasites, and remain free from infection.

What conclusion can be drawn about the relationship between the clownfish and the sea anemone?

A. It is mutually beneficial to both creatures and allows for harmonious living.
B. It is parasitic in nature and often leads to the destruction of one of the two creatures.
C. In every pairing, one of the two creatures ends up as more of a beneficiary than the other, which leads to disharmony.
D. Separating the two would mean imminent death; therefore, the relationship is not only beneficial but also necessary.

12. Historically, the study of creativity has concentrated on persons known for their innovation. Early creativity studies focused on creative "geniuses," such as Einstein, Mozart, or Shakespeare. This type of creativity is known as "Big C" creativity. However, as research on creativity progressed, a corresponding interest in how people could be creative in smaller ways— on an everyday basis—emerged in the discipline. Scholars began to investigate how ordinary tasks, such as cleaning, driving particular familiar routes, and completing work and schoolwork, could be conducted in innovative ways. This focus of creativity research has been labeled "little c" creativity.

    Ultimately, what conclusion can be drawn about creativity?

    A. It is not possible to conduct research on creativity because it is such an elusive trait.
    B. Creativity is only tracked in "Big C" cases where geniuses are concerned.
    C. Because creativity can now be found in even the mundane, it is no longer a subject worthy of study.
    D. Creativity is multifaceted and can be found in various areas of a person's daily life.

13. The current tests for measuring IQ, or an individual's intelligence quotient, were developed during the early and mid-twentieth century. Their use was popularized by Terman, who designed specific tests for use in the U.S. Army. Some psychologists today assert that the traditional system of measuring IQ should remain the sole method of assessing intelligence. Historically, the test has been constructed based on the assumption that there exists one general intelligence factor that impacts an individual's intellectual capacity.

    The validity of this assumption has been challenged by other psychologists. In particular, Howard Gardner has emphasized that a unified conception of intelligence based on a single factor remains highly limited and unnecessarily constraining. Gardner has postulated an alternative theory concerning the existence of multiple intelligences. He posits that individuals can possess intelligence in particular areas, including linguistic intelligence, spiritual intelligence, spatial intelligence, intrapersonal intelligence, interpersonal intelligence, musical intelligence, mathematical intelligence, and kinesthetic intelligence, among others.

Gardner asserts that individuals can be extremely intelligent and exhibit talent in one area, while failing to demonstrate the same level of prowess in another area. His theory has been discussed widely, although efforts to obtain empirical evidence to support his ideas remain in process.

What conclusion can be drawn about intelligence based on Howard Gardner's findings?

A. The IQ test, while flawed, remains the most important tool we have to test intelligence.
B. Intelligence is not limited to one's ability to take a test; instead, there are multiple intelligences that a person may exhibit in any given area.
C. Intelligence is elusive and difficult to measure or determine; therefore, the IQ test has questionable meaning.
D. Intelligence can only be determined through a series of tests; therefore, students should be heavily tested in every subject area.

14. Literary scholars have frequently compared the characteristics of poetry written by both the first and second generation of Romantic poets. Poets such as William Wordsworth established the foundations of the exaltation of the imagination that later influenced writers such as John Keats and Percy Bysshe Shelley. The first generation of poets was attempting to advocate for the importance of artistry and creativity. The second generation of poets built on this foundation and went even further in their speculations about what creativity could achieve, especially perhaps in a political sense. However, the second generation was also negatively impacted by their observation of the French Revolution, and this experience tempered their idealism.

What conclusion can be drawn about the influence of the French Revolution on Romantic poets?

A. It divided the British and American Romantic poets into two very distinct movements.
B. It shifted the tone and dimmed the idealism of the Romantic movement.
C. The Revolution caused the Romantics to abandon their ideals and take up arms against tyranny.
D. It forced Romantics to cling even more to their ideals and to shun the reality of war.

15. Austrian-born Sigmund Freud, a psychoanalytic psychologist, lived from the mid-nineteenth to the mid-twentieth century. The psychoanalytic approach refers to the school of thought that unconscious memories or desires guide our emotions and actions. In personality theory, this equates to events from childhood shaping the individual self without a person's conscious awareness. These specific childhood events continue to exert a strong influence over our lives and dominate our emotions. If you are a life-of-the-party, extroverted personality, perhaps you had a healthy

upbringing; however, quiet, deep-thinker types can be just as functional. How your caregivers responded to your natural urges will determine your level of mental health, according to the psychoanalytic approach.

Freud believed that as a child, an individual's actions are driven by hidden impulses—and that repression or denial of those impulses by parents or society can lead to fixations or personality disorders. Alternatively, if the child's impulses are accepted as normative to his or her development, then a functional adult behavioral pattern should take root. Now, by no means should parents allow every impulse to dictate behavior; each of us has a "censor," which Freud referred to as the "superego." This element of the psyche is largely helpful and acts as a conscience. However, if we let the superego dominate our personality, Freud believed, it could lead to repression and inauthentic behavior.

Freud often worked with highly distressed female clients, repressed in their natural modes of expression; this is how he developed many of his theories, which some people believe are not very scientific. By today's standards, they are not, but Freud's idea that unconscious urges drive our behavior was revolutionary for his time.

Based on information given in the passage, which of the following can be concluded about the psychoanalytic approach?

A. Psychoanalysis discounts the role of desire in individuals' actions.
B. Early psychoanalytic theory guides most psychological treatments today.
C. The psychoanalytic approach is not as credible today as it was in the past.
D. The psychoanalytic approach is best used with female patients only.

Answer Key

1. B		**9.** C	
2. C		**10.** A	
3. A		**11.** A	
4. D		**12.** D	
5. C		**13.** B	
6. B		**14.** B	
7. A		**15.** C	
8. D			

Answers and Explanations

1. **(B)** The question asks you to determine what influence the respective musicians had on music. The author uses words like *expanded*, *transformed*, and *altered* to indicate the influence they had. *Revolutionize* is a synonym of these terms and best represents the intended inference. Although it may be tempting to identify the term *invented* with *revolutionize*, the second half of choice A creates an extreme that does not exist in the passage. The musicians did not create new genres; instead, they worked within their genres to expand them. In addition, the passage in no way indicates that the musicians fell out of public favor, so choice A is incorrect. The passage does not discuss societal concerns either, so choice C can be eliminated. Not only does the passage not argue that the musicians invented new genres, as discussed above, but it also does not address any inspirational effects the musicians may or may not have had on other musicians. Choice D is therefore incorrect.

2. **(C)** The author notes that Morse was interested in both painting and science—this implies that Morse was not pigeonholed into any one field. His interests were well rounded. The author also claims that Morse "began to think and act for himself at quite a young age," which suggests that Morse was an independent person. Since the author establishes Morse as a child who liked to think for himself, choice A can be eliminated because it suggests that Morse was dependent by nature. While the author does mention more than one interest that Morse had, Morse was able to achieve success in painting at an early age, which eliminates choice B. Regarding choice D, the author does state that Morse was independent, but there is no mention of how he might prioritize his family over his independence.

3. **(A)** The question asks you to identify the statement that best identifies traits of the Montessori program based on the tightrope description given in the passage. In the passage, example and practice are highlighted as methodologies used to help children learn to walk properly. Regarding choice B, although the tightrope walking exercise may be considered unusual by some, the focus of the passage is on the methodology used by Montessori, not on people's response to it. The passage also explains that the exercise helps to improve students' sense of balance, not to prevent boredom. Choice C is incorrect, because the passage never addresses any negative attitude Dr. Montessori might have had toward students, nor does it identify Montessori education with rigidity or strictness. Choice D is also incorrect because, like choices B and C, it addresses a topic that is not discussed in the passage.

4. **(D)** The second paragraph states that the line is drawn on the floor so that children do not have a danger of falling while walking the line. One can infer that learning is less likely when children are afraid of falling. Although this passage discusses learning through demonstration, the author does not suggest that children can learn only through demonstration. Therefore, choice C is incorrect.

5. **(C)** Using the word "however" after stating that "some laypersons think the two genres are somewhat similar" indicates that the author believes the opposite: they are not that similar. This eliminates choices A and B, which contend that the two genres are quite similar. Choice D is incorrect because the author does not make a judgment regarding which players may or may not be the better musicians. Instead, the focus is on the differences between the two musical genres.

6. **(B)** Although the passage does not state that Queen Isabella was open-minded about new ideas, it can be inferred that she was because she believed in Columbus's vision and eventually supported his expedition. Choice A is not correct because Columbus had to convince her to support his journey. If she had believed in Ptolemy's ideas wholeheartedly, she most likely would not have needed to be convinced.

7. **(A)** Based on the passage, we can conclude that the king lacked enough support for Columbus's

vision to support it. Choices C and D are incorrect, because the passage suggests that the king had the resources to be a financial backer, and it does not discuss the king's relationship with Queen Isabella.

8. (D) This passage supports the idea that good highway systems are needed for business and local economies to thrive. If roads are in disrepair and funding for improvements is scarce, people will not be able to access the businesses along these roads. This decline in business activity is likely to negatively affect the local economy.

9. (C) The question asks you to draw a conclusion based on information presented in the second paragraph. The paragraph states that the importance of highways lies in their ability to help transfer goods from one to place to another. Choices B and D do not address the importance of highways and therefore can be eliminated.

10. (A) The first half of the second sentence states that Freud believed that dreams revealed unconscious motives. That passage does not state whether or not Freud was the first to study dreams, only that he was the first to develop a theory of the unconscious.

11. (A) The two creatures do not destroy each other, so choice B can be eliminated. The crucial component of the relationship is harmony; each of the creatures benefits equally from the other, thus eliminating choice C as well.

12. (D) The passage draws attention to the complexity of creativity and puts to rest old assumptions about how creativity should be defined. Choice D is therefore the correct answer.

13. (B) The question asks you to identify a conclusion about intelligence that could be drawn based on Gardner's findings. Gardner lists multiple areas in which people can be intelligent and believed that intelligence could manifest in a multitude of ways. Choice A does not address the traits of intelligence and instead focuses on the test, so it can be eliminated.

14. (B) The author specifically addresses a difference between first- and second-generation Romantic writers, noting that the second generation built on the foundation of the first generation, but that the influence of the French Revolution served to restrain their original idealism. In this light, choice B is the logical conclusion. The other choices fail to acknowledge correctly the split between the generations and misinterpret the effect on the Romantics' idealism.

15. (C) In the first paragraph, the author states that, according to the psychoanalytic approach, events from childhood exert a strong influence on people's lives. Later in the passage, the author states that Freud's ideas are not considered scientific by today's standards. Therefore, it can be concluded that the psychoanalytic approach is not as credible today as it was in the past.

CHAPTER 5

Identifying Purpose

Identifying Purpose questions test your understanding of the purpose of a passage or part of a passage. The answer choices for Purpose questions usually start with the word "to." A question might ask, for example, "Why does the author mention X?" The answer choices would all give reasons for why the particular detail might have been mentioned.

Purpose questions can ask about specific parts of a passage, or they may ask about the purpose of the passage as a whole. The example below asks about a specific detail, whereas the example that follows it asks about the entire passage.

Percy Bysshe Shelley was one of the second-generation Romantic poets. Along with John Keats and Lord Byron, Shelley was considered one of the most masterful poets of his generation.

Shelley was born in England in 1792, as a member of the aristocracy. He was educated at two prestigious English schools, Eton College and Oxford University. Shelley believed that poets were visionaries who could serve as societal leaders because of the creative power of their imaginations. The second generation of Romantic poets, in particular, believed that poets were going to help change the world. Shelley's generation believed that, through the imagination, anything was possible. They believed that they could use the creative power of the mind to change the government and even change the world. Shelley's poems reflect this belief. He was a truly idealistic thinker, and he claimed that poets were the "unacknowledged legislators of the world." The poet's creative vision could let him or her see things that other people could not.

Shelley's ideas were heavily influenced by the politics of his time. He grew up at a time when governments were under transformation. In fact, he came of age in the shadow of the French Revolution. This war was very violent, and since France was so close to England, Shelley was acutely aware of the violence that was occurring there. That may have led him to concentrate even more on his belief that artists were able to change the world and improve living conditions.

Shelley's poem "Mont Blanc" focuses on the Romantic notion of the sublime. The Romantic poets believed that when people interacted with Nature, it sometimes caused them to be in a state of wonder—or it caused them to be awestruck. For example, when a person gazed at a mountain, the huge size of the mountain could cause the person to become speechless with wonder. This was the effect that the sublime quality of Nature could have on a viewer.

In "Mont Blanc," Shelley describes the mountain in a way that attempts to explain its effects on the viewer's mind. According to Shelley, the mountain itself causes the viewer's thoughts to enter a kind of strange trance, and to be affected in a way that resembles how a poet or an artist feels whenever he or she is caught in the midst of a creative inspiration. In the poem, Shelley draws a comparison between the effect of the mountain on the viewer and the power that the imagination has over the artist's mind.

Why does the author mention the English schools of Eton College and Oxford University?

A. To give a description of Shelley's background
B. To present a critique of Shelley's education
C. To explain why Shelley disappointed his father
D. To describe why Shelley disliked aristocrats

The correct answer is **A**. The author mentions the English schools of Eton College and Oxford University to give a description of Shelley's background. Only wealthy students, such as those in the aristocracy, usually went to these schools.

The next passage is an example of a question that asks about the author's purpose in the full passage.

The current tests for measuring IQ, or an individual's intelligence quotient, were developed during the early and mid-twentieth century. Their use was popularized by Terman, who designed specific tests for use in the U.S. Army. Some psychologists today assert that the traditional system of measuring IQ should remain the sole method of assessing intelligence. Historically, the test has been constructed based on the assumption that there exists one general intelligence factor that impacts an individual's intellectual capacity.

The validity of this assumption has been challenged by other psychologists. In particular, Howard Gardner has emphasized that a unified conception of intelligence based on a single factor remains highly limited and unnecessarily constraining. Gardner has postulated an alternative theory concerning the existence of multiple intelligences. He posits that individuals can possess intelligence in particular areas, including linguistic intelligence, spiritual intelligence, spatial intelligence, intrapersonal intelligence, interpersonal intelligence, musical intelligence, mathematical intelligence, and kinesthetic intelligence, among others. Gardner asserts that individuals can be extremely intelligent and exhibit talent in one area, while failing to demonstrate the same level of prowess in another area. His theory has been discussed widely, although efforts to obtain empirical evidence to support his ideas remain in process.

What statement best describes the author's purpose in this passage?

A. The author is trying to prove that Gardner's theory is superior to the traditional method of measuring IQ.
B. The author believes that the traditional method of measuring IQ remains the best.
C. The author is comparing Gardner's theory to the traditional method of measuring IQ.
D. The author is demonstrating why IQ cannot be measured scientifically.

The correct answer is **C**. In this passage the author is comparing Gardner's theory to the traditional method of measuring IQ, but he does not favor either approach. Choices A and B can therefore be ruled out. Although the author points out that Gardner's theory has not been proven with empirical evidence, the passage does not state that IQ can never be measured with such evidence, so choice D is incorrect.

Additional examples of Purpose questions are given below. In each of these, the correct answer explains the *reason* an author mentions a particular element in the passage.

Literary scholars have frequently compared the characteristics of poetry written by both the first and second generation of Romantic poets. Poets such as William Wordsworth established the foundations of the exaltation of the imagination that later influenced writers such as John Keats and Percy Bysshe Shelley. The first generation of poets was attempting to advocate for the importance of artistry and creativity. The second generation of poets built on this foundation and went even further in their speculations about what creativity could achieve, especially perhaps in a political sense. However, the second generation was also negatively impacted by their observation of the French Revolution, and this experience tempered their idealism.

The author mentions that the second generation was negatively impacted by their observations of the French Revolution most likely to accomplish which of the following?

A. To make the assertion that the second generation was cynical and bitter
B. To posit that the second generation purposely differentiated themselves from the first
C. To explain why the second generation was less idealistic than the first
D. To support the claim that they were not as prolific as the first generation

The correct answer is **C**. The author mentions how the second generation's observation of the French Revolution negatively impacted their perspectives in order to explain why the second generation was less idealistic than the first. Choice B is incorrect because the second generation's intention was not to differentiate themselves from their predecessors.

Let's look another example.

As one of the most prolific female poets in nineteenth-century America, today Emily Dickinson is a household name. However, during her lifetime, she lived as a recluse and wrote most of her poetry from the solitude of her bedroom. She presents a unique perspective from this time period, when few women wrote about the themes she discusses. For this reason, critics are frequently interested in her perspective as a female author even beyond the contributions she made as an American nineteenth-century writer.

The author mentions the dual classification of Emily Dickinson most likely to demonstrate which of the following?

A. As an author, Dickinson can be classified by either focus or genre, but not both.
B. As an author, Dickinson can fit into more than one general classification.
C. Writers should be classified according to their personal practices.
D. Writers should be classified according to how much writing they do.

The correct answer is **B**. The passage mentions that some literary scholars are more interested in Dickinson's perspective as a female author than they are in her contributions as a nineteenth-century writer. This discussion reveals that Dickinson has been and can be classified in more than one manner.

Now consider this passage.

The best method of treating individuals facing psychological difficulties is a blend of cognitive-behavioral therapy and medication. This approach not only serves to address the patient's potential chemical imbalances, but it also emancipates the patient by allowing him or her some autonomy in dealing with the issues associated with a possible malaise.

Cognitive-behavioral therapy requires the patient to examine his or her own behavior and to make moderations in a rational and well-thought-out manner. If a person's chemical makeup is preventing him or her from being able to carry out such a responsibility, then medication can help alleviate specific symptoms to allow the patient to deal with the underlying emotional and psychological issues in an effective manner. Nevertheless, psychologists have wide-ranging opinions on how to help these patients cope with challenges such as depression or anxiety.

Some trained professionals assert that medication alone can best serve psychological patients. Other psychologists believe that the utilization of Freud's psychoanalytic approach represents the best method for assisting persons with these emotional symptoms. Some counselors believe that each person's set of individual circumstances should be considered. Other counselors depend on the characteristics of behaviorism to modify the patients' behavior so that their behavioral patterns become more effective. Overall, however, many professionals agree that the combination of cognitive-behavioral therapy and medication will ultimately best serve the patient.

The author notes that "cognitive-behavioral therapy requires the patient to examine his or her own behavior" primarily for which of the following reasons?

A. To advocate for the superiority of this therapeutic approach
B. To emphasize the negative aspects of this therapeutic approach
C. To describe a positive characteristic of this treatment strategy
D. To explain why this option is an inferior treatment method

The correct answer is **C**. The sentence is explaining a positive characteristic of this type of therapeutic approach. The next sentence describes how this course of treatment corresponds well with medication as adjunct treatment if necessary to alleviate specific symptoms. Choice A is incorrect because the sentence's primary function is to describe a beneficial aspect of this approach, not to advocate for its superiority.

Review Questions

1. Christopher Columbus was particularly influenced by the maps of the ancient geographer Ptolemy. Ptolemy argued that the world was round, which went against the belief of the day that the world was flat. Columbus sided with Ptolemy on this question and set out to prove that it was so.

   At the time it was widely held that sailing west from Europe would lead to certain death. Believing that the world was round, Columbus thought that one who sailed west would wind up in the east. Other scientists of the day rejected this idea, so Columbus wrote to a respected Italian scholar, Paolo Toscanelli, to ask for his opinion on the matter.

   Toscanelli supported the idea of Columbus's trip and sent word back to Columbus in 1474. After receiving Toscanelli's encouragement, Columbus focused all of his thoughts and plans on traveling westward. To make the journey, he would require the help of a generous financial backer, so he went to seek the aid of the king of Portugal. Columbus asked the king for ships and sailors to make the journey. In return, he promised to bring back wealth and to help to convert natives living on the lands to the Church. Portugal refused, and Columbus approached Italy unsuccessfully as well. He went to Spain next.

   Queen Isabella of Spain agreed to support the journey. It took some time for Columbus to convince her, but he did succeed, and she paid for the trip. Part of what led the queen to believe in Columbus was the way that he focused on his goal for such a long time with great intent. He spent the best years of his life working toward his dream, remaining persistent and determined. Legend has it that even during his first voyage, members of his crew became frightened and uncertain, wanting to return home, but Columbus pressed on. The eventual discovery of the Americas was the reward for his commitment.

   More than 500 years later, the geography of the world is often taken for granted, but Columbus was an early visionary whose results proved at least some of his theories correct.

   What is the author's purpose in writing this passage?

   A. To compare and contrast the theories of Ptolemy and Columbus
   B. To dispute the claim that Columbus discovered the Americas
   C. To offer the reader glimpses into the regrets of Columbus
   D. To argue that Columbus was a persistent and committed explorer

2. The English town of Stratford-upon-Avon is visited yearly by tourists wanting to view the birthplace of William Shakespeare. William's father, John Shakespeare, bought the family home on Henley Street, and it is here that William is believed to have been born in 1564. Shakespeare's birth home remained in his family until the early 1800s, and it is now a public museum.

   Shakespeare attended school at the King Edward VI Grammar School, which occupied the first floor of a building known as the Guildhall. It was in this Guildhall that Shakespeare first experienced theater, when he saw a theatrical performance given by a group of traveling actors. The Royal Shakespeare Company still performs in the town at the Royal Shakespeare and Swan Theaters.

   Close to the Guildhall is the site of a house known as New Place, which was bought by Shakespeare himself. Here Shakespeare lived during the later part of his life, until his death in 1616. Although he spent most of his career in London, with trips back to Stratford, he moved permanently to New Place in the last years of his life and is believed to have written some of his later works there. Only the foundations of the New Place house now remain.

   In the town of Shottery, one mile from Stratford, is the cottage where Shakespeare's wife, Anne Hathaway, was born. The Hathaway cottage, now also a museum, is actually a large, thatch-roofed farmhouse with sprawling gardens where Shakespeare is believed to have developed his relationship with Anne. They married in 1582 and had three children.

   Why does the author mention William Shakespeare's wife in a passage about Stratford-upon-Avon?

   A. Because Shakespeare's wife's parents favored the town
   B. Because Anne Hathaway was an important founder of the town
   C. Because William Shakespeare preferred Shottery to Stratford
   D. Because Hathaway was born nearby, and her cottage is now a local museum

3. One of the most important gymnastic exercises in the original Montessori school approach is that of the "line." For this exercise, a line is drawn in chalk or paint on the floor. Instead of one line, there may also be two lines drawn. The children are taught to walk on these lines like tightrope walkers, placing their feet one in front of the other.

   To keep their balance, the children must make efforts similar to those of real tightrope walkers, except that they have no danger of falling, since the lines are drawn only on the floor. The teacher herself performs the exercise first, showing clearly how she places her feet, and the children imitate her without her even needing to speak. At first it is only certain children who follow her, and when she has shown them how to walk the line, she leaves, letting the exercise develop on its own.

   The children for the most part continue to walk, following with great care the movement they have seen, and making efforts to keep their balance so they don't fall. Gradually the other children come closer and watch and try the exercise. In a short time, the entire line is covered with children balancing themselves and continuing to walk around, watching their feet attentively.

Music may be used at this point. It should be a very simple march, without an obvious rhythm. It should simply accompany and support the efforts of the children.

When children learn to master their balance in this way, Dr. Montessori believed, they can bring the act of walking to a remarkable standard of perfection.

For what reason does the author focus all five paragraphs on *walking the line*?

A. The main idea of the passage is to explain the importance of this exercise.
B. Walking the line is the most important aspect of a Montessori education.
C. The concept is a difficult one to grasp and needs extensive explanation.
D. The passage's genre is nonfiction, so it includes detailed instructions.

4. Public highways are used constantly with little thought of how important they are to the everyday life of a community. It is understandable that most people think about their local public highway only when it affects their own activities. People usually don't focus on highway improvements unless the subject is brought to their attention by increased taxes or advertising.

Highway improvements are an important issue, however. It is important for the economies of most communities to keep highways in good repair. Products purchased in one location are often manufactured in other locations, and safe highways are required to transport the products to their final destination. Good transportation facilities contribute greatly to community prosperity.

The type and amount of the highway improvement needed in any area depends on the traffic in that area. In low-population areas, the amount of traffic on local roads is likely to be small, and highways will not require as much work. But as an area develops, the use of public highways increases, and maintenance demands increase. In small towns, residents are also more able to adapt to the condition of the roads. A road shutdown does not have the same impact on business as it would in busy areas. In large districts with many activities, however, roads must be usable year-round in order for business progress to continue.

In planning improvements of highway systems, several different types of traffic may be encountered. These range from business traffic to agricultural shipping to residential transportation. Improvement activities must meet the requirements of all classes of traffic, the most important being provided for first. Those improvements of lesser importance can be performed as soon as finances permit.

What is the author's purpose in writing this passage?

A. To advise city planners about how to build and maintain highways
B. To prove that areas with low populations do not need highways
C. To highlight the necessity of highway improvements in daily life
D. To provide an objective view of how rural highways function

5. Personality is the combination of traits that make up an individual's sense of self. Traits can range from descriptors of behavior, such as "calm" or "emotional," to modes of experiencing the world, such as "thinking" or "sensing." One Swiss theorist named Carl Jung influenced the development of the now well-known Myers-Briggs personalities, which number sixteen. These sixteen personalities consist of some combination of four dimensions: introversion–extroversion, sensing–intuiting, thinking–feeling, and judging–perceiving.

What is the author's purpose in writing this passage?

A. To share a biography about a famous theorist
B. To provide additional details about a topic
C. To introduce and define a particular topic
D. To argue that a topic is of prominent importance

6. Imagine living in the year 1800. The railroads then were very scarce. Gas lights were not yet invented, and electric lights were not even dreamed of. Even kerosene wasn't used at that point. This was the world into which Samuel Morse, the inventor of the telegraph, was born.

Samuel Morse was born in Charlestown, Massachusetts, shortly before the turn of the century, in 1791. When he was seven years old, he was sent to boarding school at Phillips Academy, Andover. While he was there, his father wrote him letters, giving him good advice. He told him about George Washington and about a British statesman named Lord Chesterfield, who was able to achieve many of his goals. Lord Chesterfield was asked once how he managed to find time for all of his pursuits, and he replied that he only ever did one thing at a time, and that he "never put off anything until tomorrow that could be done today."

Morse worked hard at school and began to think and act for himself at quite a young age. His biggest accomplishment was in painting, and he established himself as a successful painter after graduating from college at Yale. But he also had an interest in science and inventions. He was passionate about the idea of discovering a way for people to send messages to each other in short periods of time.

In the early 1800s, it took a long time to receive news of any sort, even important news. Whole countries had to wait weeks to hear word of the outcomes of faraway wars. The mail was carried by stagecoach. In emergency situations, such as when ships were lost at sea, there was no way to send requests for help. Electricity had been discovered, but little application had been made of it up until that point. This was about to change when Morse set his mind to his invention.

On October 1, 1832, Morse was sailing to America from a trip overseas on a ship called the *Sully*. He became preoccupied with the thought of inventing a machine that would later become the telegraph. Morse thought about the telegraph night and day. As he sat upon the deck of the ship after dinner one night, he took out a little notebook and began to create a plan.

If a message could be sent ten miles without dropping, he wrote, "I could make it go around the globe." He said this over and over again during the years after his trip.

One morning at the breakfast table, Morse showed his plan to some of the other *Sully* passengers. Five years later, when the model of the telegraph was built, it was exactly like the one shown that morning to the passengers on the *Sully*.

Once he arrived in America, Morse worked for twelve long years to get people to notice his invention. Though some supported the idea of the telegraph, many people scoffed at it. Morse persisted, and eventually a bill was passed by Congress in 1842. It authorized the funds needed to build the first trial telegraph line.

After two years, the telegraph line was complete. Morse and his colleagues tested it in May 1844. The device worked, and the telegraph became a huge success. Morse's persistence had finally paid off.

Why do the first few paragraphs sketch a biography of Morse's early life?

A. Because the main idea of the passage is the early life of Samuel Morse
B. Because the passage is written in narrative form, with events presented chronologically
C. Because it was when Morse was young that he invented the telegraph
D. Because the author wants to demonstrate that Morse's discovery was random

7. Percy Bysshe Shelley was one of the second-generation Romantic poets. Along with John Keats and Lord Byron, Shelley was considered one of the most masterful poets of his generation.

Shelley was born in England in 1792, as a member of the aristocracy. He was educated at two prestigious English schools, Eton College and Oxford University. Shelley believed that poets were visionaries who could serve as societal leaders because of the creative power of their imaginations. The second generation of Romantic poets, in particular, believed that poets were going to help change the world. Shelley's generation believed that, through the imagination, anything was possible. They believed that they could use the creative power of the mind to change the government and even change the world. Shelley's poems reflect this belief. He was a truly idealistic thinker, and he claimed that poets were the "unacknowledged legislators of the world." The poet's creative vision could let him or her see things that other people could not.

Shelley's ideas were heavily influenced by the politics of his time. He grew up at a time when governments were under transformation. In fact, he came of age in the shadow of the French Revolution. This war was very violent, and since France was so close to England, Shelley was acutely aware of the violence that was occurring there. That may have led him to concentrate even more on his belief that artists were able to change the world and improve living conditions.

Shelley's poem "Mont Blanc" focuses on the Romantic notion of the sublime. The Romantic poets believed that when people interacted with Nature, it sometimes caused them to be in a state of wonder—or it caused them to be awestruck. For example, when a person gazed at a mountain, the huge size of the mountain could cause the person to become speechless with wonder. This was the effect that the sublime quality of Nature could have on a viewer.

In "Mont Blanc," Shelley describes the mountain in a way that attempts to explain its effects on the viewer's mind. According to Shelley, the mountain itself causes the viewer's thoughts to enter a kind of strange trance, and to be affected in a way that resembles how a poet or an artist feels whenever he or she is caught in the midst of a creative inspiration. In the poem, Shelley draws a comparison between the effect of the mountain on the viewer and the power that the imagination has over the artist's mind.

Why does the author mention the French Revolution?

A. To explain a historical event that affected Shelley's beliefs
B. To show why Shelley included violence in his poems
C. To illustrate how Shelley achieved a poetic effect
D. To describe why Shelley disliked the French so strongly

8. The Beatles influenced the genre of rock and roll just as Beethoven expanded the genre of the symphony. John Lennon, Paul McCartney, George Harrison, and Ringo Starr expanded the public's understanding of their musical genre and reclassified it as an anthem for rebellion. Their music transformed into the hippies' theme songs of the sixties. Beethoven similarly altered the public's understanding of the symphony. His addition of a chorus in the last movement of the Ninth Symphony attests to this feat.

Which of the following reflects the primary purpose of the passage?

A. To describe the Beatles' contribution to rock music
B. To explain Beethoven's influence on the Beatles
C. To describe how the Beatles and Beethoven affected their genres
D. To delineate the terms of the Beatles' musical genius

9. Athletes are extremely aware of how physical motion and its properties can affect the human body as well as the outcomes of competitions. Figure skating, for example, involves concentric motion for spins. Skaters learn how to use their arms to bring in their centers of gravity. In the same way that runners adopt a certain leg stance or swimmers use their arms to move quickly through the water, skaters also use their knowledge of physics to improve their skating.

Why does the passage mention concentric motion?

A. To suggest that a certain leg stance can impact a skater's motion
B. To differentiate it from paracentric motion, which skiers use
C. To show how skaters use their knowledge of physical motion
D. To suggest that skaters have a better sense of physical motion than other athletes

10. Bees are a natural part of the pollination cycle of plants. Many plants require the assistance of bees in order to transfer their pollen so that flowers can be produced. Bees travel from flower to flower, and minuscule grains of pollen attach to the bees' legs. The pollen travels much more efficiently via bees than it might if it had to rely on the wind, for example. In this manner, bees assist in the natural pollination cycle through the action of gathering nectar from flowers. Bees are a critical component of this process; without them, plants would face much greater challenges in their reproduction.

The passage mentions "through the action of gathering nectar from flowers" in order to do which of the following?

A. To provide a critique of the manner in which bees go about creating honey
B. To illustrate the fact that a great deal of pollen gets mixed into the nectar that bees gather
C. To suggest that nectar is the main ingredient involved in the bees' creation of honey
D. To explain the primary action through which bees contribute to the pollination process

Arguably, the most well-known Siamese cat is the seal point. The dark brown ears, face, and tail are famous markers of this popular breed of cat. Many cats that appear in popular culture, including the mischievous Siamese cats in Disney animated films, are patterned after this type of Siamese. However, cat aficionados are well aware that other types of Siamese cats also exist. Two of these include the blue point and the snowshoe. Snowshoe Siamese are characterized by the white markings on their paws along with the dark "boots": these markings earn them their name, and make the cats look as though they have been walking in the snow. Blue point Siamese cats do not have dark brown "points"; rather, their ears, paws, tails, and noses are characterized by bluish patches on their fur. Some Siamese cats are even hairless. They exhibit the darker pigment on their noses, tails, ears, and paws, similar to their fur-covered counterparts of the same breed. However, hairless Siamese cats exhibit these "points" on their skin instead of their fur. This type of Siamese is rather rare and not very well known. Despite the contrasts between the external appearances of these varying types of Siamese, all Siamese cats are known for being vocal, loyal, and rather mischievous.

The next three questions are based on this passage.

11. Which of the following best states the purpose of the passage?

   A. To assert that the seal point is the most well-known type of Siamese cat
   B. To provide a physical description of different types of Siamese cats
   C. To propose that snowshoe Siamese tend to live in colder environments
   D. To indicate that all Siamese cats in popular culture have seal point markings

12. The author mentions the Siamese cats in Disney animated films for which of the following reasons?

   A. To support the idea that seal points appear frequently in popular culture
   B. To provide a contrast between how seal points and blue points are presented
   C. To explain how Siamese cats are construed as being mischievous
   D. To explain how seal point Siamese are typically portrayed in popular culture

13. The author notes that "all Siamese cats are known for being vocal, loyal, and mischievous" in order to accomplish which of the following?

   A. To provide a contrast between blue point and snowshoe Siamese
   B. To make a generalization about all cats of this breed
   C. To indicate that the different types have distinct personalities
   D. To explain differences among the three types of Siamese cats

14. Aficionados of classical music frequently appreciate the characteristics of jazz, and some laypersons think the two genres are somewhat similar. However, jazz musicians are noted for their improvisational abilities, whereas classically trained musicians are often very reliant upon printed music. Although musicians in both genres must be very well versed in scales and various musical keys, jazz musicians must possess impeccable knowledge of this material in order to be able to perform and fulfill the requirements of their chosen genre.

   The author of the passage mentions jazz players' improvisational abilities in order to do which of the following?

   A. To demonstrate their classical music skills
   B. To differentiate them from classical players
   C. To provide evidence of the merits of their performance
   D. To explain how they receive their training

15. The acoustics of various performance venues emerge as the result of careful planning and extensive decision making. Sound travels differently when it moves through air, and the objects it encounters in a particular

environment strongly impact the way that listeners hear the sound. Venues that are designed primarily to house symphony orchestra performances require vastly different acoustic designs than do venues that cater to more intimate performances. Engineers must take into account a wide variety of variables during the design process, including vibration, sound, ultrasound, and infrasound.

A sound wave consists of a fundamental, followed by a series of sequential overtones. The way that listeners perceive these sound waves is impacted by the material used in the listening environment, the physical layout of the environment, the position of the stage relative to the audience's seating, and even the height of the ceiling. Many acoustic engineers also must take into consideration the manner in which transducers impact listening. Transducers include loudspeakers, microphones, and sonar projectors. The addition of these tools to an acoustic environment can strongly influence and transform how audience members in different locations in the room perceive any sound being transmitted.

Which of the following most likely reflects the primary purpose of the passage?

A. To indicate that a new type of material should be used to improve acoustics in performance venues
B. To indicate that unexpected elements can impact the way people hear sounds
C. To illustrate how the purpose for which a performance hall is intended impacts its acoustic design
D. To explain some of the factors that acoustic engineers consider in designing performance venues

Answer Key

1. D		**9.** C	
2. D		**10.** D	
3. A		**11.** B	
4. C		**12.** A	
5. C		**13.** B	
6. B		**14.** B	
7. A		**15.** D	
8. C			

Answers and Explanations

1. **(D)** Ptolemy is only briefly mentioned in the passage's first paragraph and is not contrasted theory-wise with Columbus; hence, choice A is incorrect. Choice B is incorrect because nowhere does the author suggest that Columbus did not discover the Americas. Finally, this passage does not concern the regrets of Columbus, but rather his discovery of the Americas, indicating that choice C is incorrect.

2. **(D)** Choices A, B, and C are incorrect because their content is neither mentioned nor suggested in the passage. Since the passage is about the town of Stratford-upon-Avon, it is appropriate to mention important buildings located nearby, which indicates that choice D is the correct answer.

3. **(A)** All paragraphs in a nonfiction passage should focus on or support the main idea of the covered subject, in this case *walking the line*. Choice B can be eliminated because of its absolute phrase *the most important*, which is not true; instead, walking the line is *one of the most important gymnastic exercises*.

4. **(C)** This passage is directed to a general audience as indicated by its first sentence, so choice A is incorrect. The first sentence of paragraph two makes the statement that highway improvements are an important issue, which is an opinion that gives away the author's purpose for writing this passage. Choice D is concerned with explaining highway function, which is not the author's purpose. Choice C is correct.

5. **(C)** The passage begins by defining the term to be discussed: *personality*. Such definitions are generally provided at the introduction of a new topic, as choice C states. Choice A is incorrect because while the passage mentions a theorist, Carl Jung, his life is not the topic of focus, as would be the case in a biography. Choice D is also incorrect because the passage offers no opinions about the subject matter.

6. **(B)** The main idea of the passage is the invention of the telegraph, not the early life of Samuel Morse, so choice A is incorrect. Choice C is also incorrect because the information in the passage leads the reader to conclude that Morse was over 40 years old when the telegraph was invented. Finally, the author demonstrates that Morse was a deep thinker and a hard worker from an early age, which would make choice D incorrect; given these qualities, his invention could not have been random. This passage is a narrative that flows chronologically, with earlier events appearing before later ones, making choice B correct.

7. **(A)** The author mentions the French Revolution to explain a historical event that affected Shelley's beliefs. The violence of this war affected Shelley and his contemporaries, possibly leading Shelley to strengthen his belief that artists could change the world. Choice C is incorrect, because the author does not talk about Shelley's poetic effects in relation to the French Revolution.

8. **(C)** The passage explains how the Beatles' compositional style challenged and expanded the genre of rock and roll. The passage uses Beethoven as an example of a musician who accomplished a similar feat in his genre.

9. **(C)** The passage mentions concentric motion to explain how skaters use their knowledge of physical motion when performing spins. Choice A is incorrect because it is not related to the passage's discussion of concentric motion.

10. **(D)** The passage describes how bees gather nectar in order to illustrate the primary action that bees take in their role in the pollination process. Choice B is incorrect because the passage does not specifically state that pollen mixes in with the nectar that is gathered.

11. **(B)** The passage provides a physical description of different types of Siamese cats. Choices A and D are incorrect because the seal point is only one type of Siamese cat discussed in the passage.

12. **(A)** The passage uses the Disney animated cats as examples of how seal points frequently appear in the popular media. Choice D is incorrect because the passage does not explain how seal points are portrayed. Other than

describing them as *mischievous*, it merely states that they appear often.

13. (B) The author ends the passage by listing characteristics common to all Siamese cats. The sentence focuses on all Siamese, so choices A, C, and D are incorrect.

14. (B) The passage mentions jazz players' improvisational abilities to differentiate them from classical players. This ability is the primary distinction that provides a contrast between jazz musicians and the abilities of their classical counterparts.

15. (D) The passage mainly explains factors that acoustic engineers have to consider to achieve their desired results in a performance venue. Choice B is incorrect because the passage focuses more on the design factors that must be considered by acoustic engineers.

CHAPTER 6
Recognizing Context

Recognizing Context questions ask about contextual issues affecting a reader's understanding of a passage. They may address three types of context: historical, cultural, and individual.

Questions pertaining to **Historical Context** test the reader's awareness of the historical context in which a passage might have been written, or the historical context affecting events presented in a passage. Here is an example:

Imagine living in the year 1800. The railroads then were very scarce. Gas lights were not yet invented, and electric lights were not even dreamed of. Even kerosene wasn't used at that point. This was the world into which Samuel Morse, the inventor of the telegraph, was born.

Samuel Morse was born in Charlestown, Massachusetts, shortly before the turn of the century, in 1791. When he was seven years old, he was sent to boarding school at Phillips Academy, Andover. While he was there, his father wrote him letters, giving him good advice. He told him about George Washington and about a British statesman named Lord Chesterfield, who was able to achieve many of his goals. Lord Chesterfield was asked once how he managed to find time for all of his pursuits, and he replied that he only ever did one thing at a time, and that he "never put off anything until tomorrow that could be done today."

Morse worked hard at school and began to think and act for himself at quite a young age. His biggest accomplishment was in painting, and he established himself as a successful painter after graduating from college at Yale. But he also had an interest in science and inventions. He was passionate about the idea of discovering a way for people to send messages to each other in short periods of time.

In the early 1800s, it took a long time to receive news of any sort, even important news. Whole countries had to wait weeks to hear word of the outcomes of faraway wars. The mail was carried by stagecoach. In emergency situations, such as when ships were lost at sea, there was no way to send requests for help. Electricity had been discovered, but little application had been made of it up until that point. This was about to change when Morse set his mind to his invention.

On October 1, 1832, Morse was sailing to America from a trip overseas on a ship called the *Sully*. He became preoccupied with the thought of inventing a machine that would later become the telegraph. Morse thought about the telegraph night and day. As he sat upon the deck of the ship after dinner one night, he took out a little notebook and began to create a plan.

If a message could be sent ten miles without dropping, he wrote, "I could make it go around the globe." He said this over and over again during the years after his trip.

One morning at the breakfast table, Morse showed his plan to some of the other *Sully* passengers. Five years later, when the model of the telegraph was built, it was exactly like the one shown that morning to the passengers on the *Sully*.

Once he arrived in America, Morse worked for twelve long years to get people to notice his invention. Though some supported the idea of the telegraph, many people scoffed at it. Morse persisted, and eventually a bill was passed by Congress in 1842. It authorized the funds needed to build the first trial telegraph line.

After two years, the telegraph line was complete. Morse and his colleagues tested it in May 1844. The device worked, and the telegraph became a huge success. Morse's persistence had finally paid off.

Which of the following historical factors led to the development of the telegraph?

A. The need to find new and productive uses for electricity
B. The need for better and faster communication
C. The need to prevent ships from sinking and other disasters
D. The need for faster ways of sending letters and packages

The correct answer is **B**. The fourth paragraph demonstrates the ways in which the lack of rapid communication made life difficult. The passage does not state that the telegraph would have any role in preventing ships from sinking, nor would it result in a more rapid way to deliver letters and other physical objects.

In the example below, the question asks about the historical context that influenced the views of Columbus.

Christopher Columbus was particularly influenced by the maps of the ancient geographer Ptolemy. Ptolemy argued that the world was round, which went against the belief of the day that the world was flat. Columbus sided with Ptolemy on this question and set out to prove that it was so.

At the time it was widely held that sailing west from Europe would lead to certain death. Believing that the world was round, Columbus thought that one who sailed west would wind up in the east. Other scientists of the day rejected this idea, so Columbus wrote to a respected Italian scholar, Paolo Toscanelli, to ask for his opinion on the matter.

Toscanelli supported the idea of Columbus's trip and sent word back to Columbus in 1474. After receiving Toscanelli's encouragement, Columbus focused all of his thoughts and plans on traveling westward. To make the journey, he would require the help of a generous financial backer, so he went to seek the aid of the king of Portugal. Columbus asked the king for ships and sailors to make the journey. In return, he promised to bring back wealth and to help to convert natives living on the lands to the Church. Portugal refused, and Columbus approached Italy unsuccessfully as well. He went to Spain next.

Queen Isabella of Spain agreed to support the journey. It took some time for Columbus to convince her, but he did succeed, and she paid for the trip. Part of what led the queen to believe in Columbus was the way that he focused on his goal for such a long time with great intent. He spent the best years of his life working toward his dream, remaining persistent and determined. Legend has it that even during his first voyage, members of his crew became frightened and uncertain, wanting to return home, but Columbus pressed on. The eventual discovery of the Americas was the reward for his commitment.

More than 500 years later, the geography of the world is often taken for granted, but Columbus was an early visionary whose results proved at least some of his theories correct.

What does the first paragraph suggest about the historical context for Columbus's ideas about the world?

A. Maps and similar charts were very rare in Columbus's day, and only those who saw them knew that the earth was round.
B. Ancient people had already sailed around the world to prove it was round, and Columbus was not the first one to do so.
C. Although some ancient geographers believed the earth was round, that knowledge was not widely respected in Columbus's day.
D. Before Columbus, geographers unanimously agreed that you could sail off the edge of the earth if you went too far.

The correct answer is **C**. Paragraph one tells us that the ancient geographer Ptolemy believed that the Earth was round, but most people in Columbus's day believed it was flat. The paragraph does not tell us how rare or common maps were, nor does it say that any ancient people had sailed around the world prior to Columbus to prove that it was round.

Here is another example concerning the effect of an historical event on British poetry:

Percy Bysshe Shelley was one of the second-generation Romantic poets. Along with John Keats and Lord Byron, Shelley was considered one of the most masterful poets of his generation.

Shelley was born in England in 1792, as a member of the aristocracy. He was educated at two prestigious English schools, Eton College and Oxford University. Shelley believed that poets were visionaries who could serve as societal leaders because of the creative power of their imaginations. The second generation of Romantic poets, in particular, believed that poets were going to help change the world. Shelley's generation believed that, through the imagination, anything was possible. They believed that they could use the creative power of the mind to change the government and even change the world. Shelley's poems reflect this belief. He was a truly idealistic thinker, and he claimed that poets were the "unacknowledged legislators of the world." The poet's creative vision could let him or her see things that other people could not.

Shelley's ideas were heavily influenced by the politics of his time. He grew up at a time when governments were under transformation. In fact, he came of age in the shadow of the French Revolution. This war was very violent, and since France was so close to England, Shelley was acutely aware of the violence that was occurring there. That may have led him to concentrate even more on his belief that artists were able to change the world and improve living conditions.

Shelley's poem "Mont Blanc" focuses on the Romantic notion of the sublime. The Romantic poets believed that when people interacted with Nature, it sometimes caused them to be in a state of wonder—or it caused them to be awestruck. For example, when a person gazed at a mountain, the huge size of the mountain could cause the person to become speechless with wonder. This was the effect that the sublime quality of Nature could have on a viewer.

In "Mont Blanc," Shelley describes the mountain in a way that attempts to explain its effects on the viewer's mind. According to Shelley, the mountain itself causes the viewer's thoughts to enter a kind of strange trance, and to be affected in a way that resembles how a poet or an artist feels whenever he or she is caught in the midst of a creative inspiration. In the poem, Shelley draws a comparison between the effect of the mountain on the viewer and the power that the imagination has over the artist's mind.

How did the context of the French Revolution most likely affect the development of Shelley's work, according to the passage?

A. It led Shelley to deemphasize the Romantic idea of the sublime.
B. It strengthened Shelley's belief in the transformative power of artists.
C. It influenced Shelley to withdraw himself from political events.
D. It caused Shelley to question the reliability of his own imagination.

The correct answer is **B**. Paragraph three states that Shelly was influenced by political, or world, events and that the French Revolution was one of those events. According to the passage, the French Revolution "may have led him to concentrate even more on his belief that artists were able to change the world and improve living conditions." The passage does not say that Shelly withdrew from politics. Instead, he used political events to shape his ideas, so choice C can be ruled out.

Like Historical Context questions, **Cultural Context questions** test the reader's understanding of how cultural beliefs might affect an issue discussed in a reading selection. The passage in the example below is followed by a question concerning cultural context.

The way that scientists have envisioned the makeup of the universe has shifted and transformed as the centuries have passed. Prior to the work of Copernicus, people believed that the earth was at the center of the universe. The idea that the earth revolved around the sun was initially taken as heresy. The progression and gradual acceptance of these originally controversial ideas paved the way for the acceptance of later discoveries by Newton and Einstein. Their theories have revolutionized the ways in which science itself is conducted today.

Which of the following statements, based on the passage, was once held as a culturally accepted belief that has since been disproven?

   A. The earth is at the center of the universe.
   B. The sun is at the center of the universe.
   C. The earth revolves around the sun.
   D. The makeup of the universe has shifted over centuries.

The correct answer is **A**. The passage states in sentence two that "prior to the work of Copernicus, people believed that the earth was at the center of the universe." The idea that the earth revolves around the sun was once taken as heresy, so choice C is the opposite of the correct answer.

Finally, **Individual Context questions** test the reader's understanding of how the author's biases and opinions affect the information conveyed. Individual context questions might ask about an author's motivation for writing a passage or an author's opinion or attitude about issues presented. An example is shown following the passage below.

Michelangelo was arguably the most talented and prolific artist to emerge from the Italian Renaissance. Not only did he spend three years on his back lying on a scaffold to create the famous paintings adorning the Sistine Chapel, but he also created a sculpture of the Biblical hero David that has been emulated for centuries. Michelangelo himself reflected that he simply took a block of marble and removed all the pieces that did not belong to the David statue. Michelangelo is considered a consummate artist because he created works in so many different media, including painting and sculpture.

Which of the following most likely characterizes the author's attitude toward Michelangelo and his art?

   A. Disregard
   B. Indifference
   C. Tolerance
   D. Admiration

The correct answer is **D**. The passage describes Michelangelo's artistic contributions with a tone that communicates an admiration of the man and his work. Choice C is incorrect because the author's tone goes beyond mere tolerance.

Review Questions

1. Christopher Columbus was particularly influenced by the maps of the ancient geographer Ptolemy. Ptolemy argued that the world was round, which went against the belief of the day that the world was flat. Columbus sided with Ptolemy on this question and set out to prove that it was so.

   At the time it was widely held that sailing west from Europe would lead to certain death. Believing that the world was round, Columbus thought that one who sailed west would wind up in the east. Other scientists of the day rejected this idea, so Columbus wrote to a respected Italian scholar, Paolo Toscanelli, to ask for his opinion on the matter.

   Toscanelli supported the idea of Columbus's trip and sent word back to Columbus in 1474. After receiving Toscanelli's encouragement, Columbus focused all of his thoughts and plans on traveling westward. To make the journey, he would require the help of a generous financial backer, so he went to seek the aid of the king of Portugal. Columbus asked the king for ships and sailors to make the journey. In return, he promised to bring back wealth and to help to convert natives living on the lands to the Church. Portugal refused, and Columbus approached Italy unsuccessfully as well. He went to Spain next.

   Queen Isabella of Spain agreed to support the journey. It took some time for Columbus to convince her, but he did succeed, and she paid for the trip. Part of what led the queen to believe in Columbus was the way that he focused on his goal for such a long time with great intent. He spent the best years of his life working toward his dream, remaining persistent and determined. Legend has it that even during his first voyage, members of his crew became frightened and uncertain, wanting to return home, but Columbus pressed on. The eventual discovery of the Americas was the reward for his commitment.

   More than 500 years later, the geography of the world is often taken for granted, but Columbus was an early visionary whose results proved at least some of his theories correct.

   Given the historical context of the passage, what were two motivations that Columbus most likely believed would convince a government to fund him?

   A. At the time science was a popular topic, and so Columbus offered new scientific discoveries as well as new wealth he might find.
   B. Columbus believed governments to be motivated both by the prospect of wealth and by the prospect of new converts to the Christian Church.
   C. Given the competitive nature of the time, Columbus offered first rights to new lands as well as any wealth he might find.
   D. Columbus knew that science and religion were important to the governments of his time, so he offered new converts and new scientific discoveries.

2. Imagine living in the year 1800. The railroads then were very scarce. Gas lights were not yet invented, and electric lights were not even dreamed of. Even kerosene wasn't used at that point. This was the world into which Samuel Morse, the inventor of the telegraph, was born.

Samuel Morse was born in Charlestown, Massachusetts, shortly before the turn of the century, in 1791. When he was seven years old, he was sent to boarding school at Phillips Academy, Andover. While he was there, his father wrote him letters, giving him good advice. He told him about George Washington and about a British statesman named Lord Chesterfield, who was able to achieve many of his goals. Lord Chesterfield was asked once how he managed to find time for all of his pursuits, and he replied that he only ever did one thing at a time, and that he "never put off anything until tomorrow that could be done today."

Morse worked hard at school and began to think and act for himself at quite a young age. His biggest accomplishment was in painting, and he established himself as a successful painter after graduating from college at Yale. But he also had an interest in science and inventions. He was passionate about the idea of discovering a way for people to send messages to each other in short periods of time.

In the early 1800s, it took a long time to receive news of any sort, even important news. Whole countries had to wait weeks to hear word of the outcomes of faraway wars. The mail was carried by stagecoach. In emergency situations, such as when ships were lost at sea, there was no way to send requests for help. Electricity had been discovered, but little application had been made of it up until that point. This was about to change when Morse set his mind to his invention.

On October 1, 1832, Morse was sailing to America from a trip overseas on a ship called the *Sully*. He became preoccupied with the thought of inventing a machine that would later become the telegraph. Morse thought about the telegraph night and day. As he sat upon the deck of the ship after dinner one night, he took out a little notebook and began to create a plan.

If a message could be sent ten miles without dropping, he wrote, "I could make it go around the globe." He said this over and over again during the years after his trip.

One morning at the breakfast table, Morse showed his plan to some of the other *Sully* passengers. Five years later, when the model of the telegraph was built, it was exactly like the one shown that morning to the passengers on the *Sully*.

Once he arrived in America, Morse worked for twelve long years to get people to notice his invention. Though some supported the idea of the telegraph, many people scoffed at it. Morse persisted, and eventually a bill was passed by Congress in 1842. It authorized the funds needed to build the first trial telegraph line.

After two years, the telegraph line was complete. Morse and his colleagues tested it in May 1844. The device worked, and the telegraph became a huge success. Morse's persistence had finally paid off.

Based on the historical context of the passage, what can the reader conclude about communication in the early 1800s and its impact on the reception of Morse's invention?

A. It was slow and unreliable to communicate with anyone who lived any distance away, so eventually Morse's invention was a welcomed success.

B. Communication was not a valued commodity; people celebrated independence from others and did not value Morse's invention.

C. Even though people knew that communication was slow, they resisted the idea of change and ultimately rejected Morse's idea.

D. People were too engrossed in the invention of electricity to delve into the possibilities of improving communication.

3. The best method of treating individuals facing psychological difficulties is a blend of cognitive-behavioral therapy and medication. This approach not only serves to address the patient's potential chemical imbalances, but it also emancipates the patient by allowing him or her some autonomy in dealing with the issues associated with a possible malaise.

Cognitive-behavioral therapy requires the patient to examine his or her own behavior and to make moderations in a rational and well-thought-out manner. If a person's chemical makeup is preventing him or her from being able to carry out such a responsibility, then medication can help alleviate specific symptoms to allow the patient to deal with the underlying emotional and psychological issues in an effective manner. Nevertheless, psychologists have wide-ranging opinions on how to help these patients cope with challenges such as depression or anxiety.

Some trained professionals assert that medication alone can best serve psychological patients. Other psychologists believe that a utilization of Freud's psychoanalytic approach represents the best method for assisting persons with these emotional symptoms. Some counselors believe that each person's set of individual circumstances should be considered. Other counselors depend on the characteristics of behaviorism to modify the patients' behavior so that their behavioral patterns become more effective. Overall, however, many professionals agree that the combination of cognitive-behavioral therapy and medication will ultimately best serve the patient.

The author's argument regarding therapy and medication is most likely motivated by which of the following beliefs?

A. Those who suffer psychological issues are best treated in hospitals that can monitor their medication intake.

B. Patients with psychological issues often respond well to only one method of treatment: either therapy or medication.

C. Medication-based treatment is the most effective option for all psychological patients.

D. Both therapy and medicine offer benefits, but using them in conjunction is most effective.

4. Austrian-born Sigmund Freud, a psychoanalytic psychologist, lived from the mid-nineteenth to the mid-twentieth century. The psychoanalytic approach refers to the school of thought that unconscious memories or desires guide our emotions and actions. In personality theory, this equates to events from childhood shaping the individual self without a person's conscious awareness. These specific childhood events continue to exert a strong influence over our lives and dominate our emotions. If you are a life-of-the-party, extroverted personality, perhaps you had a healthy upbringing; however, quiet, deep-thinker types can be just as functional. How your caregivers responded to your natural urges will determine your level of mental health, according to the psychoanalytic approach.

Freud believed that as a child, an individual's actions are driven by hidden impulses—and that repression or denial of those impulses by parents or society can lead to fixations or personality disorders. Alternatively, if the child's impulses are accepted as normative to his or her development, then a functional adult behavioral pattern should take root. Now, by no means should parents allow every impulse to dictate behavior; each of us has a "censor," which Freud referred to as the "superego." This element of the psyche is largely helpful and acts as a conscience. However, if we let the superego dominate our personality, Freud believed, it could lead to repression and inauthentic behavior.

Freud often worked with highly distressed female clients, repressed in their natural modes of expression; this is how he developed many of his theories, which some people believe are not very scientific. By today's standards, they are not, but Freud's idea that unconscious urges drive our behavior was revolutionary for his time.

In the passage, which of the following most likely reflects the author's belief about Freud?

A. He may have had original ideas, but his theories are not taken seriously by the scientific field today.
B. He was a revolutionary who continues to shape the field of psychology in fundamental ways.
C. He was a psychologist who cared little for his patients and whose contributions were detrimental to his field.
D. His contributions to psychology have proven to be seminal and grounded in scientific fact.

The way that scientists have envisioned the makeup of the universe has shifted and transformed as the centuries have passed. Prior to the work of Copernicus, people believed that the earth was at the center of the universe. The idea that the earth revolved around the sun was initially taken as heresy. The progression and gradual acceptance of these originally controversial ideas paved the way for the acceptance of later discoveries by Newton and Einstein. Their theories have revolutionized the ways in which science itself is conducted today.

The next two questions are based on this passage.

5. What is the author's attitude toward scientific theory?

   A. Skeptical regarding its potential pitfalls
   B. Condescending about its inability to produce quick answers
   C. Jovial about the possibilities that scientific theory presents
   D. Earnestly appreciative of the work science has accomplished

6. The passage suggests which of the following about the historical impact of the acceptance of Copernicus's discovery?

   A. It paved the way for the acceptance of controversial ideas by Newton and Einstein.
   B. It demonstrated to other scientists how the Church would respond to challenging theories.
   C. It revolutionized how science is conducted today in comparison with past centuries.
   D. It transformed the structure of the Catholic Church and undermined its authority.

7. One of the most important gymnastic exercises in the original Montessori school approach is that of the "line." For this exercise, a line is drawn in chalk or paint on the floor. Instead of one line, there may also be two lines drawn. The children are taught to walk on these lines like tightrope walkers, placing their feet one in front of the other.

   To keep their balance, the children must make efforts similar to those of real tightrope walkers, except that they have no danger of falling, since the lines are drawn only on the floor. The teacher herself performs the exercise first, showing clearly how she places her feet, and the children imitate her without her even needing to speak. At first it is only certain children who follow her, and when she has shown them how to walk the line, she leaves, letting the exercise develop on its own.

   The children for the most part continue to walk, following with great care the movement they have seen, and making efforts to keep their balance so they don't fall. Gradually the other children come closer and watch and try the exercise. In a short time, the entire line is covered with children balancing themselves and continuing to walk around, watching their feet attentively.

   Music may be used at this point. It should be a very simple march, without an obvious rhythm. It should simply accompany and support the efforts of the children. When children learn to master their balance in this way, Dr. Montessori believed, they can bring the act of walking to a remarkable standard of perfection.

   What cultural belief about how children learn is expressed by this passage?

   A. Children learn through individual instruction.
   B. Children learn through rhythmic exercises.
   C. Children learn through rote memorization.
   D. Children learn through imitating others.

8. Historians typically rely upon the first-person narratives of famous historical figures to serve as evidence to support their interpretations of past events. During the past couple of decades in scholarly research, however, an increasing amount of interest has been paid to the viewpoints and writings of everyday people who are not well known. This interest has stemmed from historians' acknowledgement that nonfamous persons have still played critical roles in history. Their perspectives represent the trials and the joys of "regular" people, whose experiences make up the bulk of history that famous figures speak about.

   Which of the following cultural beliefs is reflected in the emergence of scholarly interest in the writings of ordinary people?

   A. Ordinary people will often reveal the ways in which famous people are inaccurate in their descriptions of important historical events.
   B. Historians have already read all the letters and diaries of famous people, and they now need new material to develop new ideas.
   C. Most people are ordinary, and their lives reveal how historical events actually affected individuals.
   D. Most famous people are men, while ordinary people are most likely to be women, and only by studying their letters and diaries can we find out what life for women was like.

9. As one of the most prolific female poets in nineteenth-century America, today Emily Dickinson is a household name. However, during her lifetime, she lived as a recluse and wrote most of her poetry from the solitude of her bedroom. She presents a unique perspective from this time period, when few women wrote about the themes she discusses. For this reason, critics are frequently interested in her perspective as a female author even beyond the contributions she made as an American nineteenth-century writer.

   What can we infer from the passage about women of the nineteenth century?

   A. Many women of the nineteenth century lived as recluses in the same way that Emily Dickinson did.
   B. Few women of the nineteenth century wrote about the ideas and topics that Emily Dickinson did.
   C. Few women of the nineteenth century were literate and knew how to read or write as Emily Dickinson did.
   D. Many women of the nineteenth century wrote about a wide range of subjects just as Emily Dickinson did.

10. Percy Bysshe Shelley was one of the second-generation Romantic poets. Along with John Keats and Lord Byron, Shelley was considered one of the most masterful poets of his generation.

    Shelley was born in England in 1792, as a member of the aristocracy. He was educated at two prestigious English schools, Eton College and Oxford University. Shelley believed that poets were visionaries who could serve as societal leaders because of the creative power of their imaginations. The second generation of Romantic poets, in particular, believed that poets were going to help change the world. Shelley's generation believed that, through the imagination, anything was possible. They believed that they could use the creative power of the mind to change the government and even change the world. Shelley's poems reflect this belief. He was a truly idealistic thinker, and he claimed that poets were the "unacknowledged legislators of the world." The poet's creative vision could let him or her see things that other people could not.

Shelley's ideas were heavily influenced by the politics of his time. He grew up at a time when governments were under transformation. In fact, he came of age in the shadow of the French Revolution. This war was very violent, and since France was so close to England, Shelley was acutely aware of the violence that was occurring there. That may have led him to concentrate even more on his belief that artists were able to change the world and improve living conditions.

Shelley's poem "Mont Blanc" focuses on the Romantic notion of the sublime. The Romantic poets believed that when people interacted with Nature, it sometimes caused them to be in a state of wonder—or it caused them to be awestruck. For example, when a person gazed at a mountain, the huge size of the mountain could cause the person to become speechless with wonder. This was the effect that the sublime quality of Nature could have on a viewer.

In "Mont Blanc," Shelley describes the mountain in a way that attempts to explain its effects on the viewer's mind. According to Shelley, the mountain itself causes the viewer's thoughts to enter a kind of strange trance, and to be affected in a way that resembles how a poet or an artist feels whenever he or she is caught in the midst of a creative inspiration. In the poem, Shelley draws a comparison between the effect of the mountain on the viewer and the power that the imagination has over the artist's mind.

Which statement below best describes the Romantic idea of the sublime?

A. The sublime is the desire to change the world for the better.
B. The sublime is the ideal of nonviolence that emerges after war.
C. The sublime is the power of imagination to make one believe anything is possible.
D. The sublime is the awe people feel at the beauty of nature.

11. When artists achieve commercial successes, their emotional mindsets can be influenced by this experience. Claude Monet was one such example of this phenomenon. Monet's innovative style earned him considerable fame and public acclaim. In addition, he was extremely prolific as an artist because of his industrious work ethic. As a result, he was successful at his craft, and his paintings reflect a more contemplative and calm perspective than those of artists whose life experiences were fraught with poverty and struggle.

According to the passage, which sentence best describes Monet's "emotional mindset" and how it influenced his work?

A. Monet's commercial success freed him to produce art that was more meditative and tranquil than that of artists who had to struggle against poverty.

B. Monet was an industrious worker who had little use for commercial success and public acclaim, so he did not let those elements influence his art.

C. Monet's early life was fraught with poverty and struggle, which is why he worked so hard to be prolific and to create commercially successful art.

D. Monet loved and pursued commercial success and public acclaim to the detriment of his art, which became dull and unexciting.

12. Michelangelo was arguably the most talented and prolific artist to emerge from the Italian Renaissance. Not only did he spend three years on his back lying on a scaffold to create the famous paintings adorning the Sistine Chapel, but he also created a sculpture of the Biblical hero David that has been emulated for centuries. Michelangelo himself reflected that he simply took a block of marble and removed all the pieces that did not belong to the David statue. Michelangelo is considered a consummate artist because he created works in so many different media, including painting and sculpture.

Which of the following statements most likely reflects the author's attitude toward Michelangelo?

A. Michelangelo himself reflected that he simply took a block of marble and removed all the pieces that did not belong to the David statue.

B. Michelangelo created a sculpture of the Biblical hero David that has been emulated for centuries.

C. Michelangelo was arguably the most talented and prolific artist to emerge from the Italian Renaissance.

D. Michelangelo spent three years on his back lying on a scaffold to create the famous paintings adorning the Sistine Chapel.

13. The Beatles influenced the genre of rock and roll just as Beethoven expanded the genre of the symphony. John Lennon, Paul McCartney, George Harrison, and Ringo Starr expanded the public's understanding of their musical genre and reclassified it as an anthem for rebellion. Their music transformed into the hippies' theme songs of the sixties. Beethoven similarly altered the public's understanding of the symphony. His addition of a chorus in the last movement of the Ninth Symphony attests to this feat.

According to information presented in the passage, which of the following cultural beliefs is most highly identified with the music of the Beatles?

A. The acceptance of rock-and-roll artists as cultural leaders

B. The association of rock and roll with themes of rebellion

C. The public view of the symphony as expressive of emotion

D. The perception of classical music as the highest form of art

14. The current tests for measuring IQ, or an individual's intelligence quotient, were developed during the early and mid-twentieth century. Their use was popularized by Terman, who designed specific tests for use in the U.S. Army. Some psychologists today assert that the traditional system of measuring IQ should remain the sole method of assessing intelligence. Historically, the test has been constructed based on the assumption that there exists one general intelligence factor that impacts an individual's intellectual capacity.

    The validity of this assumption has been challenged by other psychologists. In particular, Howard Gardner has emphasized that a unified conception of intelligence based on a single factor remains highly limited and unnecessarily constraining. Gardner has postulated an alternative theory concerning the existence of multiple intelligences. He posits that individuals can possess intelligence in particular areas, including linguistic intelligence, spiritual intelligence, spatial intelligence, intrapersonal intelligence, interpersonal intelligence, musical intelligence, mathematical intelligence, and kinesthetic intelligence, among others. Gardner asserts that individuals can be extremely intelligent and exhibit talent in one area, while failing to demonstrate the same level of prowess in another area. His theory has been discussed widely, although efforts to obtain empirical evidence to support his ideas remain in process.

    Which of the following best describes the historical context in which traditional IQ tests were developed?

    A. At the time the tests were developed, it was believed that an individual's intelligence quotient was influenced by some factors more than others.
    B. At the time the tests were developed, it was believed that a conception of intelligence based on a single factor was unnecessarily constraining.
    C. At the time the tests were developed, it was assumed that an individual's intellectual capacity was influenced by multiple intelligences.
    D. At the time the tests were developed, it was assumed that an individual's intellectual capacity was influenced by one general intelligence factor.

15. The physician William Harvey was the first who discovered and demonstrated the true mechanism of the heart's action. No one before his time conceived that the movement of the blood was entirely due to the mechanical action of the heart as a pump. There were all sorts of speculations about the matter, but nobody had formed this conception. Harvey is as clear as possible about it. He says the movement of the blood is entirely due to the contractions of the walls of the heart—that it is the propelling apparatus—and all recent investigation tends to show that he was perfectly right.

Which of the following most likely reflects the historical context in which William Harvey developed his ideas regarding the action of the heart?

A. It was widely accepted that blood circulation was due to the action of the heart.
B. Medical practitioners were uncertain about whether blood moved in the body.
C. The medical community did not yet believe that blood circulated due to the heart.
D. Doctors and scientists concentrated more research on the heart than on other organs.

Answer Key

1.	B	**9.**	B
2.	A	**10.**	D
3.	D	**11.**	A
4.	A	**12.**	C
5.	D	**13.**	B
6.	A	**14.**	D
7.	D	**15.**	C
8.	C		

Answer and Explanations

1. (B) Columbus needed funding for his project, but no one was going to support him without some type of incentive. He offered wealth and religious converts to various governments until one of them—Spain—finally said yes. Because he offered these as an incentive for support, it is logical to deduce that governments would possibly be motivated by his offers.

   Choice A is incorrect because science is only discussed as an introduction to the motivations of Columbus and why he might be interested in sailing around the world. Choice C is incorrect because the passage never discusses competition or land rights. Regarding choice D, scientific progress may have been an instigator for Columbus, but the passage does not indicate that it was one for the governments of the time.

2. (A) The question asks you to identify what can be concluded about communication in the early 1800s and its impact on the reception of Morse's invention. In paragraph four, the passage claims that "it took a long time to receive any news" and that "whole countries had to wait weeks to hear word of the outcomes of faraway wars." The mail was carried by stagecoach on land, which was why it took so long to travel. Also, at sea there was no reliable method of communication in case of emergency. And while some may have rejected Morse at first, he eventually met with success.

   Choice B is incorrect because the passage never suggests that communication was not valued, and Morse's invention was accepted eventually. Choice C is also incorrect in its conclusion that Morse never met with success.

3. (D) The author concedes the benefits of both therapy and medication and acknowledges their merits independently. But he or she states in the first sentence that "the best method of treating individuals . . . is a blend of cognitive-behavioral therapy and medication."

Choice A is incorrect because the topic of the passage is therapy and medication; the benefits or detriments of hospitals are not discussed in the passage. While the author does mention the merits of both treatments, he or she states twice that the combination of the two best serves the patient, so choice B can be ruled out. Similar to choice B, choice C is incorrect because the author does not view medication-based treatment as most effective. Instead, he or she indicates that medication is not the only viable option and states that "many professionals agree" that using both methods is most effective.

4. (A) The question asks you to determine the author's most likely belief about Freud. While the author addresses Freud specifically as a revolutionary, he also provides the caveat that "by today's standards," Freud's theories are not scientific. Therefore, the author credits Freud for originality but ultimately labels him as lacking scientific support.

The author does think that Freud was a revolutionary, but he is quick to note at the end of the passage that Freud's theories would not be taken seriously by the scientific community today, so choice B is incorrect. Since the author notes that Freud is a revolutionary, choice C can be eliminated. Finally, choice D is incorrect because the author states that Freud's theories are not regarded as scientific by modern standards.

5. (D) The question asks you to identify the author's attitude toward scientific theory. The author's choice of phrases such as *envisioned*, *paved the way*, and *revolutionized* indicate a sincere belief in and appreciation for the positive effects of scientific theory.

Choice A is too negative and is not supported by any of the word choices the author makes. Choice B is also incorrect for a reason similar to choice A. The author uses positive words in the passage, and *condescending* indicates a negative attitude. Choice C contains a positive-tone word; however, the degree of positivity in *jovial* is too high. The author's word choices indicate an *appreciation* for scientific theory, not happiness about it.

6. (A) The passage suggests that acceptance of Copernicus's theories allowed for easier acceptance of later ideas by Newton and Einstein. Choice C is incorrect because this sentence is attributable to Newton's and Einstein's discoveries.

7. (D) The passage shows how the children initially imitate the teacher and then each other as they learn how to walk along the line. Although they may do this to music, the passage is clear in stating that the music does not have a distinct rhythm, which eliminates choice B.

8. (C) The last sentence states that material from ordinary individuals often reflects how most people experienced historical events. The author does not address whether most famous people are men, ruling out choice D. We also are not told how much material from famous people is available to historians or how accurate that material is, so choices A and B can be eliminated.

9. (B) The third sentence of the passage makes it clear that few women addressed the ideas that Emily Dickinson did. The passage does not state whether many other women of the time were recluses, or how widespread literacy was among women of the nineteenth century.

10. (D) The fourth paragraph of the passage states that the sublime is a state of wonder or awe that people experience at the sight of nature. The desire to change the world, an aversion to violence, and the power of imagination are all attributed to Romanticism in the passage but do not define the sublime.

11. (A) The fourth sentence implies that Monet's commercial success gave him security and enabled him to take a more contemplative and calm approach to art than that taken by artists who lacked financial security. The passage does not address whether Monet's early life was marked by poverty and struggle, so choice C is incorrect.

12. (C) The author's attitude is reflected in choice C. Choices A, B, and D reflect statements of fact regarding Michelangelo's accomplishments, so they are incorrect.

13. (B) The music of the Beatles is most highly identified with the association between rock and roll and themes of rebellion. According to the passage, the Beatles helped to reclassify rock and roll into "an anthem for rebellion." Choices A, C, and D are not mentioned in the passage.

14. (D) In discussing the development of traditional IQ tests, at the end of paragraph one, the passage states, "Historically, the test has been constructed based on the assumption that there exists one general intelligence factor that impacts an individual's intellectual capacity." Choice D is therefore correct.

15. (C) The passage states that Harvey was the first to discover that blood circulated through the body due to the action of the heart. "No one before his time conceived that the movement of the blood was entirely due to the mechanical action of the heart as a pump," the passage states. Choice C provides the best description of this historical context. Choice A is the opposite of the correct answer.

CHAPTER 7

Fact vs. Opinion

Fact vs. Opinion questions ask you to determine whether a portion of text is based on fact or the author's opinion. Some texts may contain a mixture of both.

Facts can be verified using empirical evidence, whereas **opinions** are based on the author's subjective views. Below are some examples of this question type.

Arguably, the most well-known Siamese cat is the seal point. The dark brown ears, face, and tail are famous markers of this popular breed of cat. Many cats that appear in popular culture, including the mischievous Siamese cats in Disney animated films, are patterned after this type of Siamese. However, cat aficionados are well aware that other types of Siamese cats also exist. Two of these include the blue point and the snowshoe. Snowshoe Siamese are characterized by the white markings on their paws along with the dark "boots": these markings earn them their name and make the cats look as though they have been walking in the snow. Blue point Siamese cats do not have dark brown "points"; rather, their ears, paws, tails, and noses are characterized by bluish patches on their fur. Some Siamese cats are even hairless. They exhibit the darker pigment on their noses, tails, ears, and paws, similar to their fur-covered counterparts of the same breed. However, hairless Siamese cats exhibit these "points" on their skin instead of their fur. This type of Siamese is rather rare and not very well known. Despite the contrasts between the external appearances of these varying types of Siamese, all Siamese cats are known for being vocal, loyal, and rather mischievous.

Which sentence or phrase in the passage refers mostly to traits of the Siamese cat that are matters of opinion rather than fact?

A. The dark brown ears, face, and tail are famous markers of this popular breed of cat.
B. Their ears, paws, tails, and noses are characterized by bluish patches on their fur.
C. All Siamese cats are known for being vocal, loyal, and rather mischievous.
D. Snowshoe Siamese are characterized by the white markings on their paws.

The correct answer is **C**. *Loyal* and *mischievous* are traits that are matters of opinion rather than physical traits. The other phrases and sentences describe traits that are physical and can be proven through observation.

Let's consider another example:

The acoustics of various performance venues emerge as the result of careful planning and extensive decision making. Sound travels differently when it moves through air, and the objects it encounters in a particular environment strongly impact the way that listeners hear the sound. Venues that are designed primarily to house symphony orchestra performances require vastly different acoustic designs than do venues that cater to more intimate performances. Engineers must take into account a wide variety of variables during the design process, including vibration, sound, ultrasound, and infrasound.

A sound wave consists of a fundamental, followed by a series of sequential overtones. The way that listeners perceive these sound waves is impacted by the material used in the listening environment, the physical layout of the environment, the position of the stage relative to the audience's seating, and even the height of the ceiling. Many acoustic engineers also must take into consideration the manner in which transducers impact listening. Transducers include loudspeakers, microphones, and sonar projectors. The addition of these tools to an acoustic environment can strongly influence and transform how audience members in different locations in the room perceive any sound being transmitted.

The author states in paragraph two that "a sound wave consists of a fundamental, followed by a series of sequential overtones." This statement can be seen as which of the following?

A. It is a fact, because the sentence after it provides evidence and support for its veracity.
B. It is an opinion, because the author is not a scientist; he is merely a music connoisseur.
C. It is a fact, because the statement can be supported with scientific data and does not reflect the author's subjective viewpoint about sound.
D. It is an opinion, because it reveals the author's feelings about sound rather than providing an objective and empirically deduced statement.

The correct answer is **C**. While both choices A and C correctly identify this statement as a fact, only choice C gives the correct support. Choice A indicates the sentence following the one quoted in the question provides support when in fact this sentence goes on to develop another idea.

Now consider this passage:

CPR, an acronym that stands for cardiopulmonary resuscitation, is a widely utilized method of attempting to save someone's life. It is especially applicable to scenarios in which a patient's heart has stopped beating. Frequently, it is also used in cases where a person is in danger of drowning.

Almost all approaches to CPR suggest that a person begin resuscitation efforts with chest compressions. To perform a chest compression, the individual places both hands flat on the patient's chest and then begins pushing down carefully but firmly, most likely at equal intervals. The compressions should be counted, so that the individual can keep track of how many compressions have been administered. The unofficial recommendation of how many chest compressions to provide is around 100 per minute.

There are many resources through which potential lifesavers can acquire training and even certification so that they can more effectively administer this lifesaving technique to a potential patient. However, the American Heart Association stresses that even if someone has not received any type of formal training, attempting to help a person who needs to be resuscitated is far better than offering no help. This is why 911 operators sometimes request that bystanders at the scene of an emergency administer CPR. The operators may even coach the bystanders verbally, over the phone. These approaches have been shown to be effective in many cases.

If a bystander at an emergency scene has received CPR training—even if the training occurred a long time ago—the bystander should attempt further techniques in addition to chest compressions, especially if the patient has been underwater. The lifesaver should start first by checking the patient's airway. He or she might also administer mouth-to-mouth rescue breathing. However, lifesavers should only perform these additional techniques if they are confident of their skills and remember their training. Otherwise, any potential lifesaver should just administer chest compressions.

Some important items to remember in administering CPR are as follows. First, the lifesaver should always check whether the patient is conscious or not. Verbal interaction or communication can be a key way of determining if a person is conscious. If the emergency is related to drowning, the lifesaver should start chest compressions. These should be conducted for about a minute or so before the lifesaver calls 911. However, if one person can perform the compressions and there is another person available who can call 911, then these steps should happen simultaneously.

For persons who are trained in CPR, one of the best ways to remember the order in which steps should be administered is to recall the memory cue CAB. This cue stands for Circulation, Airway, Breathing. The goal of CPR is to help an unresponsive person to start breathing on his or her own. First, use chest compressions to restore circulation. This is the C of CAB. Second, check the patient's airway for possible blockages. The A in CAB stands for airway. Finally, administer rescue breathing. This is, of course, the B of CAB.

The author states that "one of the best ways to remember the order in which steps should be administered is to recall the memory cue CAB." This statement can best be described by which of the following?

A. It is a fact, because CAB is a short word and is easy to remember.
B. It is an opinion, because the author is unable to determine what is objectively "best" for all people.
C. It is a fact, because empirical research has been conducted to prove the author's statement.
D. It is an opinion, because the author introduces it with the phrase, "in my opinion."

The correct answer is **B**. While choices B and D both identify this statement correctly as an opinion, only choice B accurately indicates why. The author never states that this is an opinion, but he or she does use the subjective word *best*, which indicates opinion.

To make sure you're comfortable with fact vs. opinion questions, let's look at two more examples:

Christopher Columbus was particularly influenced by the maps of the ancient geographer Ptolemy. Ptolemy argued that the world was round, which went against the belief of the day that the world was flat. Columbus sided with Ptolemy on this question and set out to prove that it was so.

At the time it was widely held that sailing west from Europe would lead to certain death. Believing that the world was round, Columbus thought that one who sailed west would wind up in the east. Other scientists of the day rejected this idea, so Columbus wrote to a respected Italian scholar, Paolo Toscanelli, to ask for his opinion on the matter.

Toscanelli supported the idea of Columbus's trip and sent word back to Columbus in 1474. After receiving Toscanelli's encouragement, Columbus focused all of his thoughts and plans on traveling westward. To make the journey, he would require the help of a generous financial backer, so he went to seek the aid of the king of Portugal. Columbus asked the king for ships and sailors to make the journey. In return, he promised to bring back wealth and to help to convert natives living on the lands to the Church. Portugal refused, and Columbus approached Italy unsuccessfully as well. He went to Spain next.

Queen Isabella of Spain agreed to support the journey. It took some time for Columbus to convince her, but he did succeed, and she paid for the trip. Part of what led the queen to believe in Columbus was the way that he focused on his goal for such a long time with great intent. He spent the best years of his life working toward his dream, remaining persistent and determined. Legend has it that even during his first voyage, members of his crew became frightened and uncertain, wanting to return home, but Columbus pressed on. The eventual discovery of the Americas was the reward for his commitment.

More than 500 years later, the geography of the world is often taken for granted, but Columbus was an early visionary whose results proved at least some of his theories correct.

The author's statement that Columbus asked the king of Portugal "for ships and sailors to make the journey" most accurately reflects which of the following?

A. It is an opinion, because the statement is based on inaccurate information.
B. It is a fact, because it expresses a subjective belief of the author.
C. It is a fact, because the statement can be supported with historical evidence.
D. It is an opinion, because it is impossible to know what Columbus asked for.

The correct answer is **C**. The question of what Columbus asked for can be documented with historical evidence, making choice D incorrect and choice C the correct answer. Choice B is incorrect, because facts express objective knowledge, not subjective beliefs.

Let's consider one more example:

Literary scholars have often speculated as to the personal characteristics of William Shakespeare. The Bard is known to many as the greatest writer the English language has ever known, but we have very few examples of his handwriting or even his own name written out in his hand. Some academics have gone so far as to speculate that Shakespeare was a pseudonym for an aristocrat. However, the majority of scholars have dismissed this proposal, and they concentrate instead on Shakespeare's thoughtful insights and dexterous construction of language.

In the passage, the author raises the idea that Shakespeare was a pseudonym for an aristocrat. Is this idea a fact or an opinion?

A. It is a fact, because scholars have been suggesting it for years.
B. It is a fact, because it has become common knowledge that Shakespeare was not real.
C. It is an opinion, because the author states some have "speculated" that Shakespeare was a pseudonym.
D. It is an opinion, because the author believes that Shakespeare does not deserve the credit for those works.

The correct answer is **C**. The idea in question has not been supported by empirical evidence; instead, some academics have merely speculated about it. Choice D can be eliminated because the passage does not express negative feelings about Shakespeare.

Review Questions

Public highways are used constantly with little thought of how important they are to the everyday life of a community. It is understandable that most people think about their local public highway only when it affects their own activities. People usually don't focus on highway improvements unless the subject is brought to their attention by increased taxes or advertising.

Highway improvements are an important issue, however. It is important for the economies of most communities to keep highways in good repair. Products purchased in one location are often manufactured in other locations, and safe highways are required to transport the products to their final destination. Good transportation facilities contribute greatly to community prosperity.

The type and amount of the highway improvement needed in any area depend on the traffic in that area. In low-population areas, the amount of traffic on local roads is likely to be small, and highways will not require as much work. But as an area develops, the use of public highways increases, and maintenance demands increase. In small towns, residents are also more able to adapt to the condition of the roads. A road shutdown does not have the same impact on business as it would in busy areas. In large districts with many activities, however, roads must be usable year-round in order for business progress to continue.

In planning improvements of highway systems, several different types of traffic may be encountered. These range from business traffic to agricultural shipping to residential transportation. Improvement activities must meet the requirements of all classes of traffic, the most important being provided for first. Those improvements of lesser importance can be performed as soon as finances permit.

The next two questions are based on this passage.

1. Read the following quotation from line 2 of the passage.

It is understandable that most people think about their local public highway only when it affects their own activities.

Which of the following statements is true concerning the quotation above?

A. This statement is an opinion, because most people probably think that it is true.
B. This statement is an opinion, because it is a viewpoint that may not be held by everyone.
C. This statement is a fact, because the claim is objective and could be proven empirically.
D. This statement is a fact, because everyone knows that people think primarily of their own interests.

2. Read the following quotation from paragraph three of the passage.

In low-population areas, the amount of traffic on local roads is likely to be small.

Which of the following statements is true regarding the quotation above?

A. This statement is a fact, because it uses a qualifier to cover any exceptions to its claim.
B. This statement is an opinion, because it is a belief that cannot be proven empirically.
C. This statement is a fact, because it has been proven through scientific experimentation.
D. This statement is an opinion, because there is evidence to support the opposite claim as well.

One of the most important gymnastic exercises in the original Montessori school approach is that of the "line." For this exercise, a line is drawn in chalk or paint on the floor. Instead of one line, there may also be two lines drawn. The children are taught to walk on these lines like tightrope walkers, placing their feet one in front of the other.

To keep their balance, the children must make efforts similar to those of real tightrope walkers, except that they have no danger of falling, since the lines are drawn only on the floor. The teacher herself performs the exercise first, showing clearly how she places her feet, and the children imitate her without her even needing to speak. At first it is only certain children who follow her, and when she has shown them how to walk the line, she leaves, letting the exercise develop on its own.

The children for the most part continue to walk, following with great care the movement they have seen, and making efforts to keep their balance so they don't fall. Gradually the other children come closer and watch and try the exercise. In a short time, the entire line is covered with children balancing themselves and continuing to walk around, watching their feet attentively.

Music may be used at this point. It should be a very simple march, without an obvious rhythm. It should simply accompany and support the efforts of the children.

When children learn to master their balance in this way, Dr. Montessori believed, they can bring the act of walking to a remarkable standard of perfection.

The next two questions are based on this passage.

3. Which of the following quotations from the passage is reflective of the author stating an opinion?

   A. The children are taught to walk on these lines like tightrope walkers, placing their feet one in front of the other.
   B. For this exercise, a line is drawn in chalk or paint on the floor.
   C. One of the most important gymnastic exercises in the original Montessori school approach is that of the "line."
   D. At first it is only certain children who follow her, and when she has shown them how to walk the line, she leaves, letting the exercise develop on its own.

4. Read the following quotation from paragraph two of the passage.

   The teacher herself performs the exercise first, showing clearly how she places her feet, and the children imitate her without her even needing to speak.

   This is an example of which of the following types of statements?

   A. It is an opinion statement, because not everyone is a visual learner.
   B. It is a factual statement, because it describes a step in the procedure for walking the line.
   C. It is an opinion statement, because the author believes that the teacher should initiate walking the line, a belief that cannot be agreed upon unanimously.
   D. It is a factual statement, because surveys to test this claim have been administered and analyzed.

Imagine living in the year 1800. The railroads then were very scarce. Gas lights were not yet invented, and electric lights were not even dreamed of. Even kerosene wasn't used at that point. This was the world into which Samuel Morse, the inventor of the telegraph, was born.

Samuel Morse was born in Charlestown, Massachusetts, shortly before the turn of the century, in 1791. When he was seven years old, he was sent to boarding school at Phillips Academy, Andover. While he was there, his father wrote him letters, giving him good advice. He told him about George Washington and about a British statesman named Lord Chesterfield, who was able to achieve many of his goals. Lord Chesterfield was asked once how he managed to find time for all of his pursuits, and he replied that he only ever did one thing at a time, and that he "never put off anything until tomorrow that could be done today."

Morse worked hard at school and began to think and act for himself at quite a young age. His biggest accomplishment was in painting, and he established himself as a successful painter after graduating from college at Yale. But he also had an interest in science and inventions. He was passionate about the idea of discovering a way for people to send messages to each other in short periods of time.

In the early 1800s, it took a long time to receive news of any sort, even important news. Whole countries had to wait weeks to hear word of the outcomes of faraway wars. The mail was carried by stagecoach. In emergency situations, such as when ships were lost at sea, there was no way to send requests for help. Electricity had been discovered, but little application had been made of it up until that point. This was about to change when Morse set his mind to his invention.

On October 1, 1832, Morse was sailing to America from a trip overseas on a ship called the *Sully*. He became preoccupied with the thought of inventing a machine that would later become the telegraph. Morse thought about the telegraph night and day. As he sat upon the deck of the ship after dinner one night, he took out a little notebook and began to create a plan.

If a message could be sent ten miles without dropping, he wrote, "I could make it go around the globe." He said this over and over again during the years after his trip.

One morning at the breakfast table, Morse showed his plan to some of the other *Sully* passengers. Five years later, when the model of the telegraph was built, it was exactly like the one shown that morning to the passengers on the *Sully*.

Once he arrived in America, Morse worked for twelve long years to get people to notice his invention. Though some supported the idea of the telegraph, many people scoffed at it. Morse persisted, and eventually a bill was passed by Congress in 1842. It authorized the funds needed to build the first trial telegraph line.

After two years, the telegraph line was complete. Morse and his colleagues tested it in May 1844. The device worked, and the telegraph became a huge success. Morse's persistence had finally paid off.

The next two questions are based on this passage.

5. Read the following quotation from the last paragraph of the passage.

    The device worked, and the telegraph became a huge success.

    This is an example of which of the following types of statements?

    A. It is a factual statement, because the success of the telegraph can be documented with evidence.
    B. It is a factual statement, because telegraphs are considered by most to be very useful.
    C. It is an opinion statement, because some people do not think that the telegraph worked very well.
    D. It is an opinion statement, because only the passage's author thinks that the telegraph was a success.

6. Which of the following quotations from the passage could be considered an opinion?

    A. Though some supported the idea of the telegraph, many people scoffed at it.
    B. "Never put off anything until tomorrow that could be done today."
    C. On October 1, 1832, Morse was sailing to America from a trip overseas on a ship called the *Sully*.
    D. Once he arrived in America, Morse worked for twelve long years to get people to notice his invention.

7. The Beatles influenced the genre of rock and roll just as Beethoven expanded the genre of the symphony. John Lennon, Paul McCartney, George Harrison, and Ringo Starr expanded the public's understanding of their musical genre and reclassified it as an anthem for rebellion. Their music transformed into the hippies' theme songs of the sixties. Beethoven similarly altered the public's understanding of the symphony. His addition of a chorus in the last movement of the Ninth Symphony attests to this feat.

    Read the following quotation from the passage.

    Beethoven similarly altered the public's understanding of the symphony.

    Which of the following is true about the above quotation?

    A. It is a factual statement, because everyone would agree that it is true.
    B. It is a factual statement, because there is a verifiable example to back it up.
    C. It is an opinion statement, because only the author thinks that Beethoven altered the public's understanding of the symphony.
    D. It is an opinion statement, because some people might not agree that Beethoven altered the public's understanding of the symphony.

8. Maslow's hierarchy postulates that human beings must have certain basic needs met before they can realize their potential by mastering more sophisticated and complex abilities. For example, people must be confident that they have reliable sources of food, clothing, and shelter before they can start to focus on needs such as being loved. This belief system serves as the foundation for early education programs like Head Start.

Read the following quotation from the passage.

For example, people must be confident that they have reliable sources of food, clothing, and shelter before they can start to focus on needs such as being loved.

Which of the following is true about the above quotation?

A. It is an opinion statement, because some people might believe that being loved should precede the obtainment of food, clothing, and shelter.

B. It is a factual statement, because it is common sense: people cannot live without food, clothing, and shelter, but they can live without being loved.

C. It is an opinion statement, because some people prefer food while others prefer love.

D. It is a factual statement, because a psychologist proposed it, and psychologists are authority figures in the area of human development.

9. Music can have a significant positive influence on individuals in many different circumstances. Persons who must spend time recuperating in the hospital are frequently soothed by the presence of soft music. Babies are trained to respond to auditory noises through the use of music. Persons going through emotional difficulties such as grief frequently listen to and create music as a means of dealing with the issues they are experiencing. Even people who simply need a short respite from the stresses of the day often use music as a calming and coping mechanism.

Read the following quotation from the passage.

Music can have a significant positive influence on individuals in many different circumstances.

Which of the following is true about the above quotation?

A. It is a factual statement, because it uses the qualifying phrase *can have*.

B. It is a factual statement, because no one would argue that music can have a negative influence.

C. It is an opinion statement, because some people might not be positively influenced by music.

D. It is an opinion statement, because only in some circumstances is music positive.

10. Athletes are extremely aware of how physical motion and its properties can affect the human body as well as the outcomes of competitions. Figure skating, for example, involves concentric motion for spins. Skaters learn how to use their arms to bring in their centers of gravity. In the same way that runners adopt a certain leg stance or swimmers use their arms to move quickly through the water, skaters also use their knowledge of physics to improve their skating.

Read the following quotation from the passage.

Athletes are extremely aware of how physical motion and its properties can affect the human body as well as the outcomes of competitions.

Which of the following revisions to the above statement would turn the statement into a fact?

A. Athletes are seldom aware of how physical motion and its properties can affect the human body as well as the outcomes of competitions.
B. All athletes are aware of how physical motion and its properties can affect the human body as well as the outcomes of competitions.
C. All athletes are extremely aware of how physical motion and its properties can affect the human body as well as the outcomes of competitions.
D. Some athletes are extremely aware of how physical motion and its properties can affect the human body as well as the outcomes of competitions.

11. Bees are a natural part of the pollination cycle of plants. Many plants require the assistance of bees in order to transfer their pollen so that flowers can be produced. Bees travel from flower to flower, and minuscule grains of pollen attach to the bees' legs. The pollen travels much more efficiently via bees than it might if it had to rely on the wind, for example. In this manner, bees assist in the natural pollination cycle through the action of gathering nectar from flowers. Bees are a critical component of this process; without them, plants would face much greater challenges in their reproduction.

Read the following quotation from the passage.

Bees are a critical component of this process; without them, plants would face much greater challenges in their reproduction.

Which of the following is true about the above quotation?

A. It is an opinion statement, because there is not enough evidence to support it.
B. It is an opinion statement, because only some people feel this way about bees.
C. It is a factual statement, because it can be verified empirically through scientific research.
D. It is a factual statement, because no one has found a way to prove or refute it.

12. As one of the most prolific female poets in nineteenth-century America, today Emily Dickinson is a household name. However, during her lifetime, she lived as a recluse and wrote most of her poetry from the solitude of her bedroom. She presents a unique perspective from this time period, when few women wrote about the themes she discusses. For this reason, critics are frequently interested in her perspective as a female author even beyond the contributions she made as an American nineteenth-century writer.

Read the following quotation from the passage.

She presents a unique perspective from this time period, when few women wrote about the themes she discusses.

Which of the following is true about the above quotation?

A. It is an opinion statement, because people have diverse feelings about Dickinson's work.
B. It is an opinion statement, because plenty of people think that Dickinson's poetry was common.
C. It is a factual statement, because people can read Emily Dickinson's poetry and decide for themselves.
D. It is a factual statement, because it can be backed up with verifiable evidence from the time period.

13. When artists achieve commercial successes, their emotional mindsets can be influenced by this experience. Claude Monet was one such example of this phenomenon. Monet's innovative style earned him considerable fame and public acclaim. In addition, he was extremely prolific as an artist because of his industrious work ethic. As a result, he was successful at his craft, and his paintings reflect a more contemplative and calm perspective than those of artists whose life experiences were fraught with poverty and struggle.

Read the following quotation from the passage.

When artists achieve commercial successes, their emotional mindsets can be influenced by this experience.

Which of the following most likely explains why the above quotation is a factual statement?

A. It is factual, because research has shown that celebrities tend to seek success.
B. It is factual, because it can be experienced with one of the senses, vision.
C. It is factual, because it can be proven by surveying a sample of celebrities.
D. It is factual, because it explains why celebrities prefer fame to struggle.

14. Arguably, the most well-known Siamese cat is the seal point. The dark brown ears, face, and tail are famous markers of this popular breed of cat. Many cats that appear in popular culture, including the mischievous Siamese cats in Disney animated films, are patterned after this type of Siamese. However, cat aficionados are well aware that other types of Siamese cats also exist. Two of these include the blue point and the snowshoe. Snowshoe Siamese are characterized by the white markings on their paws along with the dark "boots": these markings earn them their name and make the cats look as though they have been walking in the snow. Blue point Siamese cats do not have dark brown "points"; rather, their ears, paws, tails, and noses are characterized by bluish patches on their fur. Some Siamese cats are even hairless. They exhibit the darker pigment on their noses, tails, ears, and paws, similar to their fur-covered counterparts of the same breed. However, hairless Siamese cats exhibit these "points" on their skin instead of their fur. This type of Siamese is rather rare and not very well known. Despite the contrasts between the external appearances of these varying types of Siamese, all Siamese cats are known for being vocal, loyal, and rather mischievous.

Which of the following quotations from the above passage contains traces of the author's opinion?

A. However, cat aficionados are well aware that other types of Siamese cats also exist.
B. Two of these include the blue point and the snowshoe.
C. Blue point Siamese cats do not have dark brown "points"; rather, their ears, paws, tails, and noses are characterized by bluish patches on their fur.
D. Some Siamese cats are even hairless.

15. The acoustics of various performance venues emerge as the result of careful planning and extensive decision making. Sound travels differently when it moves through air, and the objects it encounters in a particular environment strongly impact the way that listeners hear the sound. Venues that are designed primarily to house symphony orchestra performances require vastly different acoustic designs than do venues that cater to more intimate performances. Engineers must take into account a wide variety of variables during the design process, including vibration, sound, ultrasound, and infrasound.

A sound wave consists of a fundamental, followed by a series of sequential overtones. The way that listeners perceive these sound waves is impacted by the material used in the listening environment, the physical layout of the environment, the position of the stage relative to the audience's seating, and even the height of the ceiling. Many acoustic engineers also must take into consideration the manner in which transducers impact listening. Transducers include loudspeakers, microphones, and sonar projectors. The addition of these tools to an acoustic environment can strongly influence and transform how audience members in different locations in the room perceive any sound being transmitted.

Read the following quotation from the passage.

Venues that are designed primarily to house symphony orchestra performances require vastly different acoustic designs than do venues that cater to more intimate performances.

This statement is best characterized by which of the following?

A. It is a fact, because it can be supported by real-life examples drawn from the field of acoustic engineering.
B. It is an opinion, because the author states a preference for orchestra venues without supporting this position.
C. It is an opinion, because the statement cannot be supported with empirical data.
D. It is a fact, because the author has attended numerous performances and has noted the acoustic differences.

Answer Key

1. B		**9.** A	
2. A		**10.** D	
3. C		**11.** C	
4. B		**12.** D	
5. A		**13.** C	
6. B		**14.** A	
7. B		**15.** A	
8. A			

Answers and Explanations

1. (B) The statement refers to the author's attitude—he or she finds this notion understandable. However, others might not agree with the author on this point, so choice A is incorrect. Choices C and D are incorrect because the statement is the author's viewpoint, not a fact.

2. (A) The author qualifies his or her statement by using the word *likely*, which indicates that there is a strong probability of low traffic on roads in sparsely populated areas. This probability can be documented with evidence, so it is a fact.

Choice C is incorrect because scientific experimentation involves manipulating variables to test a particular outcome.

3. (C) Choices A and B reflect procedures in walking the line and are factual, so they are both incorrect. Choice D may not be able to be proven with 100 percent accuracy in all situations, but it is not an opinion because it is not based on an attitude, subjective thought, or emotion. Choice C reflects a value judgment through its use of the word *important*, which can be refuted by anyone who believes that

other exercises are more valuable than walking the line.

4. (B) The statement is a fact, which eliminates choices A and C. The statement describes a step in the exercise, so choice B is correct.

5. (A) In some cases, it is a matter of opinion whether something is or is not a *success*; however, in this sentence, the assertion is not based on a value judgment, but on an observable fact: the telegraph worked, which meant that Morse's intention was realized, and the widespread use of the telegraph can be documented with historical evidence. Thus, choices C and D are incorrect.

6. (B) Some people claim to work better under pressure and thrive on "putting things off" to the last minute; therefore, choice B is reflective of an opinion. Choices A, C, and D are facts that can be historically documented, so they are incorrect.

7. (B) While this statement looks like an opinion from the outset because people could technically argue against the validity of the statement, the statement is actually a fact. The music can be compared with other music from the time, and a conclusion can be drawn: the symphony was not like other symphonies of the time period, based on its inclusion of a chorus. This change altered the public's understanding of the symphony, so choice B is correct.

8. (A) The quotation is based on a postulation made by Maslow, not on experimental data, statistical research, or clearly observable information; therefore, it is an opinion. Choice B is incorrect because *common sense* is not a reliable enough factor on which to base truth. Choice C deals with preferences rather than viewpoints and is also incorrect.

9. (A) When statements include qualifiers such as *can have* or *may have*, they are not absolute; therefore, the author is not claiming that music will always have a positive influence, but that

it *possibly* can. That statement can be verified and stands as a fact rather than an opinion.

10. (D) Referring to athletes as a group, without using a preceding qualifier such as *some* or *many*, suggests that *all* athletes are extremely aware of how physical motion can affect their bodies. This is not necessarily the case, however, so it would be impossible to prove. Choice D revises the sentence using the qualifying phrase *some athletes*, which turns the statement into a verifiable fact.

11. (C) This statement is a fact because it can be proven through scientific research; thus, choices A and B are incorrect. Choice D is incorrect because a fact is a statement that can be proven, not a statement that hasn't yet been proven or disproven.

12. (D) *Unique* means special or rare, which Dickinson's poetry was since there was so little poetry written by other women of the time period. The unique status of her poetry can be verified by evidence from the time period; therefore, the statement is a fact, eliminating choices A and B.

13. (C) A fact is a statement that can be proven using empirical evidence. This statement could be proven in several ways; conducting a survey of celebrities would be one of them.

14. (A) Not each and every cat expert, or aficionado, is necessarily well aware that there are different types of Siamese cats. Therefore, choice A is based on the author's opinion. Choices B, C, and D are facts that can be readily observed.

15. (A) This quotation from the passage can be backed up by real-life examples from the field of acoustic engineering. The author provides some explanation of the different design variables that must be taken into account, and the differences could be further documented with case studies from actual venues, so choice A is correct.

CHAPTER 8

Identifying Text Structures and Writing Styles

Identifying Text Structures and Writing Styles questions may ask about the type of writing that a passage represents, the author's rhetorical intent in writing a passage, and the type of text structure reflected in a passage.

Types of Writing

Passages may represent four different **types of writing:** technical, narrative, persuasive, and expository.

- **Technical writing** conveys complex or difficult subject matter in a specific manner with great accuracy.

- **Narrative writing** conveys a series of events.

- **Persuasive writing** attempts to convince the reader of a particular point of view.

- **Expository writing** describes a topic and may even review its features in detail.

The questions that accompany the following two passages ask you to identify the types of writing reflected in the passage:

Maslow's hierarchy postulates that human beings must have certain basic needs met before they can realize their potential by mastering more sophisticated and complex abilities. For example, people must be confident that they have reliable sources of food, clothing, and shelter before they can start to focus on needs such as being loved. This belief system serves as the foundation for early education programs like Head Start.

The above passage is reflective of which of the following types of writing?

A. Narrative
B. Persuasive
C. Technical
D. Expository

The correct answer is **D**. This passage is an example of expository writing, which describes a subject and explains its features. Choice A is incorrect because narrative writing tells a story or relates a series of events. Choice B is incorrect because persuasive writing attempts to persuade the reader to accept a particular point of view or take a certain action. Choice C is incorrect because technical writing explains highly complex topics in an accurate and often formally structured manner.

Let's look at another example.

Dear Dean Jeffries,

I am writing to oppose the imposition of an administrative fee for the use of the main student parking lot located at 765 Liberty Street on the west campus. This administrative fee would be detrimental for students and for the university. The student parking lot is currently used by students who live off campus and must park their cars in order to attend school. Since on-campus housing is highly limited and there is no public transportation located close to campus, most students must live off-campus and must drive or share rides with others, thus necessitating parking when they come to school. The main parking lot is the most convenient to campus buildings, so it attracts the greatest amount of traffic. Imposing a fee for the use of this lot would pose a financial hardship for many off-campus students, who are already paying higher rental fees for apartments outside the campus housing system.

The fee would also have a negative impact on the university, if imposed as proposed. The fee is higher than parking fees found at any other local college or university. Students who have to incur substantial costs for parking might tend to drive less to school, missing more classes and performing less well. This could affect the university's reputation, since poorly performing students are less likely to attract top faculty to the teaching staff. Students might also choose to transfer to other schools where on-campus housing is more widely available, thus avoiding parking costs altogether and increasing enrollment at local competitor colleges. This could further negatively affect the university's standing among top programs in the area. In sum, the parking fee is a poor idea and would not serve the interests of university students or the school.

Sincerely,

Rolinda Wallach

The above letter is reflective of which of the following types of writing?

A. Expository
B. Persuasive
C. Narrative
D. Technical

The correct answer is **B**. The author's intent is to persuade. Choice A is incorrect because the author does not simply give information; she also requests a change in behavior. Choice C is incorrect because the author does not relay a story or describe a series of events. Choice D is incorrect because the writing addresses a parking issue and is not technical in nature.

Rhetorical Intent

Closely related to the four types of writing is the concept of rhetorical intent. An author's **rhetorical intent** may be to inform, to persuade, to entertain, or to express feelings.

- **Informational writing** is designed to give the reader information about a particular topic.

- **Persuasive writing** attempts to convince the reader to accept a perspective or to take a certain action.

- **Entertainment writing** is designed to provide entertainment.

- **Expressive writing** serves the purpose of conveying the author's feelings or bringing up certain feelings in the reader.

The questions that accompany the following two passages ask you to identify the author's rhetorical intent:

> Maslow's hierarchy postulates that human beings must have certain basic needs met before they can realize their potential by mastering more sophisticated and complex abilities. For example, people must be confident that they have reliable sources of food, clothing, and shelter before they can start to focus on needs such as being loved. This belief system serves as the foundation for early education programs like Head Start.

> Which of the following is the author's intent in the passage?

A. To inform
B. To entertain
C. To persuade
D. To express feelings

The correct answer is **A**. The author's intent is to inform. Choice B is incorrect because the author does not attempt to engage the reader in an entertaining or captivating manner. Choice C is incorrect because the author does not make an argument and attempt to convince the reader to believe a particular idea or take a certain action. Choice D is incorrect because the author does not attempt to express feelings or bring out emotions in the reader; instead, the passage is written from an objective, neutral perspective.

Now consider this example:

> To All Restaurant Staff:

> It has come to my attention that some employees have been using the kitchen's silver serving platters to serve large parties when the porcelain serving platters are all in use. This causes a problem with serving some of our VIP guests, who may arrive unexpectedly or with short notice. Please refrain from using the silver serving platters unless they have been specifically designated to serve a reserved party. The list of reservations can be found on the back bulletin board for any given night; silver service will be marked next to a reservation with a circled S.

Additional porcelain serving platters are currently on order to ensure that we have adequate servingware to accommodate all of our guests.

Thank you for helping us to serve our VIP patrons with the level of professionalism they have come to know and expect.

George Gario,

Proprietor

Which of the following is the author's intent in the memo?

A. To entertain
B. To describe
C. To persuade
D. To express feelings

The correct answer is **C**. The author's intent is to persuade. Choice A is incorrect because the author does not attempt to engage the reader in an entertaining or captivating manner. Choice B is incorrect because the author does not simply give information without also requesting a change in behavior. Choice D is incorrect because while the author does hope to appeal to the reader's feelings, he does this only for the purpose of moving the reader to action.

Text Structure

Along with reflecting four different types of writing and four rhetorical intentions, TEAS Reading passages may reflect five **types of text structure:** sequence, problem-solution, comparison-contrast, cause-effect, and description.

- **Sequence text structures** convey ideas in order or describe steps in a process.
- **Problem-solution text structures** present a problem and provide a solution to solve that problem.
- **Comparison-contrast text structures** discuss the similarities and differences between two or more elements.
- **Cause-effect text structures** explain an outcome as the result of a particular cause, or they show how one factor leads to a certain outcome.
- **Description text structures** merely describe topics or events in a general way.

The following examples ask you to identify the text structures in each passage.

Athletes are extremely aware of how physical motion and its properties can affect the human body as well as the outcomes of competitions. Figure skating, for example, involves concentric motion for spins. Skaters learn how to use their arms to bring in their centers of gravity. In the same way that runners adopt a certain leg stance or swimmers use their arms to move quickly through the water, skaters also use their knowledge of physics to improve their skating.

Which of the following text structures is used in the last sentence of the above passage?

A. Comparison-contrast
B. Cause-effect
C. Sequence
D. Problem-solution

The correct answer is **A**. Comparison-contrast text structures highlight similarities and differences between or among entities. Choice B is incorrect because a cause-effect text structure focuses on how one factor or variable produces a specific outcome. Choice C is incorrect because a sequence text structure describes steps in a process or presents information in chronological form. Choice D is incorrect because a problem-solution text structure presents a problem and then provides a solution to that problem.

Consider this next passage:

In the animal kingdom, many symbiotic relationships exist between two species that take actions known to be mutually beneficial for both parties. In the water, clownfish have such a relationship with sea anemones. The fish are one of the only species that can swim unharmed in the anemone's waving tentacles, as typically the tentacles would sting any animal that swam near it. However, the clownfish is immune to the sting of the tentacles and is therefore protected by them; in return, its presence helps the anemone stay clean, avoid attack by parasites, and remain free from infection.

Which of the following text structures is used to organize the above passage?

A. Description
B. Sequence
C. Comparison-contrast
D. Problem-solution

The correct answer is **A**. In this passage, the clownfish and sea anemone's relationship is described. Choice B is incorrect because a sequence text structure describes steps in a process or presents information in chronological form. Choice C is incorrect because comparison-contrast text structures highlight similarities and differences between or among entities. Choice D is incorrect because a problem-solution text structure presents a problem and then provides a solution to that problem.

Let's look at one final example related to text structure:

Arguably, the most well-known Siamese cat is the seal point. The dark brown ears, face, and tail are famous markers of this popular breed of cat. Many cats that appear in popular culture, including the mischievous Siamese cats in Disney animated films, are patterned after this type of Siamese. However, cat aficionados are well aware that other types of Siamese cats also exist. Two of these include the blue point and the snowshoe. Snowshoe Siamese are characterized by the white markings on their paws along with the dark "boots": these markings earn them their name and make the cats look as though they have been walking in the snow. Blue point Siamese cats do not have dark brown "points"; rather, their ears, paws, tails, and noses are characterized by bluish patches on their fur. Some Siamese cats are even hairless. They exhibit the darker pigment on their noses, tails, ears, and paws similar to their fur-covered counterparts of the same breed. However, hairless Siamese cats exhibit these "points" on their skin instead of their fur. This type of Siamese is rather rare and not very well known. Despite the contrasts between the external appearances of these varying types of Siamese, all Siamese cats are known for being vocal, loyal, and rather mischievous.

Which of the following text structures is used to organize the above passage?

A. Sequence
B. Cause-effect
C. Comparison-contrast
D. Problem-solution

The correct answer is **C**. In the passage, the author compares different types of Siamese cats. Choice A is incorrect because a passage with a sequence text structure describes steps in a process or presents information in chronological form. Choice B is incorrect because a cause-effect text structure focuses on how one factor or variable produces a specific outcome. Choice D is incorrect because a problem-solution text structure presents a problem and then provides a solution to that problem.

Review Questions

Saltwater fish and freshwater fish are related, but their natural environments prove rather distinctive. In terms of being kept as pets, freshwater fish require less maintenance. They live in water that can be adapted from tap water, and they can be kept in many different types of containers in addition to aquariums. Saltwater fish, on the other hand, require a specific type of salt-infused water. Careful watch of the pH balance of the water must also be maintained.

The next two questions are based on this passage.

1. The author's description of saltwater and freshwater fish is reflective of which of the following types of text structures?

   A. Sequence
   B. Problem-solution
   C. Cause-effect
   D. Comparison-contrast

2. The above passage is reflective of which of the following types of writing?

   A. Technical
   B. Expository
   C. Narrative
   D. Persuasive

To All Department Supervisors:

The Acme Records Retrieval System will be undergoing scheduled maintenance this Friday, from 4:00 p.m. to midnight. Please inform all department personnel of the system outage so that researchers can make alternative arrangements to access necessary data.

An archived copy of the Core Business Records Database will be accessible in the Web Services department office from 4:00 p.m. to 8:00 p.m. on Friday. However, this database contains only core records data and is limited in its scope.

Please direct any questions to Marcus Sampson, Web Services Maintenance Officer, at (617) 555-0004.

The next two questions are based on this memo.

3. Which of the following is the author's intent in the memo?

   A. To entertain
   B. To express feelings
   C. To persuade
   D. To inform

4. The organizational structure of the above memo is best characterized as which of the following?

   A. Comparison-contrast
   B. Cause-effect
   C. Problem-solution
   D. Sequence

The acoustics of various performance venues emerge as the result of careful planning and extensive decision making. Sound travels differently when it moves through air, and the objects it encounters in a particular environment strongly impact the way that listeners hear the sound.

Venues that are designed primarily to house symphony orchestra performances require vastly different acoustic designs than do venues that cater to more intimate performances. Engineers must take into account a wide variety of variables during the design process, including vibration, sound, ultrasound, and infrasound.

A sound wave consists of a fundamental, followed by a series of sequential overtones. The way that listeners perceive these sound waves is impacted by the material used in the listening environment, the physical layout of the environment, the position of the stage relative to the audience's seating, and even the height of the ceiling. Many acoustic engineers also must take into consideration the manner in which transducers impact listening. Transducers include loudspeakers, microphones, and sonar projectors. The addition of these tools to an acoustic environment can strongly influence and transform how audience members in different locations in the room perceive any sound being transmitted.

The next two questions are based on this passage.

5. Which of the following text structures is used to organize the above passage?

   A. Description
   B. Sequence
   C. Problem-solution
   D. Comparison-contrast

6. Which of the following is the author's intent in the passage?

   A. To persuade
   B. To entertain
   C. To inform
   D. To express feelings

Aficionados of classical music frequently appreciate the characteristics of jazz, and some laypersons think the two genres are somewhat similar. However, jazz musicians are noted for their improvisational abilities, whereas classically trained musicians are often very reliant upon printed music. Although musicians in both genres must be very well versed in scales and various musical keys, jazz musicians must possess impeccable knowledge of this material in order to be able to perform and fulfill the requirements of their chosen genre.

The next two questions are based on this passage.

7. The above passage is reflective of which of the following types of writing?

   A. Narrative
   B. Expository
   C. Technical
   D. Persuasive

8. Which of the following text structures is used to organize the above passage?

   A. Comparison-contrast
   B. Description
   C. Sequence
   D. Problem-solution

9. When artists achieve commercial successes, their emotional mindsets can be influenced by this experience. Claude Monet was one such example of this phenomenon. Monet's innovative style earned him considerable fame and public acclaim. In addition, he was extremely prolific as an artist because of his industrious work ethic. As a result, he was successful at his craft, and his paintings reflect a more contemplative and calm perspective than those of artists whose life experiences were fraught with poverty and struggle.

   Which of the following is the author's intent in the passage?

   A. To persuade
   B. To entertain
   C. To inform
   D. To express feelings

As one of the most prolific female poets in nineteenth-century America, today Emily Dickinson is a household name. However, during her lifetime, she lived as a recluse and wrote most of her poetry from the solitude of her bedroom. She presents a unique perspective from this time period, when few women wrote about the themes she discusses. For this reason, critics are frequently interested in her perspective as a female author even beyond the contributions she made as an American nineteenth-century writer.

The next two questions are based on this passage.

10. Which of the following text structures is used to organize the last two lines of the above passage?

    A. Problem-solution
    B. Cause-effect
    C. Description
    D. Comparison-contrast

11. Which of the following is the author's intent in the passage?

    A. To persuade
    B. To entertain
    C. To express feelings
    D. To inform

Literary scholars have often speculated as to the personal characteristics of William Shakespeare. The Bard is known to many as the greatest writer the English language has ever known, but we have very few examples of his handwriting or even his own name written out in his hand. Some academics have gone so far as to speculate that Shakespeare was a pseudonym for an aristocrat. However, the majority of scholars have dismissed this proposal, and they concentrate instead on Shakespeare's thoughtful insights and dexterous construction of language.

The next two questions are based on this passage.

12. Which of the following text structures is used to organize the above passage?

    A. Cause-effect
    B. Sequence
    C. Description
    D. Comparison-contrast

13. The above passage is reflective of which of the following types of writing?

    A. Narrative
    B. Expository
    C. Technical
    D. Persuasive

14. The physician William Harvey was the first who discovered and demonstrated the true mechanism of the heart's action. No one before his time conceived that the movement of the blood was entirely due to the mechanical action of the heart as a pump. There were all sorts of speculations about the matter, but nobody had formed this conception. Harvey is as clear as possible about it. He says the movement of the blood is entirely due to the contractions of the walls of the heart—that it is the propelling apparatus—and all recent investigation tends to show that he was perfectly right.

    Which of the following is the author's intent in the passage?

    A. To inform
    B. To entertain
    C. To express feelings
    D. To persuade

15. To All Restaurant Staff:

    It has come to my attention that some employees have been using the kitchen's silver serving platters to serve large parties when the porcelain serving platters are all in use. This causes a problem with serving some of our VIP guests, who may arrive unexpectedly or with short notice. Please refrain from using the silver serving platters unless they have been specifically designated to serve a reserved party. The list of reservations can be found on the back bulletin board for any given night; silver service will be marked next to a reservation with a circled S.

Additional porcelain serving platters are currently on order to ensure that we have adequate servingware to accommodate all of our guests.

Thank you for helping us to serve our VIP patrons with the level of professionalism they have come to know and expect.

George Gario,

Proprietor

Which of the following text structures is used to organize the above memo?

A. Description
B. Sequence
C. Comparison-contrast
D. Problem-solution

Answer Key

1.	D	**9.**	A
2.	B	**10.**	B
3.	D	**11.**	D
4.	C	**12.**	C
5.	A	**13.**	B
6.	C	**14.**	A
7.	B	**15.**	D
8.	A		

Answers and Explanations

1. (D) In the passage, the author compares and contrasts the environmental needs of freshwater and saltwater fish. Choice A is incorrect because a sequence text structure describes steps in a process or presents information in chronological form. Choice B is incorrect because a problem-solution text structure presents a problem and then provides a solution to that problem. Choice C is incorrect because a cause-effect text structure focuses on how one factor or variable produces a specific outcome.

2. (B) This passage is an example of expository writing, which describes a subject and explains

its features. Choice A is incorrect because technical writing explains highly complex topics in an accurate and often formally structured manner. Choice C is incorrect because narrative writing tells a story or relates a series of events. Choice D is incorrect because persuasive writing attempts to convince the reader to accept a particular position or take a certain action.

3. (D) This memo offers details regarding a database shutdown, so the author's intent is to inform. Choice A is incorrect because the author does not attempt to engage the reader in an entertaining or captivating manner. Choice B is incorrect because the author does not attempt to express feelings or bring out emotions in the reader; instead, the memo is written from an objective, neutral perspective. Choice C is incorrect because the author does not make an argument and attempt to convince the reader to accept a particular position or take a certain action.

4. (C) In the memo, the author presents a problem for department supervisors: the record retrieval system will be down. He also presents a possible solution: an alternative database may be used. Choice A is incorrect because a comparison-contrast text structure focuses on highlighting the similarities and differences between or among entities. Choice B is incorrect because a cause-effect text structure focuses on how one factor or variable produces a specific outcome. Choice D is incorrect because a sequence text structure describes steps in a process or presents information in chronological form.

5. (A) In this passage, the author describes acoustics. Choice B is incorrect because a sequence text structure describes steps in a process or presents information in chronological form. Choice C is incorrect because a problem-solution text structure presents a problem and then provides a solution to that problem. Choice D is incorrect because a comparison-contrast text structure focuses on highlighting the similarities and differences between or among entities.

6. (C) The author's intent in this passage is to inform. Choice A is incorrect because the author does not make an argument and attempt to convince the reader to accept a particular position or take a certain action. Choice B is incorrect because the author does not attempt to engage the reader in an entertaining or captivating manner. Choice D is incorrect because the author does not attempt to express feelings or bring out emotions in the reader.

7. (B) This passage is an example of expository writing, which describes a subject and explains its features. Choice A is incorrect because narrative writing tells a story or relates a series of events. Choice C is incorrect because technical writing explains highly complex topics in an accurate and often formally structured manner.

Choice D is incorrect because persuasive writing attempts to persuade the reader to accept a particular position or take a certain action.

8. (A) In the passage, the author compares and contrasts jazz and classical musicians. Choice B is incorrect because a passage with a description text structure simply provides information about an entity. Choice C is incorrect because a sequence text structure describes steps in a process or presents information in chronological form. Choice D is incorrect because a problem-solution text structure presents a problem and then provides a solution to that problem.

9. (A) The author makes an argument in this passage by presenting a central claim and providing evidence to support that claim. In doing so, he or she attempts to convince the reader to accept a particular position, namely that *when artists achieve commercial successes, their emotional mindsets can be influenced by this experience*. Choice B is incorrect because the author does not attempt to engage the reader in an entertaining or captivating manner. Choice C is incorrect because the author is not simply offering information to describe a phenomenon; the description that is provided is given to support the author's point. Choice D is incorrect because the author does not attempt to express feelings or evoke emotions in the reader; instead, the passage is written from an objective, neutral perspective.

10. (B) In the last two lines of this passage, the author shows a cause-effect relationship between two factors. First, the author notes that Dickinson's perspective is unique; *for this reason*, the author explains, critics are often more interested in her point of view as a female author. Choice A is incorrect because a problem-solution text structure presents a problem and then provides a solution to that problem. Choice C is incorrect because description text structures merely present information about a subject. Choice D is incorrect because comparison-contrast text structures highlight similarities and differences between or among entities.

11. (D) The author's intent is to inform. Choice A is incorrect because the author does not make an argument and attempt to convince the reader to believe a particular point of view or take a

certain action. The author instead presents facts about Dickinson's life and work and the interests of the scholars who study her. Choice B is incorrect because the author does not attempt to engage the reader in an entertaining or captivating manner. Choice C is incorrect because the author does not attempt to express feelings or bring out emotions in the reader; instead, the passage is written from an objective, neutral perspective.

12. (C) In the passage, the author uses a descriptive text structure to present information about Shakespeare. Choice A is incorrect because cause-effect text structures focus on how one factor or variable produces a specific outcome. Choice B is incorrect because a sequence text structure describes steps in a process or presents information in chronological form. Choice D is incorrect because a comparison-contrast text structure focuses on highlighting the similarities and differences between or among entities.

13. (B) This passage is an example of expository writing, which describes a subject and explains its features. Choice A is incorrect because narrative writing tells a story or relates a series of events. Choice C is incorrect because technical writing explains highly complex topics in an accurate and often formally structured manner. Choice D is incorrect because persuasive writing attempts to persuade the reader to accept a particular position or take a certain action.

14. (A) The author's intent here is to inform. Choice B is incorrect because the author does not attempt to engage the reader in an entertaining or captivating manner. Choice C is incorrect because the author does not attempt to express feelings or bring out emotions in the reader; instead, the passage is written from an objective, neutral perspective. Choice D is incorrect because the author does not make an argument and attempt to convince the reader to accept a particular position or take a certain action.

15. (D) In the passage, the author presents a problem; he also presents solutions. Choice A is incorrect because a description text structure simply provides information about a subject. Choice B is incorrect because a sequence text structure describes steps in a process or presents information in chronological form. Choice C is incorrect because a comparison-contrast text structure focuses on highlighting the similarities and differences between or among entities.

CHAPTER 9

Vocabulary

Vocabulary questions on the TEAS ask you to define the meaning of a vocabulary word based on the context of the passage. The chosen vocabulary word is often one that might have an unusual meaning or might be interpreted as having several meanings. The correct meaning must be clarified based on your understanding of the surrounding text. Here is an example:

> Shelley was born in England in 1792, as a member of the aristocracy. He was educated at two prestigious English schools, Eton College and Oxford University.

> Based on context, which of the following is the definition of the underlined word in the sentences above?

> A. A worker's union
> B. A Republican consortium
> C. The upper class
> D. A lower socioeconomic class

The correct answer is **C**. The word *aristocracy* means the wealthy or the upper class of a society. The context clue about Shelley's education at *prestigious* schools indicates that his family was wealthy enough to afford such select schools, so choice A is correct.

The sentences are about education and not employment or labor, so we can rule out choice A. Choice B can also be eliminated because, like with choice A, there is no discussion of politics or political groups in the sentences surrounding the word. Finally, choice D is the opposite of the correct answer. The context clues lead the reader to believe that Shelley was wealthy. The phrase *lower socioeconomic class* would indicate someone who was poor and thus unable to afford expensive schooling.

The following example includes a selection from the same passage on Shelley:

> Shelley's ideas were heavily influenced by the politics of his time. He grew up at a time when governments were under transformation. In fact, he came of age in the shadow of the French Revolution. This war was very violent, and since France was so close to England, Shelley was acutely aware of the violence that was occurring there.

Based on context, which of the following is the definition of the underlined word in the passage above?

A. Change
B. Suspicion
C. Surveillance
D. Regrowth

The correct answer is **A.** *Change*, which can be synonymous with *transformation*, is the best fit with the context of this passage. *Transformation* is followed in the next sentence by the mention of a revolution, which would indicate a shift or change in governments. Therefore, the context clues given indicate that the author was describing the transforming or changing political landscape of the time.

Choice B can be eliminated because *suspicion* indicates doubt or skepticism. The paragraph does not discuss doubt or skepticism either on the part of the government or on Shelley's part. Choice C, *surveillance*, indicates that the governments were being watched closely by an entity or person. While this may have been true historically, there are no surrounding context clues in the passage to support this interpretation. Finally, choice D is incorrect because *regrowth* would mean that the governments were destroyed or eliminated and would need to be built again. There is nothing in the passage to suggest that this was the case.

Let's look at another example.

As one of the most prolific female poets in nineteenth-century America, today Emily Dickinson is a household name. However, during her lifetime, she lived as a recluse and wrote most of her poetry from the solitude of her bedroom. She presents a unique perspective from this time period, when few women wrote about the themes she discusses. For this reason, critics are frequently interested in her perspective as a female author even beyond the contributions she made as an American nineteenth-century writer.

Based on the context of the passage above, which of the following is the definition of the underlined word?

A. Happiness
B. Misery
C. Crowdedness
D. Privacy

The correct answer is **D.** In this question, the author uses the word *solitude* to describe the atmosphere of Dickinson's writing space, her bedroom. Since the passage previously describes Dickinson as a *recluse*—a person who prefers to be alone—it is logical to conclude that Dickinson would prefer a space of *privacy* that would allow her to be alone.

Choice A is incorrect because *happiness* is irrelevant to the topic. The passage does not comment on Dickinson's moods but rather on how she lived her life. Regarding choice B, the passage specifically states that Dickinson preferred to be alone: she was a recluse. This preference does not indicate *misery*. Choice C is also incorrect because *crowdedness* is the opposite of reclusiveness, which the passage has already established that Dickinson preferred.

The next two passages contain additional examples of vocabulary words similar to those that might be tested.

> Gardner has postulated an alternative theory concerning the existence of multiple intelligences. He posits that individuals can possess intelligence in particular areas, including linguistic intelligence, spiritual intelligence, spatial intelligence, intrapersonal intelligence, interpersonal intelligence, musical intelligence, mathematical intelligence, and kinesthetic intelligence, among others. Gardner asserts that individuals can be extremely intelligent and exhibit talent in one area, while failing to demonstrate the same level of prowess in another area.

> Based on the context of the passage above, which of the following is the definition of the underlined word?

> A. Claims
> B. Questions
> C. Evades
> D. Disagrees

The correct answer is **A**. The word *posits* indicates that someone, in this case Howard Gardner, has made a *claim* or argument about a particular topic. The preceding and following sentences contain similar words, such as *postulated* and *asserts*, which also indicate a claim or argument.

Choice B is incorrect because if the word *posits* were replaced by the word *questioned*, the new sentence would indicate that Gardner was unsure of the statement that followed. However, the statement was his idea, so choice B does not make sense in this context. Choice C is incorrect because the purpose of the paragraph is to identify what Gardner thinks about IQ measurement; a person who has an opinion or argument on the subject would not logically be portrayed as *evading* the topic. Similar to choice B, choice D can be eliminated because if it were used to replace the word *posits*, the sentence would have the opposite of its intended meaning. Gardner does believe that people have multiple intelligences, so saying that he *disagrees* with the information in the statement would not make sense here.

Now consider this final passage:

> The best method of treating individuals facing psychological difficulties is a blend of cognitive-behavioral therapy and medication. This approach not only serves to address the patient's potential chemical imbalances, but it also emancipates the patient by allowing him or her some autonomy in dealing with the issues associated with a possible malaise.

Based on the context of the passage above, which of the following is the definition of the underlined word?

A. Traps
B. Inspires
C. Frees
D. Confuses

The correct answer is **C**. Discussion of the patient's *emancipation* is immediately followed by mention of the patient's *autonomy* or independence. A person who is independent is *free*, so choice C is correct. Choice A is incorrect because it is the opposite of the meaning indicated. A patient cannot be *autonomous* if he or she is *trapped*. Choice B is incorrect because the passage does not describe the *inspiration* that therapy and medicine can produce. The focus is instead on the well-being of the patient and his or her ability to take ownership in dealing with psychological issues. Choice D is incorrect because if you plug *confuses* into the sentence to replace *emancipates*, the sentence no longer makes sense.

Review Questions

1. Shelley's ideas were heavily influenced by the politics of his time. He grew up at a time when governments were under transformation. In fact, he came of age in the shadow of the French Revolution.

   Based on the context of the passage above, which of the following is the definition of the underlined phrase?

   A. Before
   B. Inferior to
   C. Under the influence of
   D. As a participant in

2. Shelley's poem "Mont Blanc" focuses on the Romantic notion of the sublime. The Romantic poets believed that when people interacted with Nature, it sometimes caused them to be in a state of wonder—or it caused them to be awestruck.

   Based on context, which of the following is the definition of the underlined word in the sentences above?

   A. Below par
   B. Truly inspirational
   C. Submerged
   D. Quietly introspective

3. Almost all approaches to CPR suggest that a person begin resuscitation efforts with chest <u>compressions</u>. To perform a chest compression, the individual places both hands flat on the patient's chest and then begins pushing down carefully but firmly, most likely at equal intervals.

   Based on context, which of the following is the definition of the underlined word in the sentences above?

   A. Actions that remove items
   B. Actions that decrease density
   C. Actions that condense files
   D. Actions that press together

4. The lifesaver should start first by checking the patient's airway. He or she might also <u>administer</u> mouth-to-mouth rescue breathing.

   Which of the following is a synonym for <u>administer</u> in the sentences above?

   A. Supervise
   B. Apply
   C. Preach
   D. Teach

5. In planning improvements of highway systems, several different types of traffic may be encountered. These range from business traffic to agricultural shipping to residential transportation. Improvement activities must meet the requirements of all <u>classes</u> of traffic, the most important being provided for first.

   Based on the context of the passage above, which of the following is the definition of the underlined word?

   A. Groups of students taught by a professor
   B. Rankings in society based on economics
   C. Groups of items with similar qualities
   D. Individuals who maintain an elegant appearance

6. To keep their balance, the children must make efforts similar to those of real tightrope walkers, except that they have no danger of falling, since the lines are drawn only on the floor. The teacher herself performs the <u>exercise</u> first, showing clearly how she places her feet, and the children imitate her without her even needing to speak.

   Based on the context, which of the following is the correct definition of the word <u>exercise</u> in the sentences above?

   A. Freedom
   B. Process
   C. Removal
   D. Physical fitness

7. Personality is the combination of traits that make up an individual's sense of self. Traits can range from descriptors of behavior, such as "calm" or "emotional," to <u>modes</u> of experiencing the world, such as "thinking" or "sensing."

   Based on context, which of the following is the definition of the underlined word in the sentences above?

   A. Ways
   B. Fashions
   C. Numbers
   D. Cuisines

8. Freud believed that as a child, an individual's actions are driven by hidden impulses—and that repression or denial of those impulses by parents or society can lead to fixations or personality disorders. Alternatively, if the child's impulses are accepted as normative to his or her development, then a functional adult behavioral pattern should <u>take root</u>.

   Based on context, which of the following is the definition of the underlined phrase in the sentences above?

   A. Grow in the ground
   B. Steal
   C. Disappear
   D. Develop

9. Freud often worked with highly distressed female clients, repressed in their natural modes of expression; this is how he developed many of his theories, which some people believe are not very scientific. By today's standards, they are not, but Freud's idea that unconscious urges drive our behavior was <u>revolutionary</u> for his time.

   Based on the context of the sentences above, which of the following is the definition of the underlined word?

   A. Referring to a political advocate
   B. Referring to an early war in American history
   C. Referring to an innovative idea
   D. Referring to overthrowing a government

10. Close to the Guildhall is the <u>site</u> of a house known as New Place, which was bought by Shakespeare himself. Here Shakespeare lived during the later part of his life, until his death in 1616.

    Based on context, which of the following is the definition of the underlined word in the sentences above?

    A. A position or location
    B. The sense of looking
    C. To officially summon
    D. To refer to as an example

11. Although Shakespeare spent most of his career in London, with trips back to Stratford, he moved permanently to his home at New Place in the last years of his life and is believed to have written some of his later works there. Only the <u>foundations</u> of the New Place house now remain.

    Based on context, which of the following is the definition of the underlined word in the sentences above?

    A. States of being established
    B. The physical bases that buildings are built upon
    C. Institutions engaged in philanthropy
    D. The conceptual underpinnings of an idea

12. Christopher Columbus was particularly influenced by the maps of the ancient geographer Ptolemy. Ptolemy argued that the world was round, which went against the belief of the day that the world was flat. Columbus sided with Ptolemy on this question and <u>set out</u> to prove that it was so.

    Based on the context of the passage above, which of the following is the definition of the underlined phrase?

    A. To reflect upon an upcoming event
    B. To act against one's own beliefs
    C. To begin sailing on a voyage abroad
    D. To begin working toward a plan

13. To make the journey westward, Columbus would require the help of a <u>generous financial backer</u>, so he went to seek the aid of the king of Portugal. Columbus asked the king for ships and sailors to make the journey.

    Based on context, which of the following is the definition of the underlined phrase in the sentences above?

    A. A person who hoards resources in secret
    B. A wealthy and resourceful travel partner
    C. A person who provides money for a cause
    D. An athlete who donates his income to charity

14. Once he arrived in America, Morse worked for twelve long years to get people to notice his invention. Though some supported the idea of the telegraph, many people <u>scoffed</u> at it. Morse persisted, and eventually a bill was passed by Congress in 1842.

    Which of the following words is the best synonym for the underlined word in the sentences above?

    A. Jeered
    B. Opined
    C. Condoned
    D. Forfeited

15. Persons going through emotional difficulties such as grief frequently listen to and create music as a means of dealing with the issues they are experiencing. Even people who simply need a short respite from the stresses of the day often use music as a calming and coping mechanism.

    Based on the context of the passage above, which of the following is the definition of the underlined word?

    A. A sudden awakening
    B. A change in perspective
    C. A way to get even
    D. A pause for relief

Answer Key

1.	C	**9.**	C
2.	B	**10.**	A
3.	D	**11.**	B
4.	B	**12.**	D
5.	C	**13.**	C
6.	B	**14.**	A
7.	A	**15.**	D
8.	D		

Answers and Explanations

1. (C) Shelly was highly aware of the French Revolution, and he grew up *under the influence* of it. While *in the shadow of* also means "being overshadowed," this is not the meaning of the phrase in this particular context, eliminating choice B.

2. (B) While *sub-* is often used as a prefix meaning "under" or "below," in such words as *subpar* or *submarine*, this is not the way the prefix is being used in this excerpt, as indicated by the second sentence, which speaks of *awe* and *wonder*. Since *sublime* is equated with causing *awe* and *wonder*, its definition in this context most nearly means *truly inspirational*.

3. (D) The common definition of *compression* is an increase (not a decrease) in density, which

eliminates choice B. The word *compression* in this context means to press down on the chest to enable circulation, so choice D is the only option that makes sense here. Choice C refers to the context of the computer field and is incorrect.

4. (B) The word *administer* typically means either "to manage" or "to apply." In this case, a person may administer, or *apply*, mouth-to-mouth breathing, deeming choice B correct and choice A incorrect. Choice C offers the word *preach*, the activity of *ministers*, which does not fit the context here.

5. (C) *Classes of traffic* refers to categories of traffic with similar qualities, such as cars or big trucking rigs, deeming choice C correct. While all of the other answer choices are definitions of *classes*

in other contexts, they are incorrect in this sentence.

6. **(B)** For this sentence, choice B is the correct answer in that "performing an exercise" refers to the process of the teacher placing her feet on the line. Choice D is one definition of *exercise*, but it does not fit in this sentence. Choice A's definition, *freedom*, does not make sense in this context, and is, therefore, incorrect. Choice C is related to the word *excise*, not *exercise*.

7. **(A)** The phrase "*modes of experiencing the world*" can be replaced with "*ways of experiencing the world*," so choice A fits the context here. While *modes* can also refer to *fashions* or *numbers*, choices B and C are not the correct definitions in this context.

8. **(D)** Choice A is incorrect, since it is a literal definition of *take root* instead of an idiom, which is figurative. Choices B and C do not fit the context and are therefore incorrect, while choice D, in the context of this passage, makes sense: a functional adult behavioral pattern should *develop*.

9. **(C)** While each of the answer choices refers to a definition of *revolutionary*, only choice C makes sense in the context of this sentence; Freud's ideas about the unconscious were *innovative* during the time he was living.

10. **(A)** The word *site* is used as a noun in this sentence, since it is preceded by the word *the*, deeming the verb definitions in choices C and D incorrect. Choices C and D are definitions of a homophone for *site*, spelled *cite*. Choice B is also the definition

of a homophone for *site* that is spelled *sight*. Hence, the correct answer is choice A.

11. **(B)** Each of these choices offers a possible definition of the word *foundations*, but only choice B makes sense, as the last sentence of the selection refers to a *house*, which is a *building*.

12. **(D)** Columbus *set out to*, or *began working toward*, proving Ptolemy correct, choice D. Choices A and B are not definitions of *set out*, and neither of them makes sense in the context of this sentence. Choice C, *to begin sailing on a voyage*, is one possible definition for *set out*, but it does not make sense in this sentence.

13. **(C)** *A person who provides money for a cause*, choice C, is a *generous financial backer*; Columbus hoped that the king of Portugal would be that person, but he was not. Choices A, B, and D do not fit the context and are therefore incorrect.

14. **(A)** This sentence contrasts the words *supported* and *scoffed*, revealing that some people supported Morse's idea, but others did not. The word *jeer* means the opposite of *support*, so choice A is the correct answer. To *opine* means to give an opinion, to *condone* means to support, and to *forfeit* means to give up. None of these definitions makes sense in the context of the sentence.

15. **(D)** A synonym for the word *respite* in this sentence would be the word *break*. *Break* could be substituted for *respite* in the sentence without a change in meaning. The word *break* means *a pause for relief*, so choice D is the correct answer.

Using Maps and Resources

Using Maps and Resources questions require you to identify information given in different types of resources. Some questions may also require you to identify the appropriate resources to consult in order to obtain specific types of information. Questions may test your ability to use a number of different skills, including following directions, reading labels and ingredient lists, analyzing outlines, identifying sources, and looking up information.

In **following directions questions**, a set of directions is given, and you are asked to identify the outcome that occurs when the directions are followed. In **reading labels and ingredient lists questions**, a nutritional label is provided or the ingredients of a recipe are listed. You might be asked to determine, for instance, whether this particular food or product would be suitable for an individual with certain dietary needs.

An example of a reading labels question is provided below:

Nutrition Facts

Serving Size 2/3 cup (55g)
Servings Per Container About 8

Amount Per Serving	
Calories 230	Calories from Fat 40

	% Daily Value*
Total Fat 8g	**12%**
Saturated Fat 1g	**5%**
Trans Fat 0g	
Cholesterol 0mg	**0%**
Sodium 160mg	**7%**
Total Carbohydrate 37g	**12%**
Dietary Fiber 4g	**16%**
Sugars 1g	
Protein 3g	
Vitamin A	10%
Vitamin C	8%
Calcium	20%
Iron	45%

*Percent Daily Values are based on a 2,000 calorie diet. Your daily value may be higher or lower depending on your calorie needs.

	Calories:	2,000	2,500
Total Fat	Less than	65g	80g
Sat Fat	Less than	20g	25g
Cholesterol	Less than	300mg	300mg
Sodium	Less than	2,400mg	2,400mg
Total Carbohydrate		300g	375g
Dietary Fiber		25g	30g

A hungry woman decides to eat four servings of the product above. Her caloric needs are 2,000 calories per day. How many calories may she still eat for the rest of the day without exceeding her caloric needs?

A. 460 calories
B. 920 calories
C. 1,770 calories
D. 1,080 calories

The correct answer is **D**. Each serving of this product contains 230 calories. The number 230 multiplied by four servings is 920 calories already consumed. To find the amount of calories left to be eaten for the day, subtract 920 from 2,000 calories. The answer is 1,080.

In **analyzing outlines questions**, an outline is given, and you must identify patterns in the headings or subheadings of the outline. Here is an example:

Chapter 10 The Major Sports

1. Baseball

    A. History
    B. Rules
    C. Notable Players

2. Basketball

    A. History
    B. Rules
    C. Notable Players

3. Football

    A. History
    B. Rules
    C. Notable Players

4. Hockey

    A. History
    B. Rules
    C. Notable Players

5. Soccer

    A. History
    B. Rules
    C. Notable Players

What is the organizational pattern reflected in the headings and subheadings above?

A. The chapter discusses the history, rules, and notable players of five major sports.
B. The chapter discusses the history of five major sports played throughout the world.
C. The chapter discusses physical education activities and their rules.
D. The chapter discusses famous athletes' careers throughout history.

The correct answer is **A**. The chapter is arranged by major sport, and each sport covers the same three subtopics. No other choice offers this organizational option.

In **identifying sources questions**, a scenario is posed, and you must identify the correct information source to use to obtain the required information. Finally, in **looking up information questions**, an information source is provided, and you are asked to look up information and answer a question identifying that information. Information sources may be presented in text form or in graphic form. **Text information sources** include memos, advertisements, book indices, tables of contents, price lists, and yellow pages listings. **Graphic information sources** include graphs, charts, diagrams, and maps, among other possibilities.

Many Using Maps and Resources questions on the TEAS fall into the category of looking up information. To answer the question, you must look up the information requested and find the answer. Even though the sources provided may be vastly different—graphs and charts, for instance, versus yellow page ads—the skill used in answering these questions is the same.

The following three examples all test your skills at looking up information found in various sources:

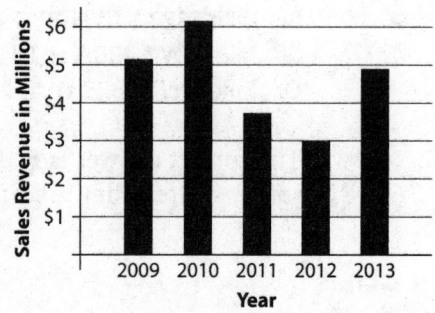

The bar graph above shows sales revenue for a business by the year. How much revenue did the business generate in 2013?

A. About $5.00
B. Almost $4,000
C. About $5,000
D. About $5,000,000

The correct answer is **D**. The bar graph compares the amount of revenue made by a business each year. The label on the left side of the graph indicates that the units are given in millions of dollars. The bar for 2013 extends to just below the 5 mark, which indicates almost 5 million dollars, or $5,000,000.

Consider this example:

Map of Lyndon B. Johnson State Park in Stonewall, Texas

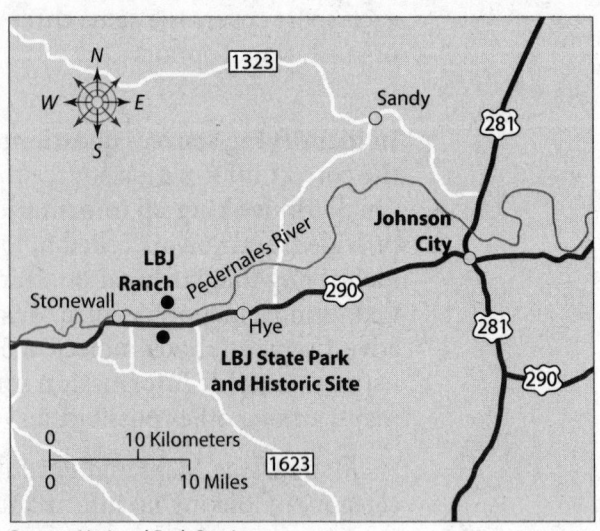

Source: National Park Service

Which of the following directions should someone who lives in the city of Sandy take in order to arrive at the LBJ State Park and Historic Site?

A. Take HWY 281 N to 290 W.
B. Take 1323 S to HWY 290 W.
C. Take HWY 290 S to HWY 281 N.
D. Take HWY 1323 W to 281 S.

The correct answer is **B**. The correct route to take is 1323 S to HWY 290 W. The other routes offer incorrect ordinal directions.

Let's look at one more example related to looking up information.

Climate

> Africa, 722–4
>
> Antarctica, 765–7
>
> Asia, 543–7
>
> Australia, 669–70
>
> Europe, 453–5, 467
>
> North America, 363, 379–81
>
> South America, 497–9

Climate changes, 203–23

A student would like to compare climate changes in the 16th and 21st centuries. On which of the following pages might she find this information?

A. Page 221
B. Page 232
C. Page 453
D. Page 723

The correct answer is **A**. Choice A is correct because page 221 falls between pages 203 and 223, under the heading of climate changes.

Review Questions

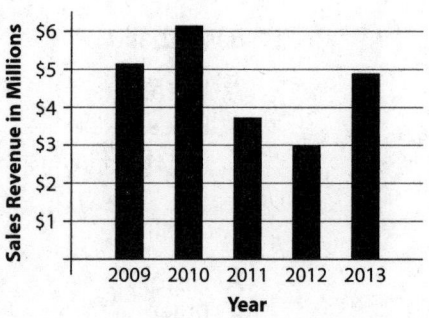

1. Based on the graph above, which of the following is true regarding sales revenue for the business shown?

    A. The revenue of the business has been increasing.
    B. The revenue of the business has been decreasing.
    C. The business has seen fluctuating revenue between 2009 and 2013.
    D. The business has brought in its best revenue in recent years.

2.

Climate

Africa, 722–4

Antarctica, 765–7

Asia, 543–7

Australia, 669–70

Europe, 453–5, 467

North America, 363, 379–81

South America, 497–9

Climate changes, 203–23

In which of the following resources would the above index most likely be found?

A. Biology textbook
B. History textbook
C. Ecology textbook
D. Chemistry textbook

3.

Chapter 10: The Major Sports

1. Baseball

   A. History
   B. Rules
   C. Notable Players

2. Basketball

   A. History
   B. Rules
   C. Notable Players

3. Football

   A. History
   B. Rules
   C. Notable Players

4. Hockey

   A. History
   B. Rules
   C. Notable Players

5. Soccer

    A. History
    B. Rules
    C. Notable Players

If the title of the above outline were changed to read "Chapter 10: Ball Sports," which of the following sections would not belong in the chapter?

    A. Hockey
    B. Football
    C. Tennis
    D. Soccer

Apple Pie

3 cups all-purpose flour

1¼ cup sugar

1 cup butter

4–5 Granny Smith apples

3 egg yolks

1 lemon

¼ cup cold water

3 Tbsp heavy cream

1 Tbsp cinnamon

The next two questions are based on this ingredients list.

4. Are the ingredients in the recipe above suitable for an individual with diabetes?

    A. Yes, because egg yolks are a staple of any diabetic diet.
    B. Yes, because diabetes is a disorder for which the body requires extra sugar ingestion.
    C. No, because diabetics are allergic to products containing fruit.
    D. No, because the ingredients include sugar, which is not appropriate for people with diabetes.

5. In which of the following cookbooks are you most likely to find a recipe using the ingredients list above?

    A. *Halloween Candies and Confections*
    B. *Egg-Based Entrees for Entertaining*
    C. *Healthy Living for Longevity*
    D. *Delicious Desserts to Die For*

Conference Registration Instructions

Time: Monday, 8:30 a.m to 10:30 a.m.

Location: Wellings Ballroom

The Society for Associated Technologies is pleased to welcome our guests for the 2015 Annual Conference in San Jose, California. Upon checking in, please settle into your rooms and enjoy a complimentary Happy Hour on the hotel's East Deck. Cocktails and light appetizers will be served both Saturday and Sunday evenings from 5–7 p.m.

Conference registration begins promptly at 8:30 on Monday morning and will run until 10:30 a.m. To register for the conference, please bring your membership ID card and payment confirmation with you to the registration area. Members with ID numbers 10000–20000 should register at Table 1; members with ID numbers 20001–30000 should register at Table 2; and members with ID numbers 30001–40000 should register at Table 3.

Members without a membership ID or payment confirmation should register in the Skylark Ballroom, located just down the corridor from the Wellings Ballroom, on the south side of the hotel. If you have questions regarding your registration, please call Liana Reyes, Registration Coordinator, at (669) 375-1700.

The next two questions are based on these instructions.

6. At which of the following tables should the member with ID number 39999 register?

   A. Table 1
   B. Table 2
   C. Table 3
   D. Table 4

7. At which of the following days and times should an attending conference member sign up for the conference?

   A. Monday morning
   B. Monday evening
   C. Thursday morning
   D. Saturday or Sunday evening

Map of Lyndon B. Johnson State Park in Stonewall, Texas

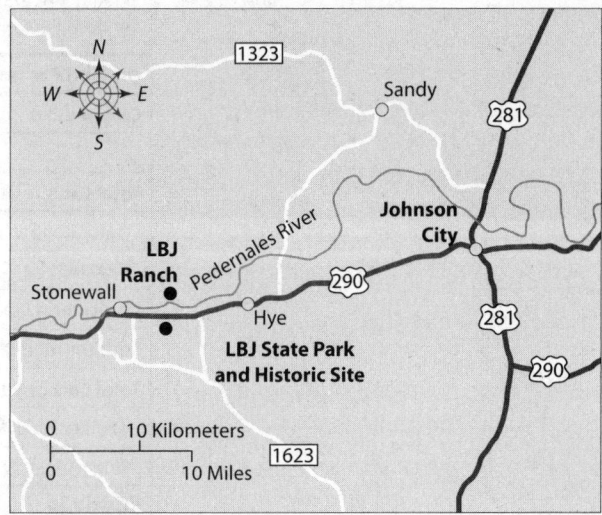

Source: National Park Service

8. In which of the following guides would you most likely find the map above?

    A. *World Atlas*
    B. *Johnson City Street Guide*
    C. *Map of California*
    D. *Texas Roads and Recreation Atlas*

9. A couple is looking for an inexpensive restaurant with tasty food. Which of the following sources would provide the couple with the desired information?

    A. A calorie counter guidebook
    B. A website of local restaurant reviews
    C. A phone book with restaurants alphabetized by name
    D. A book about recipes on a budget

10. A woman is concerned that her dog's leg might be broken. Which resource should the woman consult?

    A. A website about pet care
    B. A zoology textbook
    C. An anatomy textbook
    D. *The Yellow Pages*, under V for veterinarian

Nutrition Facts	
Serving Size 2/3 cup (55g)	
Servings Per Container About 8	

Amount Per Serving	
Calories 230	Calories from Fat 40

	% Daily Value*
Total Fat 8g	**12%**
Saturated Fat 1g	**5%**
Trans Fat 0g	
Cholesterol 0mg	**0%**
Sodium 160mg	**7%**
Total Carbohydrate 37g	**12%**
Dietary Fiber 4g	**16%**
Sugars 1g	
Protein 3g	
Vitamin A	10%
Vitamin C	8%
Calcium	20%
Iron	45%

*Percent Daily Values are based on a 2,000 calorie diet. Your daily value may be higher or lower depending on your calorie needs.

	Calories:	2,000	2,500
Total Fat	Less than	65g	80g
Sat Fat	Less than	20g	25g
Cholesterol	Less than	300mg	300mg
Sodium	Less than	2,400mg	2,400mg
Total Carbohydrate		300g	375g
Dietary Fiber		25g	30g

11. A man who recently suffered from gallstones was instructed by his doctor to consume no more than 1 percent of his daily value of total fat in one meal. The man eats a 2,000-calorie diet each day. Is the above product a suitable choice for the man?

    A. No, because each serving of the product contains 12 percent of daily fat value, which highly exceeds the man's needs.
    B. Yes, because the product contains zero cholesterol, which is beneficial to a patient suffering from gallstones.
    C. Yes, because the food offers iron, which is considered to be an essential part of a balanced diet.
    D. No, because the product contains 230 calories, which is more than the man should consume in one meal.

Units Produced by Teams A – E

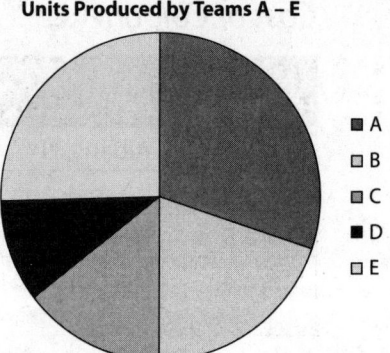

The next two questions are based on this pie chart.

12. Which of the following teams produced the most units?

    A. Team A
    B. Team B
    C. Team C
    D. Team D

13. About how many units were produced without Team E?

    A. Four-fifths of the units
    B. Half of the units
    C. Three-fourths of the units
    D. One-fourth of the units

Cost of Cologne

Company	City	Price per Case of 10	Shipping and Handling
Store 1	Albany, NY	$130.00	$15.00/case
Store 2	Washington, DC	$120.00	$20.00/case
Store 3	New York, NY	$150.00	Free shipping on all orders
Store 4	Hartford, CT	$135.00	$15.00/case (free in-state shipping)

The next two questions are based on this price list.

14. A man from Connecticut is interested in purchasing 50 bottles of cologne to give as gifts to his male employees this year. How much will he pay in total if he purchases the cologne from Store 4?

    A. $650.00
    B. $675.00
    C. $690.00
    D. $750.00

15. A woman from New York is interested in stocking her store with 90 bottles of cologne. Which store would save her the most money?

    A. Store 1
    B. Store 2
    C. Store 3
    D. Store 4

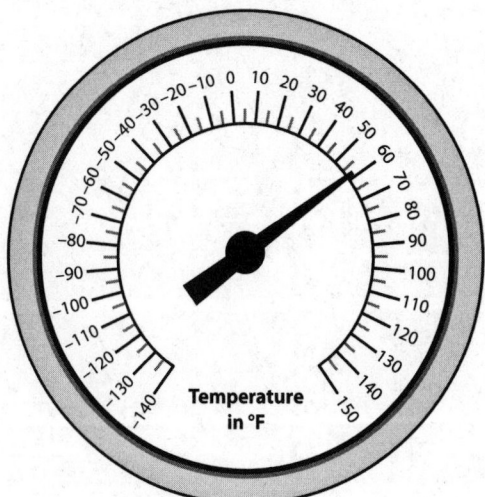

16. A temperature of approximately how many degrees is represented on the thermometer?

    A. Between 110 and 110 degrees
    B. Between 60 and 65 degrees
    C. Between 55 and 60 degrees
    D. Between 50 and 55 degrees

17. Which of the following resources would be most helpful for finding the length of a car?

    A. A protractor
    B. A ruler
    C. A yardstick
    D. A calculator

Marcia decided to run a trail 3.5 miles every other day, and to run a different path 3.9 miles on her off days. The chart below demonstrates the number of miles she ran over two weeks' time.

Sunday	Monday	Tuesday	Wednesday	Thursday	Friday	Saturday
3.5	3.9	3.5	3.9	3.9	3.5	3.9
3.5	3.9	3.5	3.9	3.9	3.5	3.9

The next three questions are based on this passage and chart.

18. How many times did Marcia run a trail, and how many times did she run a path?

    A. Marcia ran a trail five times and a path nine times.
    B. Marcia ran a trail six times and a path eight times.
    C. Marcia ran a trail eight times and a path six times.
    D. Marcia ran a trail seven times and a path seven times.

19. Which of the following is a true statement, based on the chart?

    A. Marcia ran the trail two more times than she ran the path.
    B. Marcia ran the path and the trail an equal number of times.
    C. Marcia ran the path two more times than she ran the trail.
    D. Marcia ran the path three more times than she ran the trail.

20. How many times did Marcia deviate from her typical routine?

    A. One
    B. Two
    C. Three
    D. Four

Answer Key

1. C		**6.** C	
2. C		**7.** A	
3. A		**8.** D	
4. D		**9.** B	
5. D		**10.** D	

11. A

12. A

13. C

14. B

15. B

16. C

17. C

18. B

19. C

20. B

Answers and Explanations

1. (C) There is no general trend within the revenue data presented in the bar graph. Choice D is incorrect because the business saw declining revenue in 2011 and 2012.

2. (C) Climate is a subtopic of the ecology discipline. Biology textbooks are concerned with life processes, while history textbooks are concerned with social and political events of the past. Chemistry textbooks are concerned with chemical processes, so choices A, B, and D are incorrect.

3. (A) Hockey does not belong in the chapter because the chapter is about ball sports; a puck is used in hockey. Balls are used in all of the other sports listed.

4. (D) Diabetics produce insufficient insulin to break down sugar, so their sugar intake should be limited; this apple pie recipe calls for 1¼ cups of sugar, which is not suitable for a diabetic.

5. (D) Apple pie is a dessert and would likely be included in a cookbook about desserts. Choice A is incorrect because apple pie is not a candy, and it is not traditionally served on Halloween. Choice B is incorrect because, while the recipe calls for eggs, apple pie is not considered an *egg-based* dish—such as quiche—and it is not an *entrée*, or main dish. Choice C is incorrect, because while apples are healthy, an apple pie made with sugar would not be considered to be a particularly healthy dish.

6. (C) The number 39999 falls between 30001 and 40000, so the member needs to register at Table 3; there is no Table 4 mentioned in the instructions.

7. (A) The instructions specifically mention 8:30 a.m.–10:30 a.m. on Monday morning as the designated conference sign-up period. While other times and days are also mentioned, they are not designated for conference sign-up.

8. (D) This map is too specific to be found in a world atlas, and it is too large-scale to be found in a city guidebook. Choice C is incorrect because this map excerpt shows points of interest in Texas, not California.

9. (B) A calorie counter guide lists food items and their corresponding calorie contents; a phone book lists businesses, including restaurants, but it does not objectively rate food taste or price. Choice D is incorrect because the couple is looking for a restaurant, not for inexpensive food to make at home.

10. (D) An animal's broken bone requires a veterinarian for treatment; all of the other options given are too broad and would be inappropriate for a dog owner to consult for help in treating such a major injury.

11. (A) The amount of total fat in this product is 12 percent of the suggested daily value, based on a 2,000-caloried diet. The man was instructed to eat less than 1 percent of his daily value of total fat in one meal, so this product is not suitable for him to consume.

12. (A) Team A shows the largest shaded area on the pie chart; thus, choice A is the correct answer.

13. (C) The shaded area for Team E on the pie chart represents approximately 25 percent, or one-fourth of the pie graph. Without this one-fourth, the rest of the teams' production makes

up 75 percent, or three-fourths of the total number of units produced.

14. (B) Since the man is purchasing the cologne from the store in his home state, Connecticut, he does not have to pay any shipping charges. An order of 5 boxes of 10 bottles of cologne each will be $135 times 5, which comes to a total of $675, choice B.

15. (B) To obtain 90 bottles of cologne, the woman would have to order nine cases. Store 2 would provide the cases at the lowest total cost, which is $140 per case, including shipping. Store 1 would charge $145 per case including shipping, while Store 3 and Store 4 would both charge $150 per case including shipping.

16. (C) The gauge of the thermometer is just under the 60 degree mark, which falls between 55 and 60 degrees.

17. (C) A car would be best measured with a yardstick, which is 3 feet, or 36 inches long; a ruler would be too small, at 12 inches. A calculator is used to calculate, while a protractor is used to measure angles.

18. (B) The chart demonstrates that Marcia ran 3.5 miles six times. The trail is 3.5 miles long, so she ran a trail six times. She ran 3.9 miles eight times, so she ran the path eight times.

19. (C) The chart demonstrates that Marcia ran the path eight times and the trail six times. Therefore, she ran the path two more times than she ran the trail.

20. (B) The chart demonstrates that Marcia deviated from her usual running schedule twice, on both Thursdays. The other days, she adhered to her usual schedule.

PART 2

Math

Math questions on the TEAS are designed to test your skills in four different areas: numbers and operations, data interpretation, measurement, and algebraic applications. In this section, we'll review some math fundamentals as well as more advanced skills you'll need to correctly answer questions involving word problems and algebra.

CHAPTER 11

Basic Operations

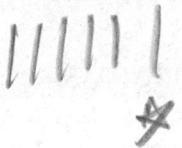

Basic operations questions on the TEAS involve addition, subtraction, multiplication, and division with whole numbers. You cannot use a calculator on the test, so you must know how to perform these operations by hand.

Multiplication Tables

The operations of multiplication and division on the TEAS generally require that you know the multiplication tables of numbers from 1 through 12 by heart. To answer the test questions in the time allotted, you'll need to be able to draw these numbers quickly from memory. Here is a multiplication table of the numbers through 12 × 12:

1	2	3	4	5	6	7	8	9	10	11	12
2	4	6	8	10	12	14	16	18	20	22	24
3	6	9	12	15	18	21	24	27	30	33	36
4	8	12	16	20	24	28	32	36	40	44	48
5	10	15	20	25	30	35	40	45	50	55	60
6	12	18	24	30	36	42	48	54	60	66	72
7	14	21	28	35	42	49	56	63	70	77	84
8	16	24	32	40	48	56	64	72	80	88	96
9	18	27	36	45	54	63	72	81	90	99	108
10	20	30	40	50	60	70	80	90	100	110	120
11	22	33	44	55	66	77	88	99	110	121	132
12	24	36	48	60	72	84	96	108	120	132	144

Order of Operations

Performing basic operations requires using the correct order of operations. In math, the **order of operations** is the set of rules that govern the sequence in which operations are performed.

The order of operations can be remembered using the phrase PEMDAS. **PEMDAS** stands for Parentheses, Exponents, Multiplication, Division, Addition, and Subtraction. Here's an example:

Simplify the expression: $4 \times (2 + 3)$.

To simplify this question, we would first perform the operation in parentheses:

$2 + 3 = 5$

Next, we would perform multiplication:

$4 \times 5 = 20$

The correct answer is **20**. When performing a series of operations, the order of operations is crucial to the accuracy of your result. If you don't follow the sequence exactly, your answer will be incorrect. In the example above, if we had multiplied 4×2 first, the answer would have been $6 + 3$, or 9, which is incorrect.

The chart below summarizes the PEMDAS rules:

	Step	Explanation
1.	**P**arentheses	Perform all operations in parentheses first.
2.	**E**xponents	Next, perform all operations involving exponents.
3.	**M**ultiplication & **D**ivision	Perform all multiplication and division in order from left to right.
4.	**A**ddition & **S**ubtraction	Perform all addition and subtraction in order from left to right.

Note that there are six letters in the word PEMDAS, and six operations to be performed, but there are only four steps in the process. This is because multiplication and division are performed together in the same step, and addition and subtraction are performed together in the step after that. Here's an example:

Simplify the expression: $5 + 7 \times 2 - 12 \div 3$.

To solve this problem, follow the rules of PEMDAS. There are no parentheses or exponents in this expression, so we'll go straight to step 3, multiplication and division. All multiplication and division must be performed first, in order from left to right, before any addition or subtraction. So, we first multiply 7×2 and divide $12 \div 3$:

$$5 + 7 \times 2 - 12 \div 3 = 5 + 14 - 4$$

Next, we perform addition and subtraction in order from left to right:

$$5 + 14 - 4 = 19 - 4$$

$$= 15$$

The correct answer is **15**. If we had multiplied 7×2 and then subtracted 12 right away, without dividing by 3 first, this would have given an incorrect answer, as shown in the example below:

Simplify the expression: $5 + 7 \times 2 - 12 \div 3$.

$$5 + 7 \times 2 - 12 \div 3 = 5 + 14 - 12 \div 3$$

$$= 19 - 12 \div 3$$

$$= 7 \div 3 \qquad \textbf{✗ INCORRECT}$$

$$= \frac{7}{3}$$

By performing the order of operations incorrectly, we reached the incorrect answer of $\frac{7}{3}$.

The correct approach is to perform all multiplication and division first, in order from left to right. Only then should you proceed to addition and subtraction, again in order from left to right:

Simplify the expression: $5 + 7 \times 2 - 12 \div 3$.

$$5 + 7 \times 2 - 12 \div 3 = 5 + 14 - 4$$

$$= 19 - 4 \qquad \textbf{✓ CORRECT}$$

$$= 15$$

Review Questions

1. $292 - 24$

Simplify the expression above. Which of the following is correct?

A. 268
B. 272
C. 278
D. 286

2. $10{,}741 \div 23$

Simplify the expression above. Which of the following is correct?

A. 365
B. 397
C. 467
D. 489

3. $8 \times (4 + 3)$

Simplify the expression above. Which of the following is correct?

A. 42
B. 35
C. 56
D. 67

4. $5{,}614 + 373$

Simplify the expression above. Which of the following is correct?

A. 5,987
B. 5,997
C. 6,017
D. 6,097

5. $17 + 6^2 - (4 + 2)$

Simplify the expression above. Which of the following is correct?

A. 23
B. 36
C. 47
D. 51

6. 324×37

Simplify the expression above. Which of the following is correct?

A. 3,240
B. 4,768
C. 11,968
D. 11,988

7. $473 - 67$

Simplify the expression above. Which of the following is correct?

A. 404
B. 406
C. 416
D. 429

8. 13,325 ÷ 5

Simplify the expression above. Which of the following is correct?

A. 400
B. 425
C. 533
D. 535

9. $3 \times 5^2 \div (9 - 4)$

Simplify the expression above. Which of the following is correct?

A. −25
B. 3
C. 15
D. 27

10. 267×45

Simplify the expression above. Which of the following is correct?

A. 2,403
B. 7,035
C. 12,015
D. 12,915

11. $2 + (4 - 5) \times (12 \div 3)$

Simplify the expression above. Which of the following is correct?

A. −2
B. 1
C. 3
D. 4

12. $3^2 \times 2 + 6 \times 4^2$

Simplify the expression above. Which of the following is correct?

A. 96
B. 114
C. 268
D. 384

13. $14 \div 7 + (1 - 5) \times 4 + 2^2$

Simplify the expression above. Which of the following is correct?

A. 22
B. 12
C. −4
D. −10

14. $5 \times (4 + 2) \div 10 + 9$

Simplify the expression above. Which of the following is correct?

A. 2
B. 12
C. 18
D. 26

15. $2^3 \times 3 \div 24 + (1 - 4)$

Simplify the expression above. Which of the following is correct?

A. −3
B. −2
C. 1
D. 14

Answer Key

1. A

2. C

3. C

4. A

5. C

6. D

7. B

8. C

9. C

10. C

11. A

12. B

13. D

14. B

15. B

Answers and Explanations

1. (A) Perform the indicated subtraction, as follows:

```
      8  12
   2  9̷  2̷
 -    2  4
 ─────────────
   2  6  8
```

To check your work, add 268 + 24. The result is the original number, 292. The correct answer is 268.

2. (C) Perform the indicated long division, as follows:

```
         467
    23)10,741
       −92
       ────
        154
       −138
       ────
        161
       −161
       ────
          0
```

To check your work, multiply 23 × 467. The result is the original number, 10,741. The correct answer is 467.

3. (C) To simplify the expression 8 × (4 + 3), use the order of operations. Following PEMDAS, first perform operations in parentheses: 4 + 3 = 7. Next, multiply 8 × 7. The correct answer is 56.

4. (A) Perform the indicated addition, as follows:

$$
\begin{array}{r}
5,\ 6\ 1\ 4 \\
+\ \ 3\ 7\ 3 \\
\hline
5,\ 9\ 8\ 7
\end{array}
$$

The correct answer is 5,987.

5. (C) To simplify the expression $17 + 6^2 - (4 + 2)$, use the correct order of operations. Following PEMDAS, first perform all operations in parentheses:

$17 + 6^2 - (4 + 2) = 17 + 6^2 - (6)$

Next, simplify all exponents:

$17 + 6^2 - (6) = 17 + (6 \times 6) - (6)$
$= 17 + (36) - (6)$

There is no multiplication or division to perform, so we move to the final step. Perform all addition and subtraction in order from left to right:

$17 + (36) - (6) = 17 + 36 - 6$
$= 53 - 6$
$= 47$

The correct answer is 47.

6. (D) Perform the indicated multiplication, as follows:

$$
\begin{array}{r}
3\ 2\ 4 \\
\times\ \ 3\ 7 \\
\hline
2,\ 2\ 6\ 8 \\
9,\ 7\ 2\ 0 \\
\hline
1\ 1,\ 9\ 8\ 8
\end{array}
$$

The correct answer is 11,988.

7. (B) Perform the indicated subtraction, as follows:

$$
\begin{array}{r}
4\ \overset{6}{\cancel{7}}\ \overset{13}{\cancel{3}} \\
-\ \ 6\ 7 \\
\hline
4\ 0\ 6
\end{array}
$$

To check your work, add 406 + 67. The result is the original number, 473. The correct answer is 406.

8. (C) Perform the indicated long division, as follows:

$$
\begin{array}{r}
533 \\
25\overline{)\ 13,325} \\
-125 \\
\hline
82 \\
-75 \\
\hline
75 \\
-75 \\
\hline
0
\end{array}
$$

To check your work, multiply 25 × 533. The result is the original number, 13,325. The correct answer is 533.

9. (C) To simplify the expression $3 \times 5^2 \div (9 - 4)$, use the order of operations. Following PEMDAS, first perform all operations in parentheses:

$3 \times 5^2 \div (9 - 4) = 3 \times 5^2 \div (5)$

Next, perform all operations involving exponents:

$3 \times 5^2 \div (5) = 3 \times 25 \div 5$

Next, perform all multiplication and division in order from left to right:

$3 \times 25 \div 5 = 75 \div 5$
$= 15$

The correct answer is 15.

10. (C) Perform the indicated multiplication, as follows:

$$
\begin{array}{r}
2\ 6\ 7 \\
\times\ \ 4\ 5 \\
\hline
1,\ 3\ 3\ 5 \\
1\ 0,\ 6\ 8\ 0 \\
\hline
1\ 2,\ 0\ 1\ 5
\end{array}
$$

The correct answer is 12,015.

11. (A) To simplify the expression $2 + (4 - 5) \times (12 \div 3)$, use the order of operations. Following PEMDAS, we first perform all operations in parentheses:

$2 + (4 - 5) \times (12 \div 3) = 2 + (-1) \times (4)$

There are no exponents in this expression, so we move to the next step. Perform all multiplication and division in order from left to right:

$2 + (-1) \times (4) = 2 + (-4)$

Finally, perform all addition and subtraction in order from left to right:

$2 + (-4) = -2$

The correct answer is −2.

12. (B) To simplify the expression $3^2 \times 2 + 6 \times 4^2$, use the order of operations. There are no parentheses in this expression, so we skip to the next step—simplify all exponents:

$3^2 \times 2 + 6 \times 4^2 = 9 \times 2 + 6 \times 16$

Next, perform all multiplication and division in order from left to right:

$9 \times 2 + 6 \times 16 = 18 + 96$

Finally, perform all addition and subtraction in order from left to right:

$18 + 96 = 114$

The correct answer is 114.

13. (D) To simplify the expression $14 \div 7 + (1 - 5) \times 4 + 2^2$, use the order of operations. Following PEMDAS, we first perform all operations in parentheses:

$14 \div 7 + (1 - 5) \times 4 + 2^2 = 14 \div 7 + (-4) \times 4 + 2^2$

Next, simplify all exponents:

$14 \div 7 + (-4) \times 4 + 2^2 = 14 \div 7 + (-4) \times 4 + 4$

Next, perform all multiplication and division in order from left to right:

$14 \div 7 + (-4) \times 4 + 4 = 2 + (-16) + 4$

Finally, perform all addition and subtraction in order from left to right:

$2 + (-16) + 4 = -10$

The correct answer is −10.

14. (B) To simplify the expression $5 \times (4 + 2) \div 10 + 9$, use the order of operations. Following PEMDAS, we first perform all operations in parentheses:

$5 \times (4 + 2) \div 10 + 9 = 5 \times (6) \div 10 + 9$

There are no exponents in this expression, so we move to the next step. Perform all multiplication and division in order from left to right:

$$
\begin{aligned}
5 \times 6 \div 10 + 9 &= 30 \div 10 + 9 \\
&= 3 + 9
\end{aligned}
$$

Finally, perform all addition and subtraction in order from left to right. The correct answer is $3 + 9$, or 12.

15. (B) To simplify the expression $2^3 \times 3 \div 24 + (1 - 4)$, use the order of operations. Following PEMDAS, we first perform all operations in parentheses:

$2^3 \times 3 \div 24 + (1 - 4) = 2^3 \times 3 \div 24 + (-3)$

Next, simplify all exponents:

$2^3 \times 3 \div 24 + (-3) = 8 \times 3 \div 24 + (-3)$

Next, perform all multiplication and division in order from left to right:

$$
\begin{aligned}
8 \times 3 \div 24 + (-3) &= 24 \div 24 + (-3) \\
&= 1 + (-3)
\end{aligned}
$$

Finally, perform all addition and subtraction in order from left to right. The correct answer is $1 - 3$, or −2.

CHAPTER 12

Fractions

Fractions questions on the TEAS test your ability to add, subtract, multiply, and divide fractions. To perform these operations, you must understand how to convert fractions to different forms.

Working with Fractions

Working with fractions requires knowledge of certain vocabulary. A fraction represents a part of a whole. **Proper fractions** consist of two numbers:

Proper Fraction

$\dfrac{1}{2}$ ◄—— Numerator
◄—— Denominator

The top number of the fraction is the **numerator**, and the bottom number is the **denominator**. In a proper fraction, the numerator is smaller than the denominator.

A fraction can also contain a numerator that is larger than the denominator. These fractions are called **improper fractions**.

Improper Fraction

$\dfrac{4}{3}$ ◄—— Numerator
◄—— Denominator

Improper fractions can be converted to a whole number plus a proper fraction. These combinations are called **mixed numbers**. The fraction above, for example, can be converted into 1 plus $\frac{1}{3}$. To write $\frac{4}{3}$ as a mixed number, we would write $1\frac{1}{3}$.

Proper Fraction	Improper Fraction	Mixed Number
$\dfrac{1}{2}$	$\dfrac{4}{3}$	$1\dfrac{1}{3}$

To perform math with fractions, we must first convert mixed numbers to improper fractions.

Comparing Fractions

When comparing fractions with the same denominator, we look at the numerator to determine which fraction is larger:

Which fraction is larger, $\frac{1}{3}$ or $\frac{2}{3}$?

In the example above, the fractions both have the same denominator, 3. When we compare the numerators, we see that $\frac{2}{3}$ is larger than $\frac{1}{3}$.

Comparing numerators works well if the fractions have the same denominator. If the fractions have different denominators, however, the comparison requires another step:

Which fraction is larger, $\frac{2}{3}$ or $\frac{5}{6}$?

In the example above, the fractions $\frac{2}{3}$ and $\frac{5}{6}$ have different denominators. To compare them, we must first change them both to fractions with the same denominator. For this, we look for the least common denominator of the two fractions.

The **least common denominator** of two fractions is the smallest number that can be divided equally by the denominators of both fractions. In this case, the number 6 is the least common denominator of the two fractions. We know this because 6 can be divided by 3 exactly 2 times, and 6 can be divided by 6 exactly 1 time. Convert both fractions to fractions over 6:

$$\frac{2}{3} = \frac{?}{6}$$

$$\frac{2}{3} \times \frac{2}{2} = \frac{4}{6}$$

Since we must multiply the denominator by 2 to produce 6, we also multiply the numerator by 2 to produce 4. The fraction $\frac{2}{3}$ is then converted to the fraction $\frac{4}{6}$. Now we can compare numerators and see that $\frac{5}{6}$ has the greatest value.

Addition

When adding fractions with the same denominator, simply add the numerators:

Simplify the expression: $\frac{1}{4} + \frac{2}{4}$.

The correct answer to this problem is $\frac{3}{4}$. We simply added the numerators, 1 + 2, to produce 3.

When adding fractions with different denominators, first convert the fractions to fractions with the same denominator:

Simplify the expression: $\frac{3}{4} + \frac{5}{6}$.

In this case, we can't simply add the numerators, because the denominators are different. To convert the fractions, we must find the least common denominator. The least common denominator is the smallest number that can be divided evenly by both 4 and 6. The number 6 won't work, because 6 cannot be divided evenly by 4. The number 12 will work, however, because it can be divided evenly by both 6 and 4.

Convert both fractions to fractions with 12 as the denominator:

$$\frac{3}{4} = \frac{?}{12}$$

$$\frac{3}{4} \times \frac{3}{3} = \frac{9}{12}$$

The fraction $\frac{3}{4}$ converts to $\frac{9}{12}$. Next, convert the fraction $\frac{5}{6}$:

$$\frac{5}{6} = \frac{?}{12}$$

$$\frac{5}{6} \times \frac{2}{2} = \frac{10}{12}$$

The fraction $\frac{5}{6}$ converts to $\frac{10}{12}$. Now we can add the numerators:

$$\frac{9}{12} + \frac{10}{12} = \frac{19}{12}$$

The sum is an improper fraction, $\frac{19}{12}$. We can also convert this to a mixed number, $1\frac{7}{12}$.

Subtraction

Subtraction of fractions works the same way as addition. When subtracting fractions with the same denominator, simply subtract the numerators:

Simplify the expression: $\dfrac{6}{8} - \dfrac{3}{8}$.

Here, the denominators are the same, so we subtract 6 − 3 to produce 3. The correct answer is $\dfrac{3}{8}$.

If the fractions have different denominators, we must convert the fractions to fractions over the same denominator:

Simplify the expression: $\dfrac{8}{12} - \dfrac{5}{8}$.

To convert the fractions, first find the least common denominator of $\dfrac{8}{12}$ and $\dfrac{5}{8}$. The least common denominator is 24. The number 24 is the smallest number that can be divided evenly by both 12 and 8. Convert both fractions to fractions over 24:

$$\frac{8}{12} = \frac{?}{24}$$

$$\frac{8}{12} \times \frac{2}{2} = \frac{16}{24}$$

The fraction $\dfrac{8}{12}$ converts to $\dfrac{16}{24}$. Next, convert the fraction $\dfrac{5}{8}$:

$$\frac{5}{8} = \frac{?}{24}$$

$$\frac{5}{8} \times \frac{3}{3} = \frac{15}{24}$$

The fraction $\dfrac{5}{8}$ converts to $\dfrac{15}{24}$. Now we can perform subtraction with the numerators:

$$\frac{16}{24} - \frac{15}{24} = \frac{1}{24}$$

The correct answer is $\dfrac{1}{24}$.

Multiplication

Multiplying fractions is relatively simple compared to adding and subtracting. This is because we don't have to convert the fractions, even if they have different denominators. To multiply fractions, multiply the numerator by the numerator and the denominator by the denominator, as follows:

Simplify the expression: $\dfrac{1}{6} \times \dfrac{3}{5}$.

These fractions have different denominators, but we can simply multiply them to get the result:

$$\frac{1}{6} \times \frac{3}{5} = \frac{1 \times 3}{6 \times 5}$$

$$= \frac{3}{30}$$

The fraction $\dfrac{3}{30}$ can be further reduced to the fraction $\dfrac{1}{10}$. This is the correct answer in its simplest form.

Division

Dividing fractions is slightly more complicated than multiplying. To divide fractions, you turn first turn the division into multiplication and then multiply as shown above. Here's an example:

Simplify the expression: $\dfrac{2}{8} \div \dfrac{3}{4}$.

When dividing fractions, you turn the divisor upside down and multiply it by the first fraction. The **divisor** is the fraction that the first fraction is being divided by:

$$\frac{2}{8} \div \left(\frac{3}{4}\right) \longleftarrow \text{Divisor}$$

In the following example, the divisor is $\dfrac{3}{4}$. Flip the divisor over, and multiply the fractions:

$$\frac{2}{8} \div \frac{3}{4} = \frac{2}{8} \times \frac{4}{3}$$

$$= \frac{2 \times 4}{8 \times 3}$$

$$= \frac{8}{24}$$

The correct answer is $\frac{8}{24}$. This can be further reduced to 1/3. The fraction 1/3 is the correct answer in its simplest form.

Fraction Summary

Here's a summary of the most important steps you need to know:

Addition Convert to fractions with the same denominator.

Add the numerators.

$$\frac{3}{4} + \frac{5}{6} = \frac{9}{12} + \frac{10}{12}$$

$$= \frac{19}{12} \text{ or } 1\frac{7}{12}$$

Subtraction Convert to fractions with the same denominator.

Subtract the numerators.

$$\frac{8}{12} - \frac{5}{8} = \frac{16}{24} - \frac{15}{24}$$

$$= \frac{1}{24}$$

Multiplication Multiply the numerators and denominators.

$$\frac{1}{6} \times \frac{3}{5} = \frac{1 \times 3}{6 \times 5}$$

$$= \frac{3}{30} \text{ or } \frac{1}{10}$$

Division Flip the divisor over.

Perform multiplication.

$$\frac{2}{8} \div \frac{3}{4} = \frac{2}{8} \times \frac{4}{3}$$

$$= \frac{2 \times 4}{8 \times 3}$$

$$= \frac{8}{24} \text{ or } \frac{1}{3}$$

Review Questions

1. $3\frac{1}{4} \times 2\frac{2}{3}$

   Simplify the expression above. Which of the following is correct?

   A. $8\frac{2}{3}$

   B. $6\frac{1}{4}$

   C. $6\frac{1}{6}$

   D. $5\frac{2}{7}$

2. $\frac{2}{3} \div \frac{5}{9}$

   Simplify the expression above. Which of the following is correct?

   A. $\frac{10}{27}$

   B. $\frac{7}{12}$

   C. $1\frac{1}{5}$

   D. $1\frac{2}{3}$

3. Which of the following lists the fractions in correct order, from least to greatest value?

   A. $\frac{2}{3}, \frac{3}{4}, \frac{7}{12}, \frac{1}{6}$

   B. $\frac{7}{12}, \frac{1}{6}, \frac{3}{4}, \frac{2}{3}$

   C. $\frac{1}{6}, \frac{7}{12}, \frac{2}{3}, \frac{3}{4}$

   D. $\frac{1}{6}, \frac{3}{4}, \frac{2}{3}, \frac{7}{12}$

4. $6\frac{1}{2} \times 3\frac{3}{8}$

Simplify the expression above. Which of the following is correct?

A. $18\frac{3}{16}$

B. $18\frac{3}{10}$

C. $20\frac{2}{5}$

D. $21\frac{15}{16}$

5. $\frac{6}{10} - \frac{1}{3}$

Simplify the expression above. Which of the following is correct?

A. $\frac{7}{30}$

B. $\frac{4}{15}$

C. $\frac{3}{10}$

D. $\frac{11}{12}$

6. $5\frac{1}{6} + 4\frac{7}{8}$

Simplify the expression above. Which of the following is correct?

A. $10\frac{1}{24}$

B. $10\frac{1}{48}$

C. $9\frac{1}{2}$

D. $9\frac{4}{7}$

7. $\dfrac{3}{8} - \dfrac{1}{4}$

Simplify the expression above. Which of the following is correct?

A. $\dfrac{3}{32}$

B. $\dfrac{1}{16}$

C. $\dfrac{1}{8}$

D. $\dfrac{1}{2}$

8. $\dfrac{6}{8} \div \dfrac{4}{10}$

Simplify the expression above. Which of the following is correct?

A. $1\dfrac{7}{8}$

B. $1\dfrac{15}{16}$

C. $2\dfrac{1}{4}$

D. $2\dfrac{3}{4}$

9. $5\dfrac{5}{6} \times 4\dfrac{2}{5}$

Simplify the expression above. Which of the following is correct?

A. $20\dfrac{1}{3}$

B. $20\dfrac{3}{10}$

C. $25\dfrac{1}{5}$

D. $25\dfrac{2}{3}$

10. $2\frac{1}{4} + 6\frac{5}{12}$

Simplify the expression above. Which of the following is correct?

A. $8\frac{3}{8}$

B. $8\frac{2}{3}$

C. $8\frac{11}{12}$

D. $8\frac{15}{16}$

11. Which of the following lists the fractions in correct order, from least to greatest value?

A. $2\frac{1}{3}, 4\frac{2}{3}, 4\frac{5}{6}, 6\frac{1}{6}$

B. $2\frac{1}{3}, 4\frac{5}{6}, 4\frac{2}{3}, 6\frac{1}{6}$

C. $2\frac{1}{3}, 4\frac{2}{3}, 6\frac{1}{6}, 4\frac{5}{6}$

D. $6\frac{1}{6}, 4\frac{2}{3}, 2\frac{1}{3}, 4\frac{5}{6}$

12. $5\frac{1}{3} - 4\frac{1}{6}$

Simplify the expression above. Which of the following is correct?

A. $\frac{7}{12}$

B. $1\frac{1}{6}$

C. $1\frac{1}{3}$

D. $1\frac{2}{3}$

13. $\dfrac{4}{9} + \dfrac{7}{10}$

Simplify the expression above. Which of the following is correct?

A. $1\dfrac{13}{90}$

B. $1\dfrac{4}{9}$

C. $1\dfrac{7}{10}$

D. $1\dfrac{13}{16}$

14. $\dfrac{6}{8} \div \dfrac{3}{12}$

Simplify the expression above. Which of the following is correct?

A. $\dfrac{7}{24}$

B. 2

C. 3

D. $3\dfrac{1}{2}$

15. $\dfrac{7}{15} - \dfrac{1}{5}$

Simplify the expression above. Which of the following is correct?

A. $\dfrac{1}{15}$

B. $\dfrac{1}{5}$

C. $\dfrac{4}{15}$

D. $\dfrac{6}{15}$

Answer Key

1. A

2. C

3. C

4. D

5. B

6. A

7. C
8. A
9. D
10. B
11. A

12. B
13. A
14. C
15. C

Answers and Explanations

1. (A) Convert the mixed numbers to improper fractions, and then multiply:

$$3\frac{1}{4} \times 2\frac{2}{3} = \frac{13}{4} \times \frac{8}{3}$$
$$= \frac{104}{12}$$
$$= 8\frac{8}{12}$$
$$= 8\frac{2}{3}$$

2. (C) Flip the divisor over and then multiply:

$$\frac{2}{3} \div \frac{5}{9} = \frac{2}{3} \times \frac{9}{5}$$
$$= \frac{18}{15}$$
$$= 1\frac{3}{15}$$
$$= 1\frac{1}{5}$$

3. (C) When the fractions are all converted to fractions over 12, they can be written as follows: $\frac{8}{12}, \frac{9}{12}, \frac{7}{12}, \frac{2}{12}$. The correct order from smallest to largest is therefore $\frac{1}{6}, \frac{7}{12}, \frac{2}{3}, \frac{3}{4}$.

4. (D) Convert the mixed numbers to improper fractions, and then multiply:

$$6\frac{1}{2} \times 3\frac{3}{8} = \frac{13}{2} \times \frac{27}{8}$$
$$= \frac{351}{16}$$
$$= 21\frac{15}{16}$$

5. (B) Find the least common denominator of the two fractions. In this case, the least common denominator is 30. Convert both fractions so that they have the same denominator, and then perform subtraction on the numerators:

$$\frac{6}{10} - \frac{1}{3} = \frac{18}{30} - \frac{10}{30}$$
$$= \frac{8}{30}$$
$$= \frac{4}{15}$$

6. (A) Convert the mixed numbers to improper fractions. Convert both fractions so that they have the same denominator, and then add the numerators:

$$5\frac{1}{6} + 4\frac{7}{8} = \frac{31}{6} + \frac{39}{8}$$
$$= \frac{124}{24} + \frac{117}{24}$$
$$= \frac{241}{24}$$
$$= 10\frac{1}{24}$$

7. (C) Find the least common denominator of the two fractions. In this case, the least common denominator is 8. Convert both fractions so that they have the same denominator, and then perform subtraction on the numerators:

$$\frac{3}{8} - \frac{1}{4} = \frac{3}{8} - \frac{2}{8}$$
$$= \frac{1}{8}$$

8. (A) Flip the divisor over and then multiply:

$$\frac{6}{8} \div \frac{4}{10} = \frac{6}{8} \times \frac{10}{4}$$

$$= \frac{60}{32}$$

$$= \frac{15}{8}$$

$$= 1\frac{7}{8}$$

9. (D) Convert the mixed numbers to improper fractions, and then multiply:

$$5\frac{5}{6} \times 4\frac{2}{5} = \frac{35}{6} \times \frac{22}{5}$$

$$= \frac{770}{30}$$

$$= 25\frac{20}{30}$$

$$= 25\frac{2}{3}$$

10. (B) Convert the mixed numbers to improper fractions. Convert both fractions so that they have the same denominator, and then add the numerators:

$$2\frac{1}{4} + 6\frac{5}{12} = \frac{9}{4} + \frac{77}{12}$$

$$= \frac{27}{12} + \frac{77}{12}$$

$$= \frac{104}{12}$$

$$= 8\frac{8}{12}$$

$$= 8\frac{2}{3}$$

11. (A) These mixed numbers begin with the whole numbers 2, 4, and 6. The fraction $\frac{2}{3}$ can be converted to $\frac{4}{6}$. The fraction $\frac{4}{6}$ is smaller than the fraction $\frac{5}{6}$, so the correct order of the fractions is $2\frac{1}{3}, 4\frac{2}{3}, 4\frac{5}{6}, 6\frac{1}{6}$.

12. (B) Convert the mixed numbers to improper fractions. Convert both fractions so that they have the same denominator, and then perform subtraction on the numerators:

$$5\frac{1}{3} - 4\frac{1}{6} = \frac{16}{3} - \frac{25}{6}$$

$$= \frac{32}{6} - \frac{25}{6}$$

$$= \frac{7}{6}$$

$$= 1\frac{1}{6}$$

13. (A) Find the least common denominator of the fractions. In this case, the least common denominator is 90. Convert both fractions so that they have the same denominator, and then add the numerators:

$$\frac{4}{9} + \frac{7}{10} = \frac{40}{90} + \frac{63}{90}$$

$$= \frac{103}{90}$$

$$= 1\frac{13}{90}$$

14. (C) Flip the divisor over and then multiply:

$$\frac{6}{8} \div \frac{3}{12} = \frac{6}{8} \times \frac{12}{3}$$

$$= \frac{72}{24}$$

$$= \frac{24}{8}$$

$$= 3$$

15. (C) Find the least common denominator of the two fractions. In this case, the least common denominator is 15. Convert both fractions so that they have the same denominator, and then perform subtraction on the numerators:

$$\frac{7}{15} - \frac{1}{5} = \frac{7}{15} - \frac{3}{15}$$

$$= \frac{4}{15}$$

CHAPTER 13

Decimals

Decimals questions on the TEAS test your ability to add, subtract, multiply, and divide decimals. You may also be asked to compare the values of decimal numbers.

Working with Decimals

A **decimal** is a number that expresses part of a whole. Decimals are similar to fractions, but instead of showing a numerator over a denominator, decimals show portions of a number using a decimal point.

Each number to the right or left of a decimal point has a certain place value. In the figure below, the numbers to the left of the decimal point are 3, 1, and 4. The number 3 is in the hundreds place, the number 1 is in the tens place, and the number 4 is in the ones place, as shown:

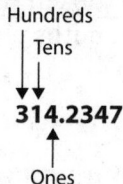

The numbers to the right of the decimal have specific place values as well. In the figure shown, the numbers to the right of the decimal are 2, 3, 4, and 7:

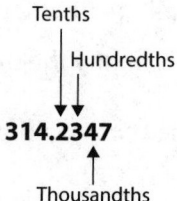

The number 2 is in the tenths place, the number 3 is in the hundredths place, the number 4 is in the thousandths place, and so on.

Comparing Decimals

To compare decimals, look at the numbers in the same place value.

Which of the following decimals is larger: 0.2 or 0.3?

In the example above, both of the decimals have numbers only in the tenths place. Since 3 is larger than 2, the decimal 0.3 is larger.

If decimal numbers contain more than one place value, look at the numbers in each place value to compare them. In the following example, both numbers have the number 2 in the tenths place:

Which of the following decimals is larger: 0.22 or 0.27?

When we look at the hundredths place, however, the numbers are different. In this case, 7 is larger than 2, so 0.27 is larger.

Here is one more example with longer decimals:

Which of the following decimals is larger: 0.22463 or 0.22419?

In this example, both of the numbers have 2 in the tenths place. Both also have 2 in the hundredths place and 4 in the thousandths place. In the ten thousandths place, however, the numbers are different. The first number has a 6 in the ten thousandths place, and the second number has a 1 in the ten thousandths place. The number 6 is greater than 1, so 0.22463 is larger.

Addition and Subtraction

To add and subtract decimals, perform addition and subtraction as you would with whole numbers. You must keep the decimal points of the two numbers lined up as you add.

Simplify the expression: 1.763 + 2.93.

Line the two numbers up by their decimals:

```
  1
  1 .7 6 3
+ 2 .9 3
  4 .6 9 3
```

Be sure to include the decimal in your answer. The correct answer is **4.693**.

When subtracting two decimals, keep the decimal points lined up as well. Here is an example:

Simplify the expression: 36.15 − 3.323.

To solve this problem, line up the decimal points as shown:

```
        5   11   4   10
    3   6̶   .1̶   5̶   0̶
  −     3   .3   2   3
    3   2   .8   2   7
```

In this case, we added a 0 to the right of the 5, so that we could subtract the 3 on the far right. Always be sure to add the decimal to your result. The correct answer is **32.827**.

Multiplication

To multiply decimals, perform multiplication as you would for whole numbers. Then count up the number of decimal places in the numbers being multiplied, and insert the decimal point correctly in your result.

Simplify the expression: 0.02×0.4.

In this case, multiply 2 times 4, which produces 8. Then, count the number of decimal places in the numbers being multiplied. The decimal 0.02 has two decimal places to the right of the decimal, 0 and 2. The number 0.4 has one decimal place to the right of the decimal, 4. Added together, there are 3 decimal places in these two numbers. So, the final answer must also have 3 decimal places. Starting with the number 8, count to the left 3 decimal places. Add zeros as you go:

0.008

This result has 3 decimal places. The correct answer is **0.008**.

Division

To divide with decimals, perform division as you normally would, paying attention to the placement of decimals. The procedure is slightly different depending on whether you are dividing by a whole number or a decimal number.

If you are dividing by a whole number, be sure to put the decimal point directly above the number being divided. Consider this example:

Simplify the expression: $16.236 \div 18$.

Set up the long division problem and divide by 18:

$$
\begin{array}{r}
.902 \\
18{\overline{\smash{\big)}\,16.236}} \\
-162 \\
\hline
3 \\
-0 \\
\hline
36 \\
-36 \\
\hline
0
\end{array}
$$

The correct answer is **0.902**.

If you are dividing by a decimal number, change the divisor to a whole number first by moving the decimal to the right. Also be sure to move the decimal the same number of places on the number being divided as well:

Simplify the expression: 270.48 ÷ 9.2.

To solve this problem, we must divide by a decimal number. Set up the long division problem:

$$9.2{\overline{\smash{\big)}\,270.48}}$$

Before going further, move the decimal points to the right one place. Do this for both numbers:

$$92{\overline{\smash{\big)}\,2{,}704.8}}$$

Now, divide as normal. Keep the decimal point in your answer directly above the decimal point in the number 2,704.8:

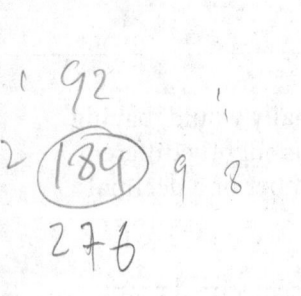

$$
\begin{array}{r}
29.4 \\
92{\overline{\smash{\big)}\,2704.8}} \\
184 \\
\hline
0864 \\
828 \\
\hline
368 \\
368
\end{array}
$$

$$
\begin{array}{r}
29.4 \\
92\overline{)\,2{,}704.8} \\
-184 \\
\hline
864 \\
-828 \\
\hline
368 \\
-368 \\
\hline
0
\end{array}
$$

The correct answer is **29.4**.

Review Questions

1. 0.11 × 0.07

Simplify the expression above. Which of the following is correct?

A. 0.00077
B. 0.0077
C. 0.077
D. 0.77

(handwritten):
0.11
×0.02
0 77
0 00
0 0 8

2. 227.65 + 320.4

Simplify the expression above. Which of the following is correct?

A. 230.85
B. 259.69
C. 547.69
D. 548.05

(handwritten): 227.65   1320.4

(handwritten circled): A. Straight

3. Which of the following lists the decimal numbers in correct order, from smallest to largest?

A. 0.0007, 0.007, 0.07, 0.7
X B. 0.007, 0.7, 0.07, 0.0007
X C. 0.7, 0.07, 0.007, 0.0007
D. 0.07, 0.0007, 0.007, 0.7

(handwritten): Start Attitude

4. 3.20 ÷ 0.40

Simplify the expression above. Which of the following is correct?

A. 0.08
B. 0.8
C. 8
D. 80

5. 12.92 − 7.6

Simplify the expression above. Which of the following is correct?

A. 5.32
B. 5.86
C. 6.32
D. 6.86

6. 41.1 × 0.06

Simplify the expression above. Which of the following is correct?

A. 0.2466
B. 2.466
C. 24.66
D. 246.6

7. Which of the following lists the decimal numbers in correct order, from largest to smallest?

A. 7.04, 6.97, 7.24, 7.54
B. 7.54, 7.24, 7.04, 6.97
C. 7.24, 7.54, 7.04, 6.97
D. 6.97, 7.04, 7.24, 7.54

8. 0.00393 + 0.0241

Simplify the expression above. Which of the following is correct?

A. 0.00634
B. 0.02803
C. 0.0634
D. 0.2803

9. 72 ÷ 0.12

Simplify the expression above. Which of the following is correct?

A. 0.06
B. 6
C. 600
D. 6,000

10. Which of the following lists the decimal numbers in correct order, from smallest to largest?

A. 0.0413, 0.0513, 0.0613, 0.0713
B. 0.0713, 0.0613, 0.0513, 0.0413
C. 0.0613, 0.0413, 0.0713, 0.0513
D. 0.0513, 0.0413, 0.0713, 0.0613

11. 0.045 − 0.0037

Simplify the expression above. Which of the following is correct?

A. 0.0008
B. 0.0413
C. 0.0467
D. 0.054

12. 5.327 + 0.0229

Simplify the expression above. Which of the following is correct?

A. 5.3499
B. 5.556
C. 5.762
D. 5.9476

13. 0.015 ÷ 0.3

Simplify the expression above. Which of the following is correct?

A. 0.00005
B. 0.0005
C. 0.005
D. 0.05

14. 0.0602 − 0.001

Simplify the expression above. Which of the following is correct?

A. 0.0502
B. 0.0592
C. 0.0601
D. 0.602

15. 0.25 × 0.075

Simplify the expression above. Which of the following is correct?

A. 0.001875
B. 0.01875
C. 0.1875
D. 1.875

Answer Key

1. B
2. D
3. A
4. C
5. A
6. B
7. B
8. B

9. C
10. A
11. B
12. A
13. D
14. B
15. B

Answers and Explanations

1. **(B)** First, multiply 11 times 7 without the decimals:

    $$11 \times 7 = 77$$

    Now, count the number of decimal places in the two numbers being multiplied. There are two decimal places in each number, for a total of four decimal places. The correct answer must also have four decimal places. Count back four decimal places from the right of 77, adding zeros if necessary, and insert a decimal. The correct answer is 0.0077.

2. **(D)** Add up the numbers, being sure to keep the decimal points aligned:

    ```
            1
        2 2 7 .6 5
      + 3 2 0 .4 0
        5 4 8 .0 5
    ```

    The correct answer is 548.05.

3. **(A)** In this set of numbers, the largest number is 0.7. It has a 7 in the tenths place, while the other numbers have zeros in the tenths place. The number 0.07 is the next largest number. It has a 7 in the hundredths place, while 0.007 and 0.0007 have zeros in the hundredths place.

    The number 0.007 is larger than 0.0007, so choice A is correct.

4. **(C)** Set up the long division problem:

    $$0.40\overline{)\,3.20}$$

    Move the decimal points two places to the right in both numbers:

    $$40\overline{)\,320}$$

    Perform long division:

    ```
              8
      40) 320
         −320
            0
    ```

    The correct answer is 8.

5. **(A)** Perform subtraction as you normally would, lining up the decimal points in the two numbers:

    ```
            12
       1  2 .9 2
     −    7 .6 0
        5   .3 2
    ```

    The correct answer is 5.32.

6. (B) First, multiply 411 times 6 without the decimals:

$411 \times 6 = 2{,}466$

Now, count the number of decimal places in the two numbers being multiplied. There is one decimal place in 41.1, and there are two decimal places in 0.06, which gives a total of three decimal places. The correct answer must also have three decimal places. Count back three decimal places from the right of 2,466 and insert a decimal. The correct answer is 2.466.

7. (B) In this set of numbers, the largest number is 7.54. It has a 7 in the tens place and a 5 in the tenths place. The other numbers with 7 in the tens place have smaller numbers in the tenths place. The number 7.24 is the next largest number. It has a 2 in the tenths place, while 7.04 has a 0 in the tenths place. The number 6.97 is the smallest of the four numbers, so B is correct.

8. (B) Add up the numbers 0.00393 and 0.0241, being sure to keep the decimal points aligned:

```
            1
  0  .0  0  3  9  3
+ 0  .0  2  4  1  0
  0  .0  2  8  0  3
```

The correct answer is 0.02803.

9. (C) First, set up the problem:

$0.12\overline{)72}$

Next, for both numbers, move the decimal points to the right two places. Add two zeros to the right of 72, to create 7,200:

$12\overline{)7{,}200}$

Now, divide as normal:

```
        600
12) 7,200
   −7,200
        0
```

The correct answer is 600.

10. (A) In this set of numbers, the only difference between the numbers is the number in the hundredths place. The numbers in the hundredths place are 4, 5, 6, and 7. So, the decimals should be placed in that order: 0.0413, 0.0513, 0.0613, and 0.0713. Choice A is correct.

11. (B) Set up the subtraction problem, lining up the two numbers based on their decimal points as shown:

```
                4  10
  0  .0  4  5̶  0̶
− 0  .0  0  3  7
  0  .0  4  1  3
```

The correct answer is 0.0413.

12. (A) Add up the numbers 5.327 and 0.0229. Be sure to line up the decimal points:

```
  5  .3  2  7  0
+ 0  .0  2  2  9
  5  .3  4  9  9
```

The correct answer is 5.3499.

13. (D) Set up the long division problem:

$0.3\overline{)0.015}$

Next, move the decimal points for both numbers one place to the right:

$0.3\overline{)0.015}$

Now, divide as normal. Keep the decimal point in your answer directly above the decimal point in the number being divided:

```
      .05
3) 00.15
   −15
     0
```

The correct answer is 0.05.

14. (B) Align the two numbers based on their decimal points and subtract:

```
              5  10
  0  .0  6̶  0̶  2
− 0  .0  0  1  0
  0  .0  5  9  2
```

The correct answer is 0.0592.

15. (B) Multiply 25 times 75 without the decimals:

$25 \times 75 = 1,875$

Next, count the number of decimal places in the two numbers being multiplied. There are two decimal places in 0.25 and three decimal places in 0.075, for a total of five decimal places. The correct answer must therefore also have five decimal places. Count back five decimal places from the right of 1,875, adding zeros if necessary, and insert a decimal. The correct answer is 0.01875.

CHAPTER 14

Percentages

Percentage questions on the TEAS test your ability to calculate percentages based on information given. You will also be asked to determine the percentage increase or decrease that is represented by a change in certain numbers. In addition, you may be asked to calculate original or final numbers when provided with information regarding a specific percentage change.

Calculating Percentages

A **percentage** is a portion of an amount. Any percentage can be expressed as a fraction over 100. Another way to write 20%, for instance, is $\frac{20}{100}$.

To take the percentage of a number, multiply that number by the percentage given. Let's look at an example:

What is 30% of 250?

To solve this problem, we must multiply 250 by 30%. To do this, first convert the percentage to a decimal number. Start with the percentage given, and move the decimal point to the left two places:

30% = 0.30

Now that we've converted the percentage to a decimal, we can multiply 250 by 0.30:

250 × 0.30 = 75.00

The correct answer is **75**.

Percentages can be numbers less than 1, and they can also be numbers greater than 100. The process for solving problems with these percentages is the same. Here's an example involving a percentage less than 1:

What is 0.10% of 170?

Notice the question did not ask for 10 percent of 170; instead, it asked for 0.10 percent. It is important to be clear about this, because the decimal point will make a big difference in your answer.

Solve this problem the same way as shown with the first example in this section. First, convert the percentage to a decimal number. Start with the percentage given, and move the decimal point two places to the left:

.10% = 0.0010

In this case, we added two zeros to the left of the 1 in order to move the decimal point two places to the left.

Next, multiply 170 by 0.0010:

$$170 \times 0.0010 = 0.1700$$

The correct answer is **0.17**.

In the following example, we'll see a problem involving a percentage that is greater than 100:

What is 400% of 12?

Although this time the percentage is a large one, we still solve the problem as we did with the first two examples in this section. First, convert the percentage to a decimal number. Start with the percentage given (400%), and move the decimal point two places to the left:

$$400\% = 4.00$$

Now, multiply 12 by 4:

$$12 \times 4 = 48$$

The correct answer is **48**.

Percentage Increase or Decrease

Another type of problem that is likely to appear on the TEAS involves the percent increase or decrease of a given quantity. Consider this example:

A sweater went on sale for 20% off its original price. The original price of the sweater was $40. What is the sale price?

To answer this question, first determine the amount of the discount. Then subtract the discount from the original price of the sweater.

The sweater originally cost $40 and went on sale for 20% off. Thus, the discount represents 20% of the original price. To calculate 20% of 40, we first convert 20% to a decimal number:

$$20\% = 0.20$$

Now, we can multiply $40 by 0.20 to determine the amount of the discount:

$$\$40 \times 0.20 = \$8.00$$

The amount of the discount is $8.00. Next, subtract $8.00 from the original price:

$$\$40.00 - \$8.00 = \$32.00$$

The sale price of the sweater is **$32.00**.

In the example above, you were given the percent decrease and asked to find the amount of the decrease. Sometimes, you may be asked to do the opposite. You may be given the amount of the decrease (or increase) and asked to find the percentage it represents:

A store increases its sales from $5,000 to $6,000 in one month. What is the percent increase in sales?

To find the percent increase, first find the amount of the increase in sales. Subtract the original sales ($5,000) from the final amount ($6,000):

$6,000 − $5,000 = $1,000

The amount of the increase in sales is $1,000. Next, to find the percent increase, divide the amount of the increase by the original amount:

$$\text{percent increase} = \frac{\text{amount of increase}}{\text{original amount}}$$

In this case, the amount of increase is $1,000, and the original amount is $5,000. Plug these values into the formula:

$$\text{percent increase} = \frac{\text{amount of increase}}{\text{original amount}}$$
$$= \frac{\$1,000}{\$5,000}$$
$$= 0.20 \text{ or } 20\%$$

The percent increase turns out to be 0.20, which can be converted to 20%. To convert a decimal to a percentage, we move the decimal point to the right two places:

$$0.20 = 20\%$$

The percent increase is **20%**.

Review Questions

1. 304.9% of 23 = _____

Which of the following completes the equation above?

A. 70.127
B. 701.27
C. 7,012.7
D. 70,127

2. A car went on sale for 80% of its original price. If the sales price of the car was $20,000, which of the following was the car's original price?

   A. $16,000
   B. $25,000
   C. $27,000
   D. $32,000

3. A bookstore inventory increases from 120,000 to 170,000 books over one year. Which of the following is the percent increase of the books? (Round the solution to the nearest tenth of a percent.)

   A. 29.4%
   B. 33.2%
   C. 41.4%
   D. 41.7%

4. The number of patients seen at a medical clinic decreased from 460 to 375 in the month of January. Which of the following is the percent decrease to the nearest tenth of a percent?

   A. 18.5%
   B. 22.7%
   C. 35.9%
   D. 81.5%

5. 23.5% of 906 = _____

Which of the following completes the equation above?

   A. 2.1291
   B. 21.291
   C. 212.91
   D. 2,129.1

6. A plumber increased his hourly rate by 10%, which added a total of $8.00 to his rate. Which of the following was the plumber's original rate?

   A. $64.00
   B. $80.00
   C. $100.00
   D. $116.00

7. 33.2% of 17.4 = _____

Which of the following completes the equation above?

   A. 0.0057768
   B. 0.057768
   C. 0.57768
   D. 5.7768

8. Which of the following represents 32% of 1,700?

   A. 5.44
   B. 54.4
   C. 544
   D. 5,440

9. The temperature in a greenhouse increases from 77 degrees to 85 degrees overnight. Which of the following is the percent increase of the temperature? (Round the solution to the nearest tenth of a percent.)

   A. 8.1%
   B. 10.4%
   C. 16.3%
   D. 21.2%

10. The number of residents at an animal shelter went down from 179 to 127 over a 6-month period. Which of the following is the percent decrease to the nearest tenth of a percent?

   A. 5.2%
   B. 13.6%
   C. 17.9%
   D. 29.1%

11. A school increased its student enrollment by 32% over a 2-year period. At the beginning of the period, a total of 7,000 students were enrolled. How many students were enrolled at the school at the end of the 2-year period?

   A. 9,240
   B. 10,060
   C. 10,350
   D. 11,480

12. 417.6% of 275 = _____

Which of the following completes the equation above?

   A. 11.484
   B. 114.84
   C. 1,148.4
   D. 11,484

13. A flock of birds increases in size from 60 birds to 200. Which of the following is the percent increase of the birds? (Round the solution to the nearest tenth of a percent.)

   A. 367.7%
   B. 233.3%
   C. 140%
   D. 70%

14. Which of the following represents 0.5% of 32?

   A. 160

   B. 16

   C. 1.6

   D. 0.16

15. A television show's audience decreased by 26% in one week. The original size of the audience was 12.5 million viewers. What was the number of viewers after one week? (Round the solution to the nearest tenth of a percent.)

   A. 3.3 million

   B. 7.6 million

   C. 9.3 million

   D. 10.4 million

Answer Key

1. A		**9.** B	
2. B		**10.** D	
3. D		**11.** A	
4. A		**12.** C	
5. C		**13.** B	
6. B		**14.** D	
7. D		**15.** C	
8. C			

Answers and Explanations

1. (A) Change the percentage to a decimal number by moving the decimal to the left two places: 304.9% = 3.049. Then multiply 23 × 3.049. The correct answer is 70.127.

2. (B) This question asks you to find the original price of the car. We know that 80% of this price is $20,000. We can use this information to find the original price. First, change the percentage to a decimal number by moving the decimal to the left two places: 80% = 0.80. Next, use the formula for calculating percentage: original price × 0.80 = $20,000. Divide $20,000 by 0.80 to find the original price. The correct answer is $25,000.

3. (D) To find the percent increase, first find the amount of the increase in books. Subtract the original number of books from the final amount: 170,000 − 120,000 = 50,000. The amount of the increase in books is 50,000. Next, to find the percent increase, divide the amount of the increase by the original number of books: 50,000 ÷ 120,000 = 0.4167. The percent increase is 0.4167, which can be converted to 41.67% and rounded up to 41.7%.

4. (A) First, find the amount of the decrease in patients seen. Subtract the final number of patients from the original number: 460 − 375 = 85. The number of patients seen decreased by 85. Now divide the amount of the decrease by the original number of patients: 85 ÷ 460 is approximately 0.1848. The percent decrease is about 0.1848, which can be converted to 18.48% and rounded up to 18.5%.

5. (C) Change the percentage to a decimal number by moving the decimal to the left two places: 23.5% = 0.235. Then multiply 906 × 0.235. The correct answer is 212.91.

6. (B) First, change the percentage to a decimal number by moving the decimal to the left two places: 10% = 0.10. Next, use the formula for calculating percentages: original rate × 0.10 = $8.00. Divide $8 by 0.10 to find the original rate. The correct answer is $80.00.

7. (D) Change the percentage to a decimal number by moving the decimal to the left two places: 33.2% = 0.332. Then multiply 17.4 × 0.332. The correct answer is 5.7768.

8. (C) Change the percentage to a decimal number by moving the decimal to the left two places: 32% = 0.32. Then multiply 1,700 × 0.32. The result is 544.

9. (B) To find the percent increase in temperature, first find the amount of the increase. Subtract the original temperature from the final temperature: 85 − 77 = 8. The temperature in the greenhouse increased by 8 degrees. Next, to find the percent increase, divide the amount of the increase by the original temperature: 8 ÷ 77 equals approximately 0.1039. The percent increase is about 0.1039, which can be converted to 10.39% and rounded up to 10.4%.

10. (D) First, find the amount of the decrease in residents at the shelter. Subtract the final number of animals from the original number: 179 − 127 = 52. The number of animals decreased by 52. Now divide the amount of the decrease by the original number of animals: 52 ÷ 179 is approximately 0.2905. The percent decrease is about 0.2905, which can be converted to 29.05% and rounded up to 29.1%.

11. (A) First, determine the amount of the increase. Then add the increased amount to the original number of enrolled students. At the beginning of the period, a total of 7,000 students were enrolled. In two years, the enrollment increased by 32%. To calculate 32% of 7,000, first convert 32% to a decimal number: 32% = 0.32. Then multiply 7,000 by 0.32 to determine the amount of the increase: 7,000 × 0.32 = 2,240. The enrollment increased by 2,240 students. Next, add 2,240 to the original number of enrolled students: 7,000 + 2,240 = 9,240. At the end of the 2-year period, the number of enrolled students was 9,240.

12. (C) Change the percentage to a decimal number by moving the decimal to the left two places: 417.6% = 4.176. Then multiply 275 × 4.176. The correct answer is 1,148.4.

13. (B) First, find the amount of the increase. Subtract the original number of birds from the final number: 200 − 60 = 140. The flock increased by 140 birds. Now divide the amount of the increase by the original number of birds: 140 ÷ 60 equals approximately 2.3334. The percent increase is about 2.3334, which can be converted to 233.34% and rounded down to 233.3%.

14. (D) The question is asking for 0.5% of 32, not 5%. Starting with the percentage of 0.5, move the decimal to the left two places: 0.5% = 0.005. In this case, you must add two zeros before the 5 to move the decimal point two places to the left. Now multiply 32 × 0.005. The result is 0.16.

15. (C) First, determine the amount of the decrease. Then subtract the decreased amount from the original number of viewers. The original size of the audience was 12.5 million viewers. In one week, the audience decreased by 26%. To calculate 26% of 12.5 million, first convert 26% to a decimal number: 26% = 0.26. Then multiply 12.5 million by 0.26 to determine the amount of the decrease: 12.5 million × 0.26 = 3.25 million. The audience decreased by 3.25 million viewers. Next, subtract 3.25 million from the original size of the audience: 12.5 million − 3.25 million = 9.25 million. After one week, the number of viewers was about 9.3 million.

CHAPTER 15

Converting Fractions, Decimals, and Percentages

Conversion questions on the TEAS test ask you to recognize equivalent values in different forms. You may be asked to convert between decimals and percentages, fractions and decimals, fractions and percentages, and vice versa.

Decimals and Percentages

In the preceding chapter, we have seen how to convert between decimals and percentages and vice versa. To convert a percentage to a decimal, move the decimal point to the left two places.

41.7% = 0.417

To convert a decimal to a percentage, move the decimal point to the right two places.

0.0635 = 6.35%

Fractions and Decimals

To convert a fraction to a decimal, divide the numerator of the fraction by the denominator:

$$\frac{5}{20} = 0.25$$

To convert a decimal to a fraction, remove the decimal point and use the remaining number as the numerator of the fraction. Here is an example:

What fraction is equivalent to 0.36?

Start by removing the decimal point and placing the number 36 in the numerator of the fraction:

$$0.36 = \frac{36}{\text{denominator}}$$

Use the following method to determine the denominator. Start with the number 1 and add a zero for every decimal place in the original number. In this case, 0.36 has two decimal places, so we start with 1 and add two zeros:

$$0.36 = \frac{36}{100}$$

Next, simplify the fraction. The fraction $\frac{36}{100}$ reduces to $\frac{9}{25}$.

Fractions and Percentages

To convert a fraction to a percentage, first convert the fraction to a decimal number. Then move the decimal to the left two places:

What percentage is equivalent to $\frac{2}{5}$?

Divide the numerator of the fraction by the denominator:

$$\frac{2}{5} = 0.40$$

Then, move the decimal two places to the right:

0.40 = 40%

The correct answer is **40%**.

To convert a percentage to a fraction, first convert the percentage to a decimal number. Then convert the decimal number to a fraction:

What fraction is equivalent to 80%?

Move the decimal to the left two places:

80% = 0.80

Then follow the steps to convert a decimal to a fraction. Place the number in the numerator of the fraction, without the decimal:

$$0.80 = \frac{80}{\text{denominator}}$$

For the denominator, start with the number 1. Then add a zero for every decimal place in the original number. The decimal 0.80 has two decimal places, so we add two zeros:

$$0.80 = \frac{80}{100}$$

This fraction simplifies to $\frac{8}{10}$, which further reduces to $\frac{4}{5}$. The correct answer is $\frac{4}{5}$.

Review Questions

1. $-7, -\dfrac{17}{3}, -7.2, -\dfrac{43}{6}$

Arrange the numbers above from least to greatest. Which of the following is correct?

A. $-7, -\dfrac{43}{6}, -7.2, -\dfrac{17}{3}$

B. $-7.2, -7, -\dfrac{43}{6}, -\dfrac{17}{3}$

C. $-7.2, -\dfrac{43}{6}, -7, -\dfrac{17}{3}$

D. $-\dfrac{43}{6}, -7, -\dfrac{17}{3}, -7.2$

2. Which of the following is equivalent to 60%?

A. $\dfrac{3}{5}$

B. $\dfrac{2}{3}$

C. $\dfrac{5}{6}$

D. $\dfrac{7}{8}$

3. Which of the following percentages is equivalent to 0.017?

A. 0.17%
B. 1.7%
C. 17%
D. 170%

4. Which of the following is the decimal equivalent of $\dfrac{3}{8}$?

A. 0.375
B. 2.667
C. 5
D. 11

5. Sarah scored 83 out of a possible 90 points on a test. Which of the following is the decimal equivalent of Sarah's score? (Round the solution to the nearest thousandth of a percent.)

A. 173
B. 7
C. 1.084
D. 0.922

6. Order the following list of numbers from least to greatest.

   $5, \dfrac{9}{2}, -1, 4.1$

   A. $-1, \dfrac{9}{2}, 4.1, 5$

   B. $5, \dfrac{9}{2}, 4.1, -1$

   C. $-1, 4.1, 5, \dfrac{9}{2}$

   D. $-1, 4.1, \dfrac{9}{2}, 5$

7. Rashid tossed a coin 12 times, and 9 times the result was heads. Which of the following is the decimal equivalent of the fraction of tosses that were heads?

   A. 0.60
   B. 0.75
   C. 1.333
   D. 3

8. Which of the following is the decimal equivalent of 834%?

   A. 0.0834
   B. 0.834
   C. 8.34
   D. 83.4

9. Which of the following percentages is equivalent to 7.237?

   A. 0.07237%
   B. 0.7237%
   C. 72.37%
   D. 723.7%

10. Which of the following is the decimal equivalent of 0.29%?

    A. 0.0029
    B. 0.29
    C. 2.9
    D. 29.0

Answer Key

1. C
2. A
3. B
4. A
5. D

6. D
7. B
8. C
9. D
10. A

Answers and Explanations

1. (C) Convert the fractions to decimals. The fraction $-\frac{17}{3}$ is equivalent to $-17 \div 3$, or approximately -5.667. The fraction $-\frac{43}{6}$ is equivalent to $-43 \div 6$, or approximately -7.167. The correct answer is $-7.2, -\frac{43}{6}, -7, -\frac{17}{3}$.

2. (A) To convert a percentage to a fraction, first convert the percentage to a decimal number. Move the decimal to the left two places: $60\% = 0.60$. Next, convert the decimal number to a fraction. Place the number in the numerator of the fraction, without the decimal:

$$0.60 = \frac{60}{\text{denominator}}$$

   For the denominator, start with the number 1 and add a zero for every decimal place in the original number:

$$0.60 = \frac{60}{100}$$

   The fraction $\frac{60}{100}$ reduces to $\frac{3}{5}$.

3. (B) To convert a decimal to a percentage, move the decimal point to the right two places: $0.017 = 1.7\%$.

4. (A) To convert a fraction to a decimal number, divide the numerator of the fraction by the denominator: $\frac{3}{8} = 0.375$.

5. (D) First, write Sarah's score as a fraction: 83 points out of 90 can be written as $\frac{83}{90}$. Now divide the numerator of the fraction by the denominator: $83 \div 90$ equals approximately 0.922.

6. (D) Convert the fraction to a decimal number. The fraction $\frac{9}{2}$ is equivalent to 4.5. The numbers, in order from least to greatest, are $-1, 4.1, \frac{9}{2}$, and 5.

7. (B) Write the number of heads as a fraction of all the coin tosses: 9 heads out of 12 throws can be written as $\frac{9}{12}$. This fraction reduces to $\frac{3}{4}$. Now divide the numerator of the reduced fraction by the denominator: $3 \div 4 = 0.75$.

8. (C) To convert a percentage to a decimal, move the decimal point to the left two places: $834\% = 8.34$.

9. (D) To convert a decimal to a percentage, move the decimal point to the right two places: $7.237 = 723.7\%$.

10. (A) To convert a percentage to a decimal, move the decimal point to the left two places: $0.29\% = 0.0029$.

CHAPTER 16

Ratios and Proportions

Ratios and proportions questions test your ability to identify ratios and to use proportions to solve problems regarding ratios.

Ratios are a means of comparing numbers. They express the relationship of one number to another. Let's look at an example:

> Adrian received 4 toys and 6 pieces of clothing for his birthday. What is the ratio of toys to pieces of clothing that Adrian received?

The ratio of toys to clothing can be expressed as 4 to 6. It can also be written as 4:6, using a colon, or as $\frac{4}{6}$ in fractional form.

To solve problems regarding ratios, we use proportions. **Proportions** are equations in which two ratios are set equal to each other.

> Brianna buys 4 pizzas for a total cost of $25.00. How much does it cost her to buy 6 more pizzas if she buys them at the same price per pizza?

To solve this problem, we set up a proportion. Create two ratios and set them equal to each other:

$$\frac{4 \text{ pizzas}}{\$25} = \frac{6 \text{ pizzas}}{c}$$

We are looking for the cost, c, of the 6 pizzas. Cross multiply $4 \times c$ and $\$25 \times 6$. Set the values equal to one another:

$$\frac{4 \text{ pizzas}}{\$25} = \frac{6 \text{ pizzas}}{c}$$
$$4 \times c = \$25 \times 6$$
$$4c = \$25 \times 6$$

Now solve for c:

$$4c = \$25 \times 6$$
$$4c = \$150$$
$$c = \frac{\$150}{4}$$
$$c = \$37.50$$

It will cost $37.50 to buy 6 pizzas at the same rate. We will discuss more about solving equations in Chapter 20, Algebra.

Review Questions

1. A sleepaway camp had 120 campers last year divided evenly into 8 squads. This year, the number of campers will rise to 165. If each squad has the same number of students as last year, how many squads will the camp have this year?

   A. 8
   B. 10
   C. 11
   D. 15

2. Merrill reads 360 pages in 180 minutes. How many pages can she read in 30 minutes if she reads at the same rate of speed?

   A. 45
   B. 60
   C. 90
   D. 120

3. A model of a skyscraper is built according to a 1:2,000 scale. If the model skyscraper measures 30 centimeters in height, which of the following is the actual height of the skyscraper?

   A. 6,000 centimeters
   B. 15,000 centimeters
   C. 60,000 centimeters
   D. 66,667 centimeters

4. The Doll Collector's Store has an inventory of 420 dolls. A total of 70 dolls are made of porcelain, and the remainder are made of plastic. Which of the following is the ratio of the plastic dolls to the total number of dolls in the store's inventory?

   A. $\dfrac{1}{6}$

   B. $\dfrac{3}{8}$

   C. $\dfrac{5}{6}$

   D. $\dfrac{7}{8}$

5. The scale on a trail map indicates that 1 centimeter on the map represents 10 miles. Lilah walks a distance of 12 miles on the trail. Which of the following represents the measure of that distance on the map?

   A. 0.6 centimeters
   B. 1.2 centimeters
   C. 6.4 centimeters
   D. 12 centimeters

6. Geraldo has 180 marbles. Of these, 120 are solid colors, and the rest are multicolored. Which of the following is the ratio of the multicolored marbles to the total number of marbles in Geraldo's collection?

A. $\dfrac{1}{3}$

B. $\dfrac{1}{2}$

C. $\dfrac{2}{3}$

D. $\dfrac{4}{5}$

7. The families on a neighborhood block have 14 dogs and 20 cats altogether. What is the ratio of dogs to cats on the block?

A. $\dfrac{7}{17}$

B. $\dfrac{10}{17}$

C. $\dfrac{7}{10}$

D. $\dfrac{10}{7}$

8. A replica of a radio tower is built based on a 1:300 scale. If the replica measures 9 inches in diameter across its base, which of the following is the diameter of the base of the radio tower?

A. 1,200 inches
B. 1,500 inches
C. 1,800 inches
D. 2,700 inches

9. An interior designer brings 16 textured fabric samples and 18 smooth fabric samples to a job site. What is the ratio of textured to smooth fabric samples that she brings?

A. $\dfrac{8}{9}$

B. $\dfrac{15}{16}$

C. $\dfrac{17}{18}$

D. $\dfrac{5}{4}$

10. A map contains a scale showing that every 1 inch on the map represents 12 kilometers. A cyclist wishes to travel a distance measuring 4 inches on the map. Which of the following represents the distance the cyclist will travel in kilometers?

    A. 3.0
    B. 4.8
    C. 30
    D. 48

Answer Key

1. C

2. B

3. C

4. C

5. B

6. A

7. C

8. D

9. A

10. D

Answers and Explanations

1. (C) Create a proportion using two ratios. The first ratio is the number of campers to squads last year: $\dfrac{120 \text{ campers}}{8 \text{ squads}}$. The second ratio is the number of campers to squads this year: $\dfrac{165 \text{ campers}}{? \text{ squads}}$. Set the ratios equal to each other:

$$\frac{120 \text{ campers}}{8 \text{ squads}} = \frac{165 \text{ campers}}{? \text{ squads}}$$

Use the letter s to represent the missing number of squads:

$$\frac{120 \text{ campers}}{8 \text{ squads}} = \frac{165 \text{ campers}}{s}$$

Cross multiply to solve for s, the missing number of squads:

$$\frac{120}{8} = \frac{165}{s}$$
$$120s = 165 \times 8$$
$$120s = 1,320$$
$$s = \frac{1,320}{120}$$
$$s = 11$$

This year, the camp will have 11 squads.

2. (B) Create a proportion using two ratios. The first ratio is the number of pages read in 180 minutes: $\dfrac{360 \text{ pages}}{180 \text{ minutes}}$. The second ratio is the number of pages read in 30 minutes: $\dfrac{? \text{ pages}}{30 \text{ minutes}}$. Set the ratios equal to each other:

$$\frac{360 \text{ pages}}{180 \text{ minutes}} = \frac{? \text{ pages}}{30 \text{ minutes}}$$

Use the letter p to represent the missing number of pages:

$$\frac{360 \text{ pages}}{180 \text{ minutes}} = \frac{p}{30 \text{ minutes}}$$

Cross multiply to solve for p:

$$\frac{360}{180} = \frac{p}{30}$$
$$180p = 360 \times 30$$
$$180p = 10,800$$
$$p = \frac{10,800}{180}$$
$$p = 60$$

Merrill can read 60 pages in 30 minutes.

3. (C) Create a proportion, setting the two ratios equal to each other:

$$\frac{1}{2,000} = \frac{30 \text{ centimeters}}{\text{actual height}}$$

Cross multiply to solve for h, the actual height:

$$\frac{1}{2,000} = \frac{30 \text{ centimeters}}{h}$$
$$1h = 2,000 \times 30$$
$$h = 60,000$$

The actual height of the skyscraper is 60,000 centimeters.

4. (C) The store has 420 dolls total. The number of porcelain dolls is 70. Subtract 70 from the total to find the number of plastic dolls: $420 - 70 = 350$. The ratio of plastic dolls to the total dolls is $\frac{350}{420}$, which reduces to $\frac{5}{6}$.

5. (B) Create a proportion, setting the two ratios equal to each other:

$$\frac{1 \text{ centimeter}}{10 \text{ miles}} = \frac{? \text{ centimeters}}{12 \text{ miles}}$$

Cross multiply to solve for c, the missing number of centimeters:

$$\frac{1}{10} = \frac{c}{12}$$
$$10c = 1 \times 12$$
$$10c = 12$$
$$c = \frac{12}{10}$$
$$c = 1.2$$

The measure of the distance on the map is 1.2 centimeters.

6. (A) Geraldo has 180 marbles total. The number of solid colored marbles is 120. Subtract 120 from the total to find the number of multicolored marbles: $180 - 120 = 60$. The ratio of multicolored marbles to the total number of marbles is $\frac{60}{180}$, which reduces to $\frac{1}{3}$.

7. (C) The ratio of dogs to cats on the block is $\frac{14}{20}$, which reduces to $\frac{7}{10}$.

8. (D) Create a proportion, setting the two ratios equal to each other:

$$\frac{1}{300} = \frac{9}{\text{diameter}}$$

Cross multiply to solve for d, the missing length of the diameter:

$$\frac{1}{300} = \frac{9}{d}$$
$$1d = 9 \times 300$$
$$d = 2,700$$

The measure of the diameter of the base is 2,700 inches.

9. (A) The ratio of textured fabrics to smooth fabrics is $\frac{16}{18}$, which reduces to $\frac{8}{9}$.

10. (D) Create a proportion, setting the two ratios equal to each other:

$$\frac{1 \text{ inch}}{12 \text{ kilometers}} = \frac{4 \text{ inches}}{? \text{ kilometers}}$$

Cross multiply to solve for k, the missing number of kilometers:

$$\frac{1}{12} = \frac{4}{k}$$
$$1k = 12 \times 4$$
$$k = 48$$

The cyclist will travel 48 kilometers.

CHAPTER 17

Word Problems

Word problems questions test your knowledge of how to solve math problems expressed mainly in words rather than numbers. Though some numbers are usually given in word problems, your main task is to translate words into numbers so you can find the solution. In previous sections in this part, we have already seen word problems related to percentages, ratios, and proportions. Other types of word problems that may appear on TEAS Math involve calculating the total cost of a set of items, calculating the final balance in a checking account, and determining the amount of an individual's take-home pay.

Calculating Total Cost

Certain word problems ask you to calculate the total cost of a purchase. These problems can be solved using addition alone. The purchase will involve a set of items, and the costs for each item must be added together. Consider this example:

> A decorator is purchasing furniture for a client's home. She buys a sofa for $688.00, a coffee table for $175.00, and two accent chairs for $204.00 each. What is the total cost of the items purchased?

> Add together the cost of all items purchased by the decorator:

> $688.00 + $175.00 + $204.00 + $204.00 = $1,271.00

The correct answer is **$1,271.00**. Be sure to add the cost of each chair ($204.00) twice, since two chairs were purchased. If you had missed the second chair and only added in $204.00 for one chair, your answer would have been $1,067.00, which is incorrect.

Calculating Account Balances

Other word problems ask you to determine the final balance of a checking account, based on adding and subtracting certain transactions. To solve these problems, start with the previous balance in the account. Then add in the amount of the deposits and any interest earned, and subtract the amount of the checks and any fees incurred.

Reconcile this checking account for the month of January 2015. The previous balance was $2,735.16. Deposits were made for $1,499.05. Checks were written for $1,336.60. There is a returned check charge of $38.00. What is the balance after reconciling this account?

In the above example, the starting balance in the account is $2,735.16. Add in the total amount of the deposits:

$$\$2,735.16 + \$1,499.05 = \$4,234.21$$

Next, subtract the total checks written:

$$\$4,234.21 - \$1,336.60 = \$2,897.61$$

Finally, subtract the returned check charge of $38.00:

$$\$2,897.61 - \$38.00 = \$2,859.61$$

The final balance in the account is **$2,859.61**.

Determining Take-Home Pay

A third type of word problem asks you to calculate the take-home pay received after certain amounts are deducted from a paycheck. These problems are solved using subtraction alone. Starting with the total amount received in the pay period, subtract each deduction given. The remainder is the take-home pay.

A hairstylist receives $1,017.00 each pay period. The deductions per pay period are federal tax $101.70, federal insurance $77.80, state tax $47.29, retirement plan $50.00, and health insurance $63.34. What is the take-home pay per pay period?

The hairstylist received $1,017.00 this pay period. Subtract the five deductions given from this amount:

$$\$1,017.00 - \$101.70 - \$77.80 - \$47.29 - \$50.00 - \$63.34 = \$676.87$$

The hairstylist's take-home pay is **$676.87**.

Review Questions

1. A warehouse worker receives $1,504.26 each pay period. The deductions per pay period are federal tax $150.42, federal insurance $115.08, state tax $69.20, retirement plan $40.00, and health insurance $175.67. Which of the following is the take-home pay per pay period?

   A. $497.62
   B. $738.16
   C. $953.89
   D. $1,007.59

2. A hardware store is having a tool sale. Customers who buy one tool at full price can purchase a second tool, of equal or lesser value, for half off the original price. A builder wants to purchase a drill for $84.98 and a jigsaw for $69.98. Which of the following is the cost of both tools?

   A. $119.97
   B. $122.47
   C. $131.24
   D. $149.96

3. Reconcile this checking account for the month of February 2015. The previous balance is $3,765.17. Deposits were made for $2,972.46. Checks were written for $2,760.95. Interest earned is $0.03, and there is a service charge of $6.95. Which of the following is the balance after reconciling this account?

   A. $2,910.20
   B. $3,546.74
   C. $3,969.76
   D. $4,516.39

4. A homeowner plans to purchase a hot tub for $5,765.00 installed. The hot tub will require an electrical upgrade costing $2,316.00. Which of the following will be the total cost of installing the hot tub if the homeowner makes the electrical upgrade?

   A. $3,449.00
   B. $6,945.00
   C. $7,081.00
   D. $8,081.00

5. A doctor has lunch in the hospital cafeteria. She orders the daily special of spaghetti with meatballs for $8.95. She then adds a side of steamed vegetables for $3.65, a bottle of water for $1.79, and an apple for $0.50. Which of the following is the cost of this lunch?

   A. $12.29
   B. $13.69
   C. $14.39
   D. $14.89

6. A dog groomer works at a pet store and earns $1,076.35 per pay period. The groomer's deductions each pay period are federal tax $107.64, federal insurance $82.34, state tax $50.01, retirement plan $60.00, and health insurance $90.77. Which of the following is the dog groomer's take-home pay per pay period?

   A. $533.77
   B. $685.59
   C. $929.82
   D. $969.37

7. Reconcile this checking account for the month of May 2015. The previous balance was $842.50. Deposits were made for $3,257.97. Checks were written for $2,463.02. There is a check printing charge of $32.00. Which of the following is the balance after reconciling this account?

    A. $762.95
    B. $1,294.04
    C. $1,605.45
    D. $1,637.45

8. A couple is having 6 bridesmaids and 6 groomsmen in their wedding party. Each bridesmaid will receive a silver-plated mirror and a perfume atomizer. Each groomsman will receive a barbecue utensil set and a pocket watch. The cost of each gift is $30.00 for the mirrors, $28.75 for the atomizers, $25.50 for the utensil sets, and $32.00 for the pocket watches. Which of the following will be the cost of gifts for the bridesmaids and groomsmen?

    A. $348.75
    B. $568.95
    C. $601.25
    D. $697.50

9. Reconcile this checking account for the month of March 2015. The previous balance was $96.55. Deposits were made for $782.47. Checks were written for $87.67. There is a returned check charge of $35.00. Which of the following is the balance after reconciling this account?

    A. $563.25
    B. $756.35
    C. $826.35
    D. $827.62

10. A fund-raising gala is planned for supporters of a healthcare foundation. Dinner costs are $50.00 for each sponsor and $62.50 for each benefactor. The foundation has sold 72 sponsor dinner tickets and 120 benefactor dinner tickets. Which of the following is the total cost of the dinner?

    A. $11,100
    B. $11,560
    C. $12,400
    D. $12,750

Answer Key

1. C		**6.**	B
2. A		**7.**	C
3. C		**8.**	D
4. D		**9.**	B
5. D		**10.**	A

Answers and Explanations

1. (C) The worker received $1,504.26 this pay period. Subtract the five deductions given from this amount:

$1,504.26 − $150.42 − $115.08 − $69.20 − $40.00 − $175.67 = $953.89

The worker's take-home pay is $953.89.

2. (A) The jigsaw is the tool of lesser value. So, it will sell for half of $69.98, or $34.99. Add together the cost of the drill and the jigsaw: $84.98 + $34.99 = $119.97. The cost of both tools is $119.97.

3. (C) The starting balance in the account is $3,765.17. Add in the total amount of the deposits:

$3,765.17 + $2,972.46 = $6,737.63

Next, subtract the total checks written:

$6,737.63 − $2,760.95 = $3,976.68

Now add the interest:

$3,976.68 + $0.03 = $3,976.71

Finally, subtract the service charge of $6.95:

$3,976.71 − $6.95 = $3,969.76

The final balance in the account is $3,969.76.

4. (D) Add together the cost of installing the hot tub and the electrical upgrade: $5,765.00 + $2,316.00 = $8,081.00. If the homeowner makes the electrical upgrade, the total cost of installing the hot tub will be $8,081.00.

5. (D) Add together the cost of the items the doctor purchased: $8.95 + $3.65 + $1.79 + $0.50 = $14.89. The total cost of the lunch is $14.89.

6. (B) The dog groomer received $1,076.35 this pay period. Subtract the five deductions given from this amount:

$1,076.35 − $107.64 − $82.34 − $50.01 − $60.00 − $90.77 = $685.59

The dog groomer's take-home pay is $685.59.

7. (C) The starting balance in the account is $842.50. Add in the total amount of the deposits:

$842.50 + $3,257.97 = $4,100.47

Next, subtract the total checks written:

$4,100.47 − $2,463.02 = $1,637.45

The, subtract the check printing charge of $32.00:

$1,637.45 − $32.00 = $1,605.45

The final balance in the account is $1,605.45.

8. (D) Add together the total costs of all of the gifts purchased. Each bridesmaid will receive a mirror costing $30.00 and an atomizer costing $28.75. The cost of each bridesmaid's gifts is $58.75. There are 6 bridesmaids, so the cost of all 6 bridesmaids' gifts is $58.75 × 6, or $352.50. Each groomsman will receive a utensil set costing $25.50 and a pocket watch costing $32.00. The cost of each groomsman's gifts is $57.50. There are 6 groomsmen, so the cost of all 6 groomsmen's gifts is $57.50 × 6, or $345.00. Added together, the total cost of gifts for the bridesmaids and groomsmen is $352.50 + $345.00, or $697.50.

9. **(B)** The starting balance in the account is $96.55. Add in the total amount of the deposits:

$96.55 + $782.47 = $879.02

Next, subtract the total checks written:

$879.02 − $87.67 = $791.35

Then, subtract the returned check charge of $35.00:

$791.35 − $35.00 = $756.35

The final balance in the account is $756.35.

10. **(A)** Add together the costs of the sponsor dinners and the benefactor dinners. Each sponsor dinner will cost $50.00, and there are 72 sponsor dinners. So, the cost of the sponsor dinners will be $50.00 × 72, or $3,600.00. Each benefactor dinner will cost $62.50, and there are 120 benefactor dinners. The cost of the benefactor dinners will be $62.50 × 120, which equals $7,500.00. The total cost of all of the dinners is $3,600 + $7,500, or $11,100.

CHAPTER 18

Measurements and Conversions

Measurements and Conversions questions ask you to make conversions between units of measurement in the metric system or the English system. You may also be asked to convert measurements from units in one system to units in the other. Some questions ask about the appropriate tool to be used to measure a particular quantity as well.

English System Conversions

The **English system** of measurement uses the following units to measure weight, volume, and length. Weight is measured in ounces, pounds, and tons. Volume is measured in ounces, cups, pints, quarts, and gallons. Length is measured in inches, feet, yards, and miles.

To convert between units in the English system, you must know the equivalent measures for each step in the measurement system. A table of equivalents is given below:

Measurement Type	Equivalents	
Weight	16 ounces	= 1 pound
	2,000 pounds	= 1 ton
Volume	8 ounces	= 1 cup
	2 cups	= 1 pint
	2 pints	= 1 quart
	4 quarts	= 1 gallon
Length	12 inches	= 1 foot
	3 feet	= 1 yard
	5,280 feet	= 1 mile

Metric System Conversions

The **metric system** also measures weight, volume, and length, but it uses a different set of units for measurement. The basic unit of weight measurement is the gram. The basic unit of volume measurement is the liter, and the basic unit of length measurement is the meter.

In the metric system, each unit of measurement starts with a prefix that indicates whether the measurement is smaller than the basic unit or larger than it.

Prefix	Measurement Compared to Basic Unit	Weight	Volume	Length
kilo-	1,000 times	kilogram (kg)	kiloliter (kL)	kilometer (km)
hecto-	100 times	hectogram (hg)	hectoliter (hL)	hectometer (hm)
deka-	10 times	dekagram (dag)	dekaliter (daL)	dekameter (dam)
Basic unit	Basic unit	gram (g)	liter (L)	meter (m)
deci-	1/10	decigram (dg)	deciliter (dL)	decimeter (dm)
centi-	1/100	centigram (cg)	centiliter (cL)	centimeter (cm)
milli-	1/1,000	milligram (mg)	milliliter (mL)	millimeter (mm)

As the table shows, each unit of measurement in the different levels of the metric system is 10 times smaller than the unit above it and 10 times larger than the unit below it. One centimeter is equal to 10 millimeters, one gram is equal to 10 decigrams, and so on.

Conversions Between Systems

To convert between measurements in the English and metric systems, you need to know the approximate equivalents between units. Some of the common equivalents are as follows:

English Measurement	Metric Equivalent
1 kilogram	Approx. 2.2 pounds
1 liter	Approx. 1 quart
2.5 centimeters	Approx. 1 inch
1 meter	Approx. 1 yard

Measurement Tools

Measurement tools tested on the TEAS can be divided into three categories, based on whether they measure weight, volume, or length. For measuring weight, **scales** are traditionally used and may have varying degrees of accuracy. For measuring volume, **pipettes** are measuring tubes or droppers used to measure small amounts of liquid with high precision, whereas measuring cups, flasks, and beakers provide less precise measurements for larger amounts of liquid. **Graduated cylinders** vary in size and are typically less precise than pipettes but more precise than measuring cups, flasks, and beakers.

For measuring length, **calipers** are the most precise measuring tool and take measurements using two points. **Rulers** are the next most precise tool, followed by **yardsticks** and **metersticks**. For measuring longer distances, **tape measures** may be used in varying sizes. **Odometers** measure the distances traveled by a vehicle and would be appropriate for measurements taken in miles or kilometers.

Review Questions

1. A powdered chemical must be measured to the nearest $\frac{1}{4}$ of a pound. Which of the following is the most appropriate measurement tool for this task?

   A. Graduated cylinder
   B. Beaker
   C. Yardstick
   D. Scale

2. Which of the following is the number of pints in 3 gallons?

   A. 8
   B. 12
   C. 16
   D. 24

3. Which of the following is an approximate metric quantity for the volume of a glass of water?

   A. 10 mL
   B. 0.1 cL
   C. 0.5 L
   D. 1 kL

4. If a piece of wood measures 25.4 centimeters in length, which of the following is the wood's approximate length in English measurement? (Note: 1 inch ≈ 2.54 centimeters)

   A. 10 inches
   B. 35.4 inches
   C. 64.52 inches
   D. 100 inches

5. Which of the following metric units of measurement is most reasonable to measure the weight of a full tube of a cream medication?

   A. Milligram (mg)
   B. Gram (g)
   C. Hectogram (hg)
   D. Kilogram (kg)

6. Which of the following is the number of centimeters in 1.46 meters?

   A. 1.46
   B. 14.6
   C. 146
   D. 1,460

7. A builder must measure a steel rod exactly 5 inches long for a building project. Which of the following measurement tools is appropriate for this task?

   A. Ruler
   B. Pipette
   C. Yardstick
   D. Odometer

8. Which of the following is the number of centimeters in 20 decimeters?

   A. 2
   B. 20
   C. 200
   D. 2,000

9. A technician must measure exactly 6 ounces of a liquid to add to a medical preparation. It is important for the measurement to be as precise as possible. Which of the following measurement tools is most appropriate for this task?

   A. Scale
   B. Beaker
   C. Caliper
   D. Graduated cylinder

10. If a container holds about 4 liters, which of the following is the container's approximate volume in English measurement? (Note: 1 liter ≈ 1 quart)

    A. 2 pints
    B. 4 pints
    C. 1 gallon
    D. 4 gallons

Answer Key

1. D		**6.** C	
2. D		**7.** A	
3. C		**8.** C	
4. A		**9.** D	
5. B		**10.** C	

Answers and Explanations

1. **(D)** A scale is the appropriate measuring tool for measuring weight. Graduated cylinders and beakers are used to measure volume, while yardsticks are used to measure length.

2. **(D)** A gallon consists of 4 quarts, and there are 2 pints in each quart. Since $4 \times 2 = 8$, there are 8 pints in each gallon. Multiply 3 gallons by 8 pints: $3 \times 8 = 24$. There are 24 pints in 3 gallons.

3. **(C)** A glass of water is best approximated by a measurement of about half a liter, or 0.5 L. The measurements of 10 mL and 0.10 cL are equal and are both too small. The measurement of 1 kL is too large.

4. **(A)** Set up a proportion to determine the missing measurement. Cross multiply to solve:

$$\frac{1 \text{ inch}}{2.54 \text{ centimeters}} = \frac{x \text{ inches}}{25.4 \text{ centimeters}}$$
$$2.54 \times x = 1 \times 25.4$$
$$2.54x = 25.4$$
$$x = \frac{25.4}{2.54}$$
$$x = 10$$

   The wood measures approximately 10 inches.

5. **(B)** A full tube of a cream medication would most likely be measured in grams. The unit of milligrams would be too small. Hectogram and kilogram units would be too large.

6. **(C)** Convert the number of meters to centimeters. One meter equals 100 centimeters. Multiply $1.46 \times 100 = 146$.

7. **(A)** A ruler would be most suited for measuring a length in inches. A yardstick would be too large, so C is incorrect.

8. **(C)** Convert decimeters to centimeters. One decimeter equals 10 centimeters. Multiply $20 \times 10 = 200$. There are 200 centimeters in 20 decimeters.

9. **(D)** The volume of a liquid is best measured by a graduated cylinder or beaker, among the choices listed here. Graduated cylinders generally provide more precise measurements than beakers, so a graduated cylinder would be the most appropriate tool for this task.

10. **(C)** Set up a proportion to determine the missing measurement. Cross multiply to solve:

$$\frac{1 \text{ liter}}{1 \text{ quart}} = \frac{4 \text{ liters}}{x \text{ quarts}}$$
$$1 \times x = 1 \times 4$$
$$x = 4$$

   The container's approximate volume is 4 quarts. There are 4 quarts in a gallon, so the container holds approximately 1 gallon.

CHAPTER 19

Data Interpretation

Data Interpretation questions ask you to interpret data given in certain types of graphs. Other questions may ask you to distinguish between dependent and independent variables in a statement or description of an event.

Reading Graphs

In the Reading chapters earlier in this book, we reviewed certain questions that involved using maps and resources. Data interpretation questions on the TEAS are similar to some of the Reading questions involving graphs that we saw earlier, except the questions may be more complex.

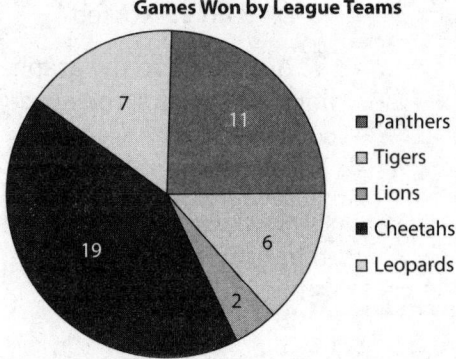

Games Won by League Teams

The graph above shows the distribution of 45 games won by teams in a soccer league during one season.

Games won by the Panthers represent what percentage of all games won that season? (Round the solution to the nearest tenth of a percent.)

A. 4.4%
B. 24.4%
C. 27.6%
D. 42.2%

To solve this problem, locate the section of the circle graph that shows games won by the Panthers. According to the key, the Panthers' section is in the top right quadrant. The Panthers won 11 out of 45 games during the season, or $\frac{11}{45}$. Divide 11 by 45 to determine the percentage: $11 \div 45$ is approximately 0.244. Convert this decimal to a percentage by moving the decimal point to the right two places. The Panthers won 24.4% of the games. The correct answer is **B**.

The **circle graph** above shows visually how a whole is divided into parts. Here is another data interpretation example involving a **line graph**, which shows change over time:

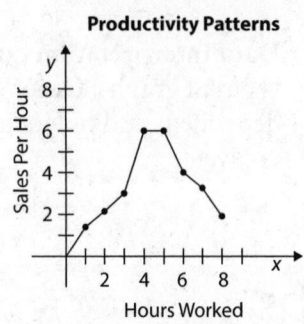

Productivity Patterns

The graph above shows the relationship between the number of hours worked by members of a sales team and the number of sales made per hour. Which of the following resulted in the highest sales per hour?

A. 2 hours worked
B. 3 hours worked
C. 6 hours worked
D. 8 hours worked

According to the graph, at 6 hours worked, the result was 4 sales per hour. At 8 hours, the number drops to 2 sales per hour, so choice **C** is correct.

Like the line graph in the example above, the **bar graph** below also shows change over time. This type of graph uses bars, rather than lines, to indicate values.

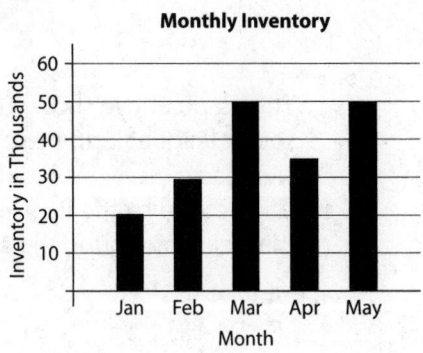

Monthly Inventory

The graph above shows the number of products held in the inventory of a warehouse over a period of five months. During which of the following months did the warehouse have more than 30,000 products in inventory?

A. January, March, and April
B. February, March, and April
C. February, March, and May
D. March, April, and May

According to the graph, the warehouse had 50,000 products in inventory during March, 35,000 during April, and 50,000 in May. Therefore, choice **D** is correct.

Dependent and Independent Variables

Some data interpretation questions ask you to identify dependent or independent variables in a given statement. The topic of dependent and independent variables is discussed in greater detail in Chapter 21. To answer Math questions regarding dependent and independent variables, you must understand the difference between the two.

Dependent and independent variables define a causal relationship between two factors. The **dependent variable** is the factor being acted upon. The **independent variable** is the factor that influences the outcome. In cause-and-effect terms, we would say that the dependent variable is the effect and the independent variable is the cause.

Certain flowering plants have more blooms with increased sunlight.

What is the independent variable in the event described above?

In the above example, the statement explains that increased sunlight causes the plants to have more blooms. Sunlight is the independent variable in the relationship, because it is the factor that influences plants to bloom. The number of blooms is the dependent variable in the relationship, because this is the outcome that results from the influence of more sunlight.

Review Questions

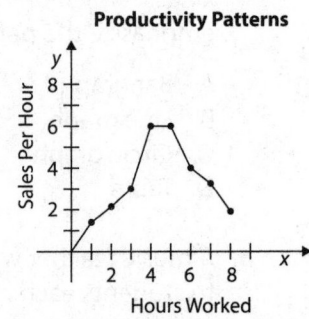

Productivity Patterns

1. The graph above shows the relationship between the number of hours worked by members of a sales team and the number of sales made per hour. Based on the information given in the graph, which of the following achieved the highest number of sales per hour?

   A. A team member who worked for 2 or 3 hours
   B. A team member who worked for 3 hours
   C. A team member who worked for 4 or 5 hours
   D. A team member who worked for 6 hours

2. Most companies increase their customers with more advertising.

   Which of the following is the dependent variable in the statement above?

   A. Marketing
   B. Customers
   C. Advertising
   D. Products

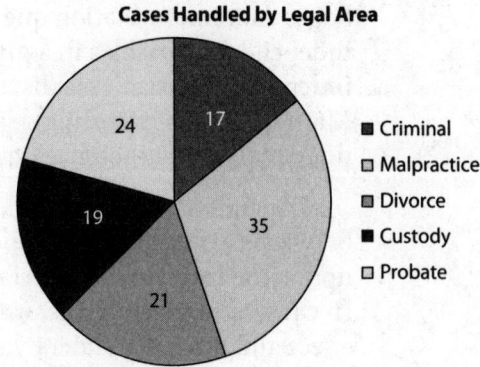

Cases Handled by Legal Area

- Criminal
- Malpractice
- Divorce
- Custody
- Probate

3. The graph above shows the distribution of 116 cases handled by a law firm in certain legal areas over a period of one year.

   Custody cases represent what percentage of all cases handled by the firm that year? (Round the solution to the nearest tenth of a percent.)

   A. 16.4%
   B. 18.1%
   C. 21.0%
   D. 30.1%

4. A scientist is presenting a report on the results of a survey that shows the number of people taking different medications to treat the same illness. Which of the following graphs should the scientist use to visually emphasize the percentage of patients taking each medication?

   A. Bar graph
   B. Line graph
   C. Circle graph
   D. Table

5. A music teacher wishes to visually compare the number of lessons taught to students each month over a period of one year. Which of the following graphs is most appropriate for the music teacher to use?

   A. Table
   B. Pie chart
   C. Scatterplot
   D. Bar graph

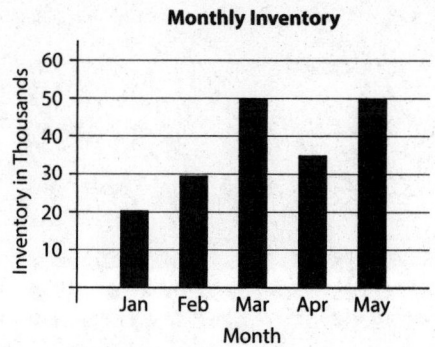

6. The graph above shows the number of products held in the inventory of a warehouse over a period of 5 months. Which of the following is the difference between the largest and smallest monthly inventories shown in the graph?

A. 15,000
B. 20,000
C. 27,000
D. 30,000

7. Stock prices usually decrease when investors panic.

Which of the following is the independent variable in the event described above?

A. Investor panic
B. Stock prices
C. Market fluctuations
D. News reports

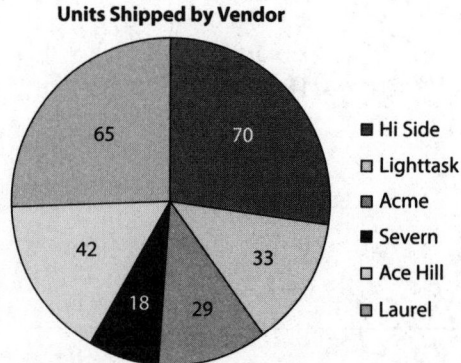

8. The graph above shows the distribution of 257 units shipped by particular vendors to a company over a 6-month period.

The units shipped by Severn represent what percentage of all units shipped by vendors during that period? (Round the solution to the nearest tenth of a percent.)

A. 5.2%
B. 6.3%
C. 7.0%
D. 27.2%

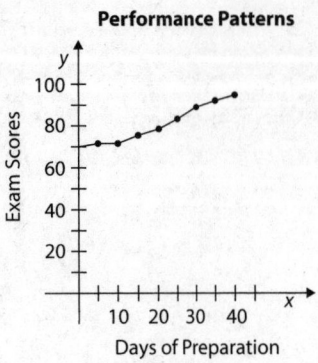

Performance Patterns

9. The graph above shows the relationship between the number of days of preparation by students studying for an exam and the exam scores received. Based on the information given in the graph, which of the following conclusions can be drawn?

A. Students needed at least 5 days of preparation to score a 70 or higher.
B. There was no score difference recorded between 5 and 10 days of preparation.
C. The highest scores were achieved by those who had 30 days of preparation.
D. Students who scored over 90 spent at least 20 days preparing for the exam.

10. People become wiser as they have more life experiences.

Which of the following is the independent variable in the event described above?

A. Life experiences
B. Recognition
C. Judgment
D. Wisdom

Answer Key

1. C	**6.** D
2. B	**7.** A
3. A	**8.** C
4. C	**9.** B
5. D	**10.** A

Answers and Explanations

1. (C) The line graph shows that the highest number of sales per hour were achieved at 4 and 5 hours worked.

2. (B) In this statement, *customers* is the dependent variable. The number of customers is influenced by the level of *advertising*, which is the independent variable.

3. (A) The firm handled 19 custody cases during the year, or $\frac{19}{116}$. Divide 19 by 116 to determine the percentage: 19 ÷ 116 is approximately 0.164. Convert this decimal to a percentage by moving the decimal point to the right two places. Custody cases represent 16.4% of all cases handled by the firm.

4. (C) A circle graph shows visually how a whole is divided into parts. It would be the best choice to use to visually emphasize the percentage of patients taking each medication.

5. (D) Bar graphs and line graphs can both be used to visually show change over time. A table would be less effective for a visual comparison because it lacks the imagery contained in a graph.

6. (D) The largest monthly inventory is 50,000 products, held in March and May. The smallest monthly inventory is 20,000 products, held in January. To find the difference between these two, use subtraction: 50,000 − 20,000 = 30,000.

7. (A) In this statement, the cause is panic of investors, and the effect is the decrease in stock prices. *Investor panic* is the independent variable, because it influences the outcome of stock price decline.

8. (C) According to the graph, Severn shipped 18 units during the 6-month period. This amounts to $\frac{18}{257}$ of the total units shipped. Divide 18 by 257 to determine the percentage: 18 ÷ 257 = 0.07. Convert this decimal to a percentage by moving the decimal point to the right two places. The units shipped by Severn represent 7% of all units shipped.

9. (B) Looking at the graph, we can see that students who prepared for 5 days scored just over 70 on the exam. Students who prepared for 10 days scored the same. Therefore, there was no difference recorded between 5 and 10 days of preparation, as choice B states. Choice A is incorrect because students who spent no days preparing scored a 70 on the exam.

10. (A) In this statement, the independent variable is *life experiences*, and the dependent variable is *wisdom*. Life experiences is the factor that causes the outcome of people gaining wisdom.

CHAPTER 20

Algebra

Algebra questions on the TEAS test your ability to simplify expressions and to solve equations containing unknown quantities. You may also be asked to solve inequalities and absolute value equations or inequalities.

Simplifying Expressions

To simplify algebraic expressions, we must combine like terms. **Like terms** in algebra are terms that contain the same variables raised to the same power (or no variables at all):

Simplify the expression: $(x^2 + 2x + 1) + (2x^2 + x + 4)$.

To simplify this expression, combine like terms. In this expression, x^2 and $2x^2$ are like terms. They both contain the variable x raised to the second power (x^2). The terms $2x$ and x are also like terms. They both contain the variable x, with no exponent.

Finally, the terms 1 and 4 are like terms. They contain no variables at all. Combine the three sets of like terms. It may be helpful to put the like terms next to each other in the equation:

$$(x^2 + 2x + 1) + (2x^2 + x + 4) = x^2 + 2x^2 + 2x + x + 1 + 4$$
$$= (x^2 + 2x^2) + (2x + x) + (1 + 4)$$
$$= 3x^2 + 3x + 5$$

The simplified expression is **$3x^2 + 3x + 5$**.

FOIL

Some expressions require you to multiply two binomials. **Binomials** contain exactly two terms, such as $x + 3$ or $2x + 5$:

Simplify the expression: $(x + 3)(2x + 5)$.

Here you are being asked to multiply the binomial $x + 3$ by the binomial $2x + 5$. To perform this multiplication, we use a process known as FOIL. The letters in **FOIL** stand for First, Outer, Inner, and Last. This tells you the order of terms to multiply in the two binomials.

First, multiply the first two terms of each binomial:

First: $x \times 2x = 2x^2$

Then, multiply the outer two terms:

Outer: $x \times 5 = 5x$

Then, multiply the inner two terms:

Inner: $3 \times 2x = 6x$

Then multiply the last two terms:

Last: $3 \times 5 = 15$

Now, add the results together:

$2x^2 + 5x + 6x + 15$

This expression can be further simplified to $\mathbf{2x^2 + 11x + 15}$.

Solving Equations

Algebra equations contain at least one unknown variable. This unknown variable is represented by a letter, such as x or y. The purpose of solving the equation is to find the value of the unknown variable.

To solve equations, we must isolate the variable on one side of the equation. Let's consider an example:

Solve the equation: $2x + 4 = 8$.

To solve this equation, we must isolate the variable x on one side of the equation. First, subtract the number 4 from both sides:

$$2x + 4 = 8$$
$$2x + 4 - 4 = 8 - 4$$
$$2x + 0 = 4$$
$$2x = 4$$

Subtracting 4 from both sides leaves only the term $2x$ on the left side of the equation. Now, divide both sides by 2 to isolate the variable x:

$$2x = 4$$
$$\frac{2x}{2} = \frac{4}{2}$$
$$x = 2$$

The value of x is **2**.

Solving Inequalities

In algebra, **inequalities** express relationships between quantities where one quantity is greater than or less than another. The symbols > and < are used to express "greater than" and "less than." A quantity may also be greater than or equal to another quantity. The symbol ≥ is used to represent "greater than or equal to," and the symbol ≤ represents "less than or equal to."

Inequality Symbols

>   greater than

<   less than

≥   greater than or equal to

≤   less than or equal to

Inequalities are solved in the same way as equations, with one exception. When multiplying or dividing both sides of an inequality by a negative number, you must reverse the direction of the inequality sign.

Solve the inequality: $-3x > 6$.

To solve this inequality, we must isolate x on one side of the equation. This means we must divide both sides of the inequality by -3. Therefore, we must reverse the direction of the inequality sign:

$$-3x > 6$$
$$\frac{-3x}{-3} < \frac{6}{-3}$$
$$x < -2$$

Notice that when we divide by -3, we change the direction of the inequality sign from greater than (>) to less than (<). The correct answer is **$x < -2$**.

Absolute Value Equations

Absolute value equations may also appear on TEAS Math. The **absolute value** of a number is the distance that number lies from zero on a number line. Absolute value is indicated by two vertical bars, as shown:

$$|x| = 5$$

If the absolute value of x equals 5, then x must lie exactly 5 units away from zero on the number line. The value of x could be positive (5) or it could be negative (−5). Both 5 and −5 lie exactly 5 units away from zero on the number line. So, the value of x is 5 or −5. Here is another example:

Solve the equation: $|x - 1| = 6$.

In this equation, the absolute value of $x - 1$ is 6. This tells us that the quantity $x - 1$ lies exactly 6 units away from zero on the number line. So, $x - 1$ could equal 6 or −6. Set up two equations and solve for both possibilities:

$$x - 1 = 6 \qquad\qquad x - 1 = -6$$
$$x - 1 + 1 = 6 + 1 \qquad x - 1 + 1 = -6 + 1$$
$$x = 7 \qquad\qquad x = -5$$

The value of x is **7 or −5**. In set notation, this would be written as {7, −5}.

Review Questions

1. $12 - \dfrac{x}{4} = 8$

Solve the equation above. Which of the following is correct?

A. $x = 6$
B. $x = 8$
C. $x = 12$
D. $x = 16$

2. $(3x + 2)(x + 1)$

Simplify the expression above. Which of the following is correct?

A. $4x + 2$
B. $3x^2 + 2$
C. $3x^2 + 5x + 2$
D. $3x^2 + 6x + 1$

3. $|x + 2| > 4$

Solve the inequality above. Which of the following is correct?

A. $x > 2$ or $x < -6$
B. $x > 4$ or $x > -6$
C. $x > 6$
D. $x < 8$

4. Cassandra's height, x, is 3 inches greater than twice her brother's height, y.

Which of the following algebraic equations best represents the statement above?

A. $x = 3x + y$
B. $x = 2y + 3$
C. $y = 2x + 3$
D. $x = 3y + 2$

5. $4(x + 7) = 2(x + 15)$

Solve the equation above. Which of the following is correct?

A. $x = 1$
B. $x = 3$
C. $x = 4$
D. $x = 8$

6. $(2x^2 + 4x - 7) - (2x^2 + 3x - 4)$

Simplify the expression above. Which of the following is correct?

A. $2x + 8$
B. $x - 3$
C. $7x - 3$
D. $4x^2 + 1$

7. The value of x is 5 less than $\dfrac{3}{4}$ the value of y.

Which of the following algebraic expressions correctly represents the sentence above?

A. $x - 5 = \dfrac{3}{4}y$

B. $y = \dfrac{3}{4}x + 5$

C. $x = 5 - \dfrac{3}{4}y$

D. $x = \dfrac{3}{4}y - 5$

8. $-4x - 9 > 3$

Solve the inequality above. Which of the following is correct?

A. $x < -3$
B. $x > 2$
C. $x < 3$
D. $x > 4$

9. $(2x^2 - 3x + 7) + (3x^2 + 2x + 6)$

Simplify the expression above. Which of the following is correct?

A. $5x^2 - x + 13$
B. $5x^2 + 5x - 1$
C. $6x^2 + x + 13$
D. $6x^2 + 5x - 1$

10. $|9-x| = 4$

Which of the following is the solution set for the equation above?

A. {5, –13}
B. {5, 13}
C. {–5, 13}
D. {–5, –13}

Answer Key

1. D	**6.** B
2. C	**7.** D
3. A	**8.** A
4. B	**9.** A
5. A	**10.** B

Answers and Explanations

1. (D) Isolate the variable x on one side of the equation. First, subtract the number 12 from both sides:

$$12 - \frac{x}{4} = 8$$

$$-\frac{x}{4} = 8 - 12$$

$$-\frac{x}{4} = -4$$

Then, multiply both sides by –4 to isolate the variable x:

$$-\frac{x}{4} = -4$$

$$-4 \times \left(-\frac{x}{4}\right) = -4 \times -4$$

$$x = 16$$

The value of x is 16.

2. (C) Use the process of FOIL to multiply the binomials $(3x + 2)(x + 1)$. First, multiply the first two terms of each binomial:

First: $3x \times x = 3x^2$

Then, multiply the outer two terms:

Outer: $3x \times 1 = 3x$

Then, multiply the inner two terms:

Inner: $2 \times x = 2x$

Then multiply the last two terms:

Last: $2 \times 1 = 2$

Now, add the results together:

$3x^2 + 3x + 2x + 2$

This expression can be further simplified to $3x^2 + 5x + 2$.

3. (A) In this inequality, the absolute value of $x + 2$ is greater than 4. This tells us that the quantity $x + 2$ lies more than 4 units away from zero on the number line. So, the value of $x + 2$ could be greater than 4, or it could be less than –4. Set up two inequalities and solve for both possibilities:

$x + 2 > 4$	$x + 2 < -4$
$x + 2 - 2 > 4 - 2$	$x + 2 - 2 < -4 - 2$
$x > 2$	$x < -6$

The solution is $x > 2$ or $x < -6$.

4. (B) Start with Cassandra's height, x. Then set up an equation:

$$x = ?$$

Cassandra's brother's height is denoted by y. Cassandra's height is equal to 3 more than twice y, which can be written as $2y + 3$. Add this expression to the equation:

$$x = 2y + 3$$

5. (A) Isolate the variable x on one side of the equation. First, perform the multiplication on both sides of the equation:

$$4(x + 7) = 2(x + 15)$$
$$4x + 28 = 2x + 30$$

Then, subtract 28 from both sides:

$$4x + 28 = 2x + 30$$
$$4x + 28 - 28 = 2x + 30 - 28$$
$$4x = 2x + 2$$

Next, subtract $2x$ from both sides:

$$4x = 2x + 2$$
$$4x - 2x = 2$$
$$2x = 2$$

Now, divide both sides by 2 to isolate the variable x:

$$2x = 2$$
$$\frac{2x}{2} = \frac{2}{2}$$
$$x = 1$$

The value of x is 1.

6. (B) To simplify this expression, combine like terms:

$$(2x^2 + 4x - 7) - (2x^2 + 3x - 4) = 2x^2 - 2x^2 + 4x - 3x - 7 - (-4)$$
$$= (2x^2 - 2x^2) + (4x - 3x) - (7 + 4)$$
$$= 0 + x - 3$$
$$= x - 3$$

The simplified expression is $x - 3$.

7. (D) Start with the value of x, and set up an equation:

$$x = ?$$

The question tells us that x is 5 less than $\frac{3}{4}$ the value of y, which can be written as $\frac{3}{4}y - 5$. Add this expression into the equation:

$$x = \frac{3}{4}y - 5$$

8. (A) To solve this inequality, we must isolate x on one side of the equation. To do this, first add 9 to both sides of the equation:

$$-4x - 9 > 3$$
$$-4x - 9 + 9 > 3 + 9$$
$$-4x > 12$$

Next, divide both sides of the equation by -4:

$$-4x > 12$$
$$\frac{-4x}{-4} < \frac{12}{-4}$$
$$x < -3$$

Because we are dividing by a negative number, we must change the direction of the inequality sign. The correct answer is therefore $x < -3$.

9. (A) To simplify this expression, combine like terms: $(2x^2 - 3x + 7) + (3x^2 + 2x + 6)$

$$(2x^2 - 3x + 7) + (3x^2 + 2x + 6) = 2x^2 + 3x^2 - 3x + 2x + 7 + 6$$
$$= (2x^2 + 3x^2) - (3x + 2x) + (7 + 6)$$
$$= 5x^2 - x + 13$$

The simplified expression is $5x^2 - x + 13$.

10. (B) In this equation, the absolute value of $9 - x$ is 4. This tells us that the quantity $9 - x$ lies exactly 4 units away from zero on the number line. So, $9 - x$ could equal 4 or -4. Set up two equations and solve for both possibilities:

$$9 - x = 4 \qquad\qquad 9 - x = -4$$
$$9 - 9 - x = 4 - 9 \qquad 9 - 9 - x = -4 - 9$$
$$-x = -5 \qquad\qquad -x = -13$$
$$x = 5 \qquad\qquad x = 13$$

The value of x is 5 or 13. In set notation, this is written as {5, 13}.

PART 3

Science

The **TEAS Science section** tests your scientific knowledge and skills in four areas: scientific reasoning, human body science, life science, and earth and physical science. In this part, we'll review scientific concepts essential for success on the test, along with key formulas you'll need to solve problems involving calculations.

CHAPTER 21

The Scientific Method

Questions concerning the **Scientific Method** test your understanding of the steps in the process of developing scientific knowledge. They also address the definitions of certain scientific terms: deductive and inductive reasoning, dependent and independent variables, experimental and control groups, and direct and inverse correlations.

Steps in the Scientific Method

There are six steps in the scientific method, and they are always conducted in the same order, as follows:

Step 1   Make an observation and identify the **problem** to be studied.

Step 2   Ask a **question** or questions about the problem.

Step 3   Formulate a **hypothesis** that attempts to answer one of the questions raised about the problem.

Step 4   Gather data and/or conduct an **experiment** to test the hypothesis.

Step 5   **Analyze** the data gathered.

Step 6   Draw a **conclusion** regarding whether or not the hypothesis is supported by the data.

Inductive versus Deductive Reasoning

Scientific progress proceeds based on logical reasoning. **Inductive reasoning** involves drawing general conclusions based on observation of specific events. If a scientist observes swans on a lake, and all of the swans that he sees are white, the scientist might conclude that *all swans are white*.

Inductive reasoning is based on observation, but it has its flaws. Suppose black swans do exist somewhere, but the scientist has never seen them. It would be incorrect for the scientist to conclude definitively that all swans are white because it is impossible for him to research all swans on the planet to verify this conclusion.

Deductive reasoning involves drawing a specific conclusion based on a general premise. A scientist might start out with the general premise that all accountants are good with numbers. She might then meet Omar, who is an accountant. The scientist would conclude that Omar is good with numbers.

When using deductive reasoning, the conclusion can only be true if the general premise is also true. If a scientist starts out with a false premise, the conclusion will be false. Here is an example:

All men are over six feet tall. Jerome is a man. Therefore, Jerome is over six feet tall.

In the argument above, the conclusion is false because the general premise is false. Some men are less than six feet tall.

Dependent and Independent Variables

Science experiments are often designed in terms of dependent and independent variables. The **dependent variable** is the outcome, or effect, being studied. The **independent variable** is the causal factor being studied.

It may help to think of the two types of variables in terms of the following diagram:

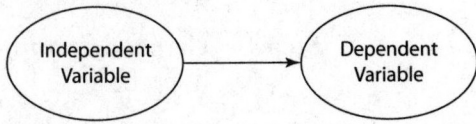

The independent variable acts on the dependent variable to produce a certain outcome. We say the dependent variable is *dependent* because it is influenced by the action of the independent variable. The independent variable, on the other hand, is free to act and is not influenced by another source, at least in terms of the design of the study.

The study described in the example below gives an example of independent and dependent variables in an experiment.

Scientists wish to investigate whether the growth of a certain plant is affected by a fertilizer. One group of 10 plants is grown with no fertilizer. A second group of 10 plants is grown with fertilizer administered at regular intervals with each watering. At the end of the study, the fertilized plants are 10 centimeters taller, on average, than the plants that received no fertilizer.

In this experiment, fertilizer is the independent variable, and plant growth is the dependent variable. The scientists are testing whether the fertilizer has an effect on plant growth.

Fertilizer   Plant growth

Independent variable   **Dependent variable**

We can conceptualize the relationship between fertilizer and plant growth visually as shown:

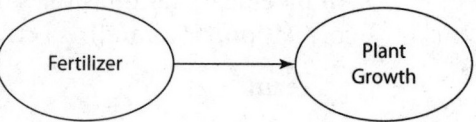

Experimental and Control Groups

Experiments are often designed with two types of test groups: experimental groups and control groups. **Experimental groups** are the test groups that receive a particular factor being tested, such as a medication or fertilizer, as in the example above. Experimental groups may also be called **treatment groups**. They are receiving the treatment being tested.

Control groups are groups that do not receive the treatment or factor being tested. Control groups may receive no factors, such as in the example above, where one group received no fertilizer. Control groups may also be given a "false" factor, known as a **placebo**. In pharmaceutical experiments, for example, placebos can take the form of pills that are made to resemble a certain medication being tested—but the placebo actually contains none of the medication itself.

Direct and Inverse Correlations

When we say that there is a correlation between two factors, this means that the factors have a relationship. A **direct correlation** shows that as one factor increases, the other factor also increases. An **inverse correlation**, by contrast, shows that as one factor increases, the other decreases:

The higher the temperature rose, the more quickly the substance melted.

In the scenario above, temperature and melting rate are directly correlated. As temperature increases, the rate of melting also increases. As temperature decreases, the rate of melting slows down.

Here is an example of inverse correlation:

As the incline on the treadmill increased, the patient's speed slowed down.

In this scenario, the level of incline and the patient's speed are inversely correlated. As the incline increases, the patient's speed decreases. Presumably as the incline decreases, the patient's speed would pick back up.

Direct correlations are also known as **positive correlations**. These terms are used interchangeably. Inverse correlations can be referred to as **negative correlations** or as **indirect correlations**. Inverse, negative, and indirect correlation all mean the same thing.

In addition, correlations can sometimes be referred to as **variations**. A direct variation is the same as a direct correlation or a positive correlation. An inverse variation is the same as an inverse correlation, a negative correlation, or an indirect correlation.

Term	Means the Same as
Positive correlation	
Direct variation	Direct correlation
Positive variation	
Negative correlation	
Indirect correlation	
Inverse variation	Inverse correlation
Negative variation	
Indirect variation	

Reading Graphs of Experimental Results

Correlations can be graphed to show the results of an experiment. The line of a line graph with a direct or positive correlation will have a positive slope:

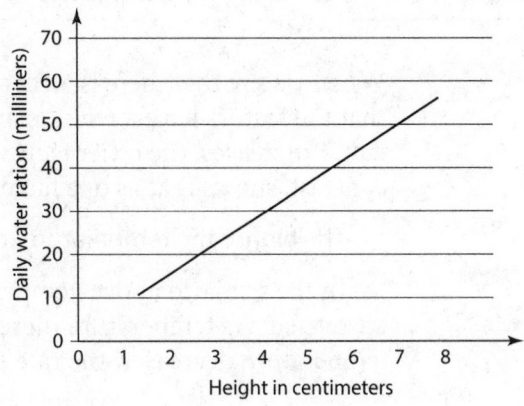

The graph above shows a line slanting upward to the right, which indicates a **positive slope**. As the daily water ration increases, the height also increases. The results of this graph show that height and daily water intake are *directly correlated*. Another way to say this is that height *varies directly* with daily water intake.

The line graph below shows an inverse correlation, or an inverse variation, which is represented by a line with a negative slope. This time, as the daily water ration increases, the height decreases.

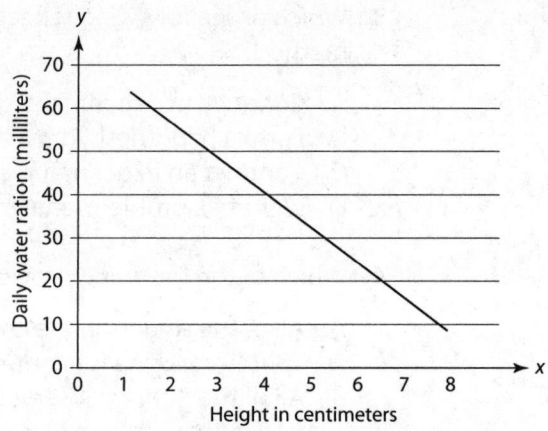

The line slanting downward to the right shows a **negative slope**. Based on the results shown in this graph, it can be concluded that height and daily water intake are *inversely correlated*. We might also say that height *varies indirectly* with the daily water intake.

Review Questions

1. A scientist studies the effect of rainfall on wood decomposition in the Amazon rainforest. In this study, rainfall is which of the following types of variables?

   A. Independent
   B. Extraneous
   C. Dependent
   D. Qualitative

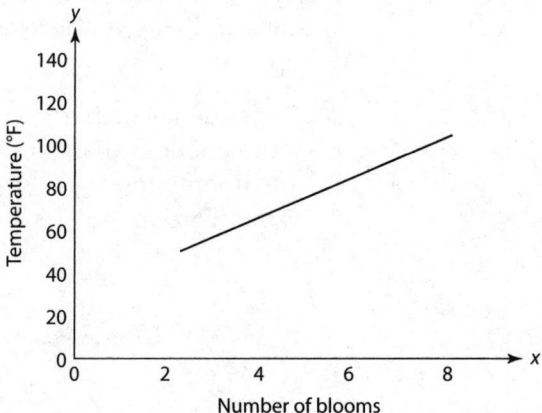

2. Based on the graph above, which of the following describes the correlation between temperature and the number of plant blooms?

   A. Linear
   B. Indirect
   C. Negative
   D. Direct

3. Which of the following reflects the correct order of steps in the scientific method?

   A. Conduct an experiment, draw a conclusion, form a hypothesis
   B. Form a hypothesis, draw a conclusion, conduct an experiment
   C. Conduct an experiment, analyze the data, draw a conclusion
   D. Identify a problem, analyze the data, form a hypothesis

4. Which of the following provides an example of inductive reasoning?

   A. All of the singers in the choir are talented. Elana is in the choir. Therefore, Elana is talented.
   B. All of the gorillas observed in the zoo have brown hair. Therefore, all gorillas have brown hair.
   C. All surgeons are detail oriented. Jorge is a surgeon. Therefore, Jorge is detail oriented.
   D. All libraries are quiet. The MacArthur Reading Room is a library. Therefore, the MacArthur Reading Room is quiet.

5. Scientists conduct an experiment to assess the effect of a certain substance, Substance A, on bacterial cell division. One group of bacteria is exposed to Substance A at regular intervals over a period of 10 days. A second group of bacteria receives no exposure to Substance A. Which of the following is the dependent variable in this study?

   A. Bacterial cell division
   B. Substance A
   C. The group of bacteria exposed to Substance A
   D. The group of bacteria with no exposure to Substance A

6. A study is conducted to determine the effect of aspirin on heart attack risk. Study participants are divided into two groups. Participants in the first group are given a low dose of aspirin daily, while participants in the second group receive no aspirin. Which of the following describes the first group?

   A. Dependent variable
   B. Independent variable
   C. Treatment group
   D. Control group

Effect of Birth Order on Birth Weight

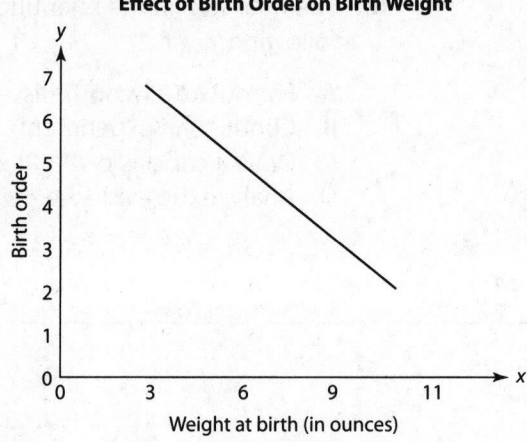

7. Based on the graph above, which of the following statements accurately describes the relationship between birth order and weight at birth?

   A. Birth order varies directly with weight at birth.
   B. Birth order varies indirectly with weight at birth.
   C. Birth order is directly correlated with weight at birth.
   D. Birth order is positively correlated with weight at birth.

8. In a pregnancy study, women in Group 1 were given a low dose of medication X daily. Women in Group 2 did not receive medication X. The pregnancy rate for the medication X users was 60%, and the pregnancy rate for the nonusers was 40%.

   Which of the following is a reasonable hypothesis related to this experiment?

   A. Women in Group 2 have higher pregnancy rates than women in Group 1.
   B. Women in Group 1 have higher pregnancy rates than women in Group 2.
   C. Therapy with medication X reduces labor time.
   D. Therapy with medication X improves pregnancy rates.

9. All humans require water to survive. Jessalyn is a human. Therefore, Jessalyn requires water to survive.

   The argument above reflects which of the following types of reasoning?

   A. Deductive
   B. Circular
   C. Inductive
   D. Ad hominem

10. The final step in the scientific method is reflected by which of the following?

   A. Formulate a hypothesis
   B. Conduct an experiment
   C. Draw a conclusion
   D. Analyze the evidence

Answer Key

1. A	**6.** C
2. D	**7.** B
3. C	**8.** D
4. B	**9.** A
5. A	**10.** C

Answers and Explanations

1. (A) Rainfall is the independent variable in this study. The scientist is examining how rainfall affects wood decomposition. Rainfall is the independent variable influencing the outcome. Wood decomposition is the dependent variable.

2. (D) The line in this graph slants upward to the right, indicating a positive slope. It therefore depicts a direct correlation. As the temperature increases, the number of blooms also increases.

3. (C) The correct order of steps in the scientific method is as follows: identify a problem, ask questions about the problem, form a hypothesis, gather data or conduct an experiment, analyze the data, and draw a conclusion.

4. (B) The argument in choice B is an example of inductive reasoning. It starts with a statement regarding specific observations: *All of the gorillas observed in the zoo have brown hair*. It then draws a general conclusion: *Therefore, all gorillas have brown hair*. Only certain gorillas have been observed—the ones in the zoo—but the conclusion refers to all gorillas in general. Choices A, C, and D are all examples of deductive reasoning.

5. (A) In this experiment, bacterial cell division is the dependent variable under study. Substance A is the independent variable. The scientists are assessing the effect that Substance A has on bacterial cell division, so Substance A is the "cause" in this instance. Bacterial cell division is the "outcome" or "effect."

6. (C) The first group is the treatment group, or experimental group. Participants in the first group receive a dose of aspirin, which is the independent variable under study. The second group is the control group, because participants in this group do not receive the factor under study.

7. (B) The graph shows that as the position in the birth order increases, the birth weight decreases. Therefore, the two factors are inversely correlated. Another way to say this would be to say that they show indirect variation, or that birth order varies indirectly with birth weight.

8. (D) The study tested the effect of medication X on pregnancy rates in women. A reasonable hypothesis related to this study would be that *therapy with medication X improves pregnancy rates*. Choices A and B are incorrect, because

the study focused on how medication X affected pregnancy rates specifically. Choice C is incorrect, because the study did not address labor time.

9. (A) The argument is an example of deductive reasoning. It starts with a general premise: *All humans require water to survive.* It then draws a specific conclusion: *Jessalyn requires water to survive.*

10. (C) The final step in the scientific method is to draw a conclusion. Scientists must analyze the evidence before drawing a conclusion, and they must conduct an experiment before analyzing the evidence, so choices D and B are incorrect.

CHAPTER 22

Bodily Organs and Systems

Questions concerning **Bodily Organs and Systems** test your knowledge of the 12 human organ systems that are essential to life. You may also be tested on specific vocabulary terms related to the understanding of anatomy.

The Skeletal System

The skeletal system serves several important functions in the body. It not only provides the framework for vital organs, but it also protects these same organs from injury. Bones are nearly as strong as steel, which allows them to act as the armor for the soft organs of the body. For example, the heart and lungs are protected by the sternum.

The body contains 206 bones. These bones can be classified into two groups. The **axial skeleton** consists of the skeleton's center and includes the skull, the vertebral column, and the rib cage. The **appendicular skeleton** consists of the arms and legs, otherwise known as **appendages**.

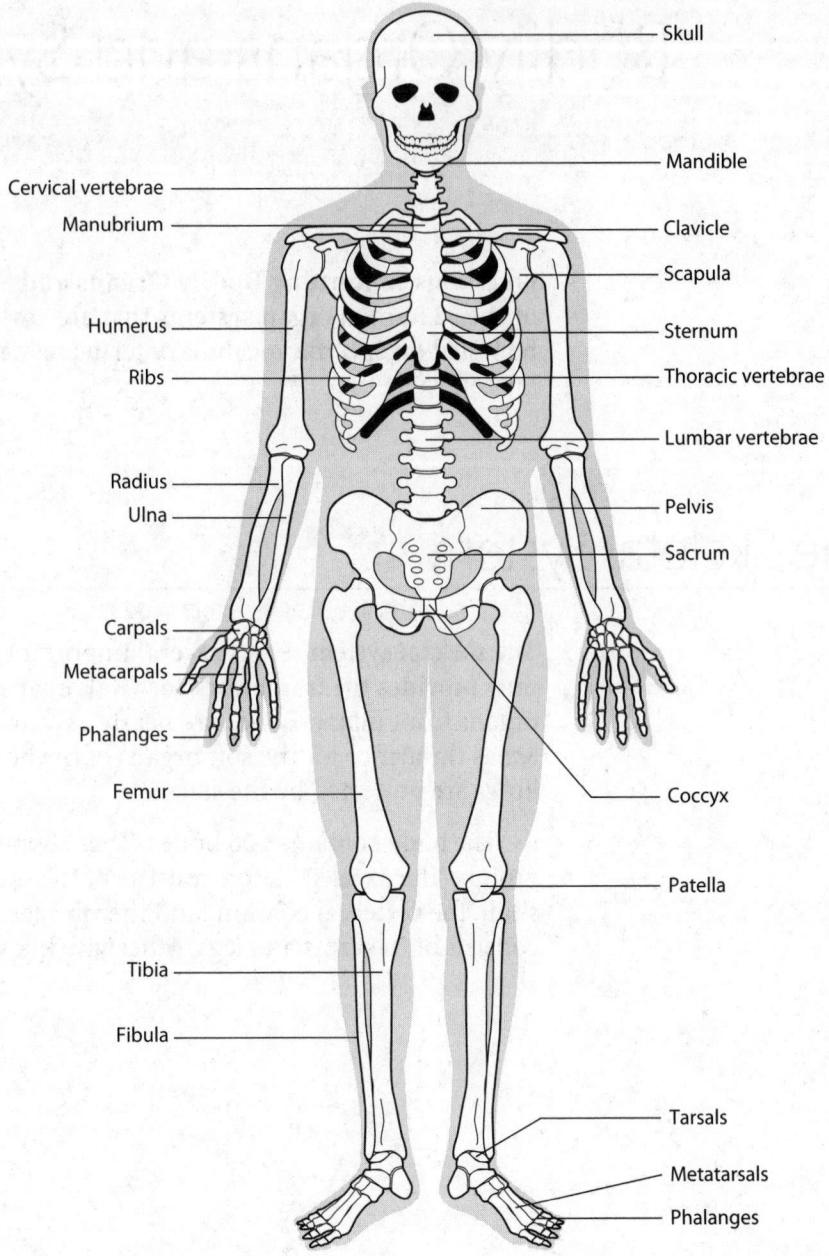

The figure above shows the **anterior**, or frontal, view of the skeleton. The **posterior** view is the back of the skeleton.

Another important function of the skeletal system is the interaction between the bones and the muscles. The muscles are attached to the bones by **tendons**, connective tissue found in the body. As the muscles contract, they pull on the bones, thus moving certain parts of the body.

The Muscular System

The muscular system is responsible for movement in the body, such as walking, chewing, and circulating blood. Another important function of this system is sustaining posture and body position.

There are three types of muscle: cardiac, smooth, and skeletal. **Cardiac muscle** pumps blood from the heart to the entire body. Its functions are controlled by the nervous system and are involuntary. **Smooth**, or **visceral**, **muscle** is found in the walls of organs, such as the stomach and intestines. These muscles help move substances through the organs. Their functions are also controlled by the nervous system and are involuntary. **Skeletal muscle** is attached to bone and provides movement to the body when the muscles pull on the bones.

Each skeletal muscle is made up of thousands of **muscle fibers**. The movement of these muscles is voluntary, meaning that you are able to control them. Skeletal muscles function by contracting or shortening their length and pulling one bone closer to another. The **origin** of a muscle is the location on the immobile bone where the muscle is connected. The **attachment** of the muscle to the mobile bone is called the **insertion**. Muscle groups are identified by several different characteristics, such as size, location, number of origins and insertions, and functions of the muscles.

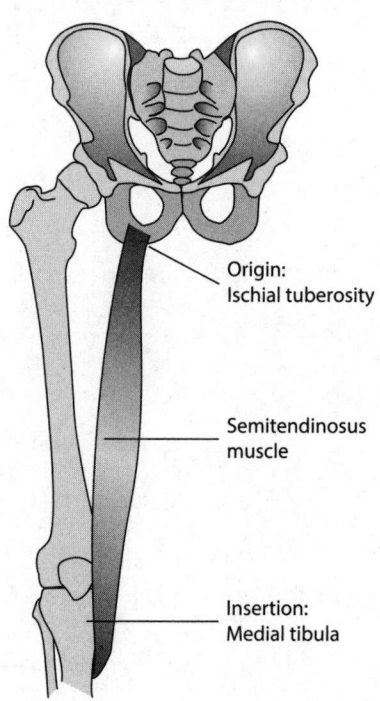

Origin:
Ischial tuberosity

Semitendinosus muscle

Insertion:
Medial tibula

The Nervous System

The nervous system coordinates the tasks of the other systems of the body and consists of the brain, spinal cord, and nerves. It regulates the body by responding to different **stimuli**, changes that occur both inside and outside of the body. It is also the source of all mental activity, such as learning and thought. The nervous system is divided into two main subparts: the **central nervous system (CNS)** and the **peripheral nervous system (PNS)**. The CNS contains the brain and spinal cord, which read information and decide on a correct response. The PNS consists of nerves that transmit messages to and from the CNS.

The peripheral nervous system can be divided even further into the **somatic** and **autonomic** systems. The somatic system responds to outside changes, while the autonomic system regulates internal changes. Both systems contain two types of **neurons**, special cells that receive and transmit chemical signals to the brain. **Afferent** or **sensory neurons** convey information from receptors in the body to the CNS. **Efferent** or **motor neurons** then bring information from the CNS back to the appropriate effectors in the body.

The neuron, pictured below, consists of a main cell body or **soma**, the center of which is the nucleus. Stemming off the cell body are **dendrites**, which receive neural impulses and convey them to the cell body. After receiving this information, an **axon** will transmit the message to another neuron. The axon is covered by a **myelin sheath**, which acts as an insulator to allow for electrical impulses to transmit into the cell.

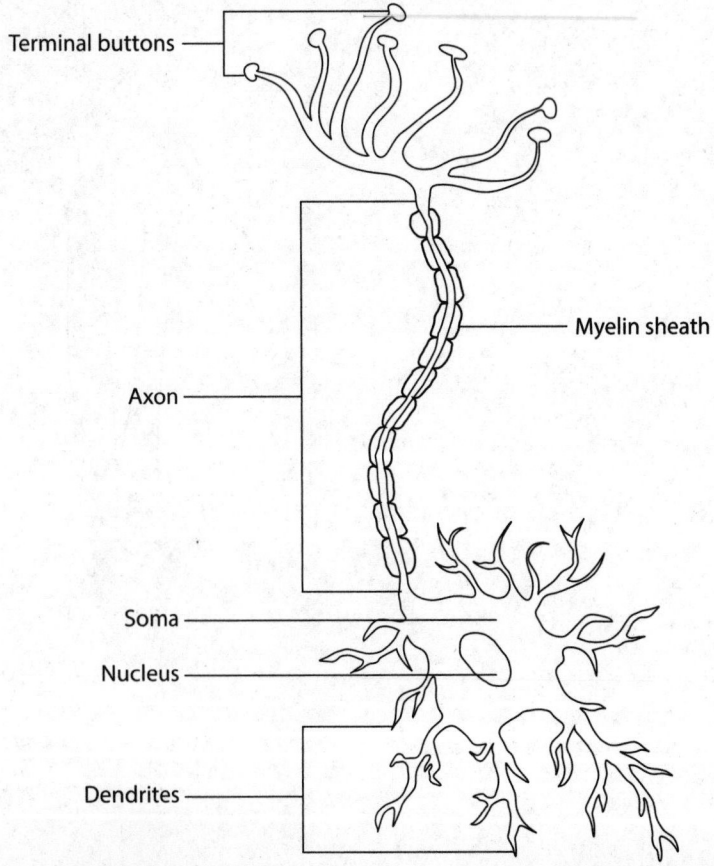

Terminal buttons

Myelin sheath

Axon

Soma

Nucleus

Dendrites

The Endocrine System

Working closely with the nervous system to maintain balance in the body, the endocrine system helps to regulate the glands and hormone production. **Hormones** are chemical messengers produced by the **endocrine glands** in the body. These glands secrete information to different parts of the body through the bloodstream to **target cells**—the particular cells they are meant to act upon. Hormones are transmitted to maintain homeostasis in the body. If the gland producing the hormone receives feedback from a system, the gland can respond appropriately by increasing or decreasing the production of that hormone.

There are several different endocrine glands located throughout the body. The **pituitary gland** is controlled by the **hypothalamus** in the brain and is responsible for much of the system's regulatory function. One particularly important hormone it produces is growth hormone. The **pineal gland** is responsible for the hormone melatonin, which influences the sleep cycle. The **thyroid gland**, located in the neck, produces hormones for regular growth and metabolic rate. The **adrenal gland** regulates metabolism and also helps the body deal with stress. The **pancreatic gland** secretes digestive enzymes that help break down food in the body. The **gonads** produce sex hormones in the body. They consist of the ovaries for women and the testes for men.

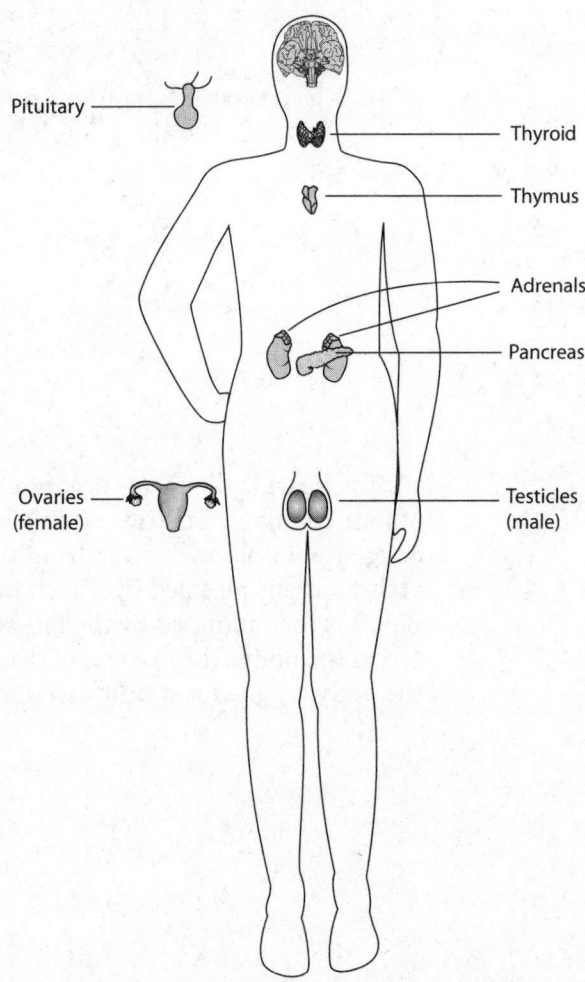

Pituitary

Ovaries
(female)

Thyroid

Thymus

Adrenals

Pancreas

Testicles
(male)

The Circulatory System

The circulatory, or cardiovascular, system transports blood pumped from the heart throughout the entire body. The blood is carried through various **blood vessels** and contains vital nutrients, oxygen, and hormones to help maintain the body's homeostasis. There are three types of blood vessels that work in conjunction with the heart to provide blood to the body. **Arteries** carry blood away from the heart. **Capillaries** transmit nutrients and waste products between arteries and **veins,** which then bring the blood back to the heart. These vessels form a network that carries the blood pumped from the heart to the body's tissues and then back to the heart again.

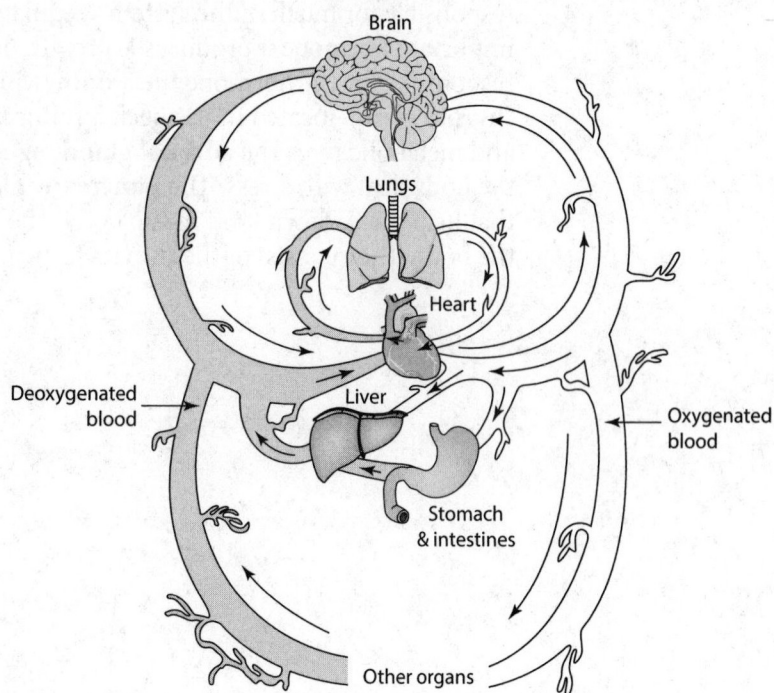

The heart is the major organ relevant to the circulatory system. It consists of four chambers and two circulatory systems. In **pulmonary circulation**, oxygen-poor blood coming from the body enters the heart through the **right atrium** and is pumped by the **right ventricle** to the lungs to receive oxygen. Blood is then pumped by the **left ventricle** to the **left atrium** and then sent out to the body. The process of delivering oxygen-rich blood to the rest of the body is called **systemic circulation**.

The heart has its own system of blood vessels that specifically circulates blood for its own function. This system is called the **coronary system**.

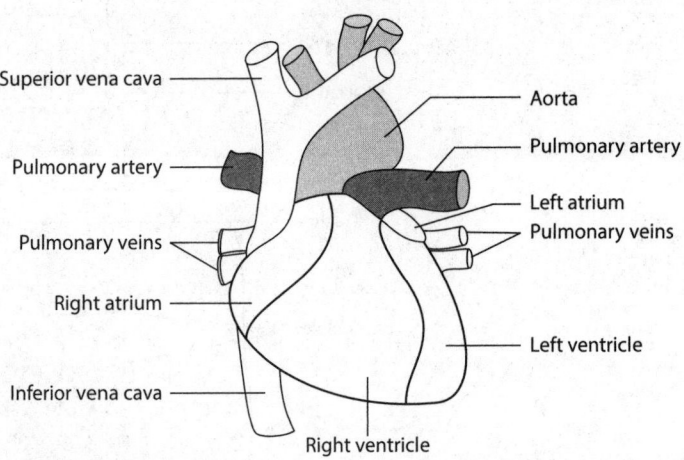

Superior vena cava

Aorta

Pulmonary artery

Pulmonary artery

Left atrium

Pulmonary veins

Pulmonary veins

Right atrium

Left ventricle

Inferior vena cava

Right ventricle

The **cardiac cycle** is the process of one heartbeat: the heart contracts and blood is forced out; then it relaxes and the heart fills with blood. The stage of contraction is called **systole**, and the stage of relaxation is called **diastole**.

The Respiratory System

The respiratory system involves bringing in oxygen through the airway to the lungs and releasing carbon dioxide. **Pulmonary ventilation** is the movement of air into and out of the lungs. **Inspiration** is the process of air coming in, while **expiration** involves air flowing out. The ventilation process begins with air entering the body through the nose or mouth and then traveling through the **pharynx**, or throat. Next, the air flows down the windpipe, or **trachea**, and enters the **bronchi**. Each lung connects to a bronchus, which breaks down into smaller and smaller bronchi within the lungs, forming a **bronchial tree**. When inside the lungs, oxygen reaches the **air sacs** and is then diffused into the blood.

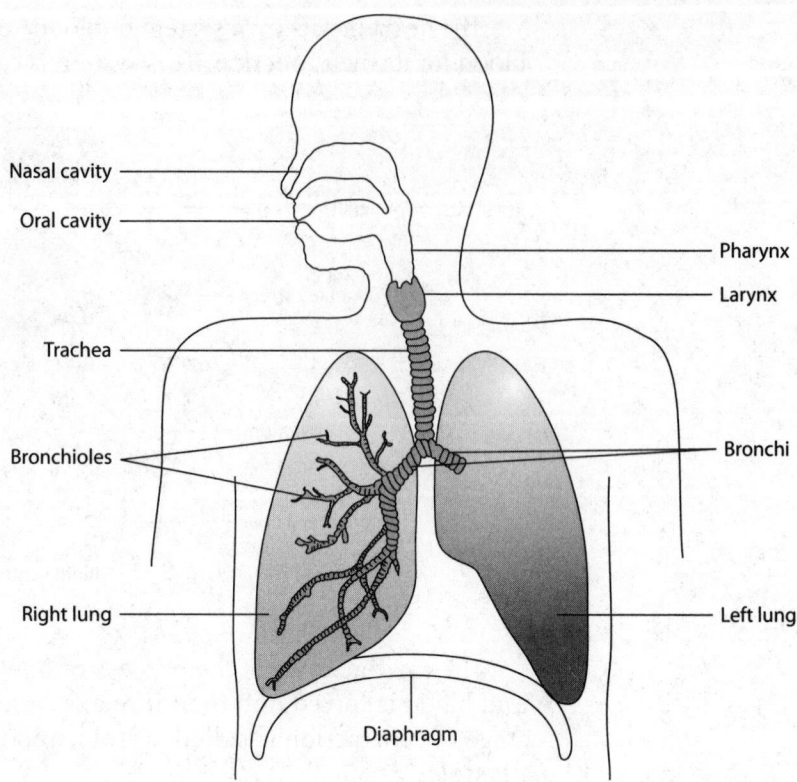

Nasal cavity

Oral cavity

Pharynx

Larynx

Trachea

Bronchioles

Bronchi

Right lung

Left lung

Diaphragm

Another process of the respiratory system is **cellular respiration**, the process by which cells get energy from nutrients. Oxygen is required for respiration, and carbon dioxide is released during this process.

The Digestive System

The digestive system involves a series of processes that break down the food we eat into structures that can be delivered and then used by the cells. Food is first **ingested** into the mouth, chewed, and then swallowed. Next, food is **digested** through **mechanical digestion**, the physical breakdown of food through chewing and mixing movements in the stomach. **Chemical digestion** breaks food down further through the use of enzymes so that the nutrients can be absorbed. The **absorption** process transports the digested food through the intestine into the circulatory system. Lastly, undigested food is **eliminated**. (For a diagram of the digestive system, see "The Process of Digestion," in Chapter 23.)

The **digestive tract**, or **gastrointestinal (GI) tract**, is about eight to nine meters long and begins with the mouth, where food enters, and ends at the anus, where waste is eliminated. In between, the GI tract is made up of various organs through which food passes and is broken down. The sequence of the GI tract includes the mouth, throat, esophagus, stomach, small intestine, and large intestine. Most digestion takes place in the small intestine.

Other vital organs necessary for the digestion and absorption of food are the **pancreas** and the **liver.** The pancreas secretes pancreatic juice, which helps to break down fats into useful nutrients for the body. The liver produces **bile**, which is important in the digestion of fats. The bile is stored in the **gallbladder** until it is needed.

The Urinary System

The urinary system has several functions; its most vital function is to regulate the volume and composition of bodily fluids. Other functions include regulating the acid–base level of blood and fluids, adjusting the amounts of sodium and water excreted in the urine, and eliminating metabolic waste. **Metabolic waste** consists of water, carbon dioxide, and nitrogenous material and is removed by the **kidneys**. The kidneys produce urine, which is then passed through the **urinary bladder**, where it is discharged from the body through the **urethra**.

The Lymphatic System

The lymphatic system has three functions. The first is that it returns excess fluid back into the blood, which helps maintain fluid balance. Second, it absorbs fats from the digestive track and deposits them in the bloodstream. Lastly, it defends the body against pathogens. The **lymph nodes** are small glands found mainly in the thorax and abdomen. These glands help prevent disease by filtering out bacteria in the **lymph,** a watery fluid formed from interstitial, or tissue, fluid. Other organs that are vital to the lymphatic system are the spleen, tonsils, and thymus. The **spleen** filters bacteria in the blood. **Tonsils**, which are located at the base of the tongue, function as a filter of interstitial fluid. The **thymus gland** is pertinent for immune responses.

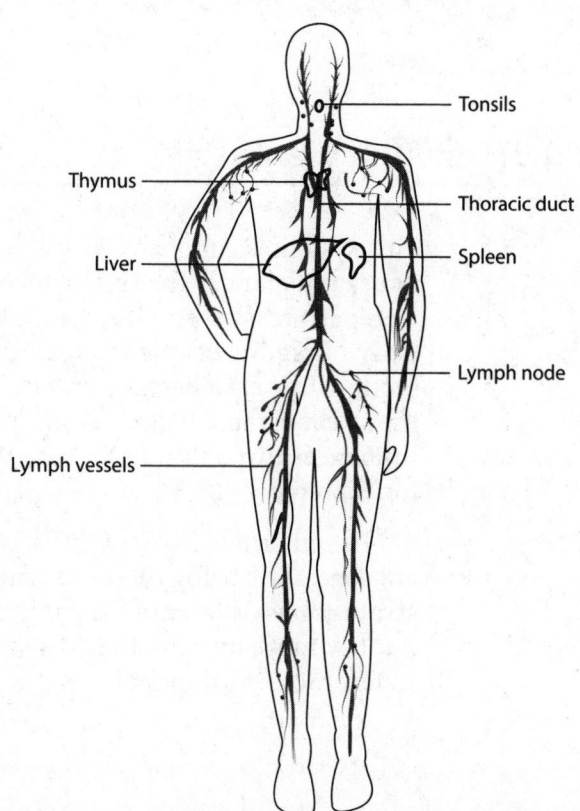

Tonsils

Thymus

Thoracic duct

Liver

Spleen

Lymph node

Lymph vessels

The Immune System

The immune system is supported by different defense mechanisms in the body that prevent disease and bacterial pathogens from developing in the body. An **immune response** occurs when the body recognizes these pathogens and creates an action against them. Harmful molecules that are recognized and elicit an immune response are called **antigens**. In response to antigens, the body makes **antibodies** to fight off specific antigen cells.

The body's first line of defense against pathogens includes the skin and various secretions, such as sweat and saliva. If pathogens successfully enter the body, often a fever or inflammation will occur to fight off an infection. **Lymphocytes**, special white blood cells, are formed in response to certain antigens. Some examples of lymphocytes include **natural killer (NK) cells**, **T cells**, and **B cells**. NK cells work against cells infected with bacteria and viruses, T cells attack body cells infected with pathogens, and B cells produce specific antibodies.

Active immunity develops from natural exposure to pathogens and an immune response. It can also be mimicked through **vaccinations**, where an individual is given a weakened antigen so the body can induce a response and build memory cells. **Passive immunity** elicits a temporary response when a person is given antibodies produced by another person or animal.

When the immune system is compromised, illness will occur with differing levels of severity. Sometimes the illness that manifests is the common cold, while other pathogens, such as cancer cells, evade immune responses.

The Integumentary System

This system is comprised of the body's protective covering: the skin, hair, nails, and glands. The skin, which averages in total size to about 20 square feet, performs several important functions. First and foremost, it is the body's first line of defense against pathogens as discussed in the previous section. The skin helps maintain body temperature through regulation of the sweat glands. It also communicates with the body regarding outside influences through sensory receptors to determine heat, cold, or pain, for example.

The outermost layer of the skin is called the **epidermis**. Epidermal cells are constantly being shed and renewed. New cells are developed in the **stratum basale** layer of the epidermis and pushed toward the top layer. As they move upward, the cells develop **keratin**, which provides a layer of waterproofing for the skin.

Hair provides protection from UV radiation and serves as a lubricant for the skin. **Sebaceous glands** secrete an oily substance called **sebum** through the hair follicles. Sebum oils the hair and skin cells and prevents water loss.

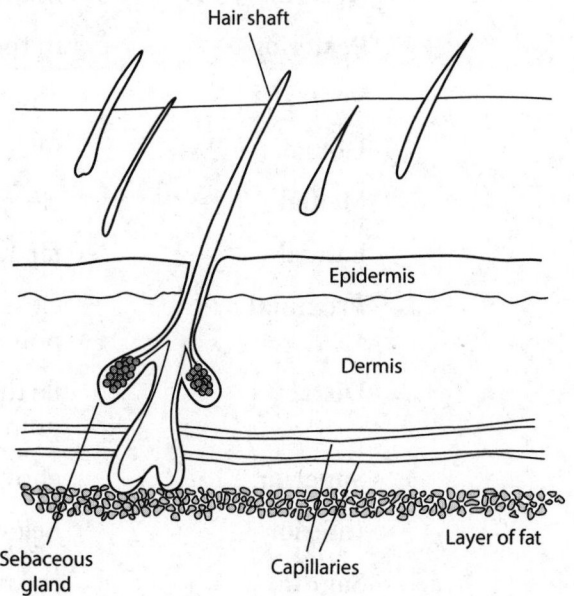

The Reproductive System

The reproductive system is regulated by hormones that influence the male and female reproductive organs and their interactions. The female gonads are the **ovaries**, a pair of small glands in the pelvic region where eggs, or **ova**, are developed. During **ovulation**, the process by which mature eggs leave the ovaries, an egg will travel through the **fallopian tubes** toward the **uterus**. If the egg is fertilized, it will remain in the **uterus**, or womb, for pregnancy. If it is not, the egg will be flushed out of the body along with the **endometrium**, a mucous membrane that builds up inside the uterine wall. This process is called the **menstrual cycle** and typically occurs every 28 days in women.

Male gonads, the **testes**, are small organs that produce the male sex cells called **sperm**. In the reproductive process, fertilization occurs when sperm and egg fuse to create a pregnancy.

Relevant Anatomical Terms

The following terms are commonly used when discussing anatomy.

Anterior	in the front or in front of
Posterior	in the back or in back of
Ventral	refers to the front of the body
Dorsal	refers to the back of the body
Medial	closer to the center line of the body
Lateral	farther from the center line of the body
Proximal	closer to the origin of a limb or attachment point
Distal	farther from the origin of a limb or attachment point
Superior	above or higher up
Inferior	below or lower down
Sagittal	the plane that divides the body vertically from right to left
Transverse	the plane that divides the body horizontally from top to bottom
Coronal (also called frontal)	the plane that divides the body vertically from front to back

Review Questions

1. Which of the following is a correct example of a part of the appendicular skeleton?

   A. Cranium
   B. Rib cage
   C. Legs
   D. Spinal cord

2. What is the main function of the nervous system?

   A. It regulates the body's movement.
   B. It maintains homeostasis in the body.
   C. It breaks down the food we eat through digestion.
   D. It coordinates the body's responses to different stimuli.

3. _____ are chemical messengers produced by the endocrine glands.

   Which of the following best completes the sentence above?

   A. Hormones
   B. Sperm cells
   C. White blood cells
   D. Antigens

4. The right atrium in the heart receives what kind of blood?

   A. Oxygen-rich blood from the left ventricle
   B. Oxygen-poor blood from the tissues
   C. Oxygen-rich blood from the right ventricle
   D. Oxygen-poor blood from the left atrium

5. Which of the following is *not* a body part involved in the respiratory system?

   A. Trachea
   B. Lungs
   C. Bronchial tree
   D. Ovaries

6. What is another name for the digestive tract?

   A. The stomach tract
   B. The food absorption tunnel
   C. The gastrointestinal tract
   D. The digestion path

7. Which of the following is a function performed by the kidneys?

   A. Remove metabolic waste
   B. Pump blood
   C. Produce sperm
   D. Secrete sweat

8. Which of the following is the body's first line of defense against pathogens?

   A. Hair
   B. Tonsils
   C. Uterus
   D. Skin

9. If a female egg is not fertilized, what happens to the egg during the menstrual cycle?

   A. It remains in the uterus.
   B. It is discharged during menstruation.
   C. It fuses together with sperm.
   D. It travels back to the ovaries.

10. Which of the following is *not* a function of the lymphatic system?

  A. It returns excess fluid back into the blood.
  B. It absorbs fats from the digestive system.
  C. It reduces the level of oxygen in the blood.
  D. It defends against pathogens.

11. If you are viewing the posterior of a skeleton, you are seeing which side of it?

  A. The front
  B. The back
  C. The side
  D. The top

12. Much of the endocrine system's activity is controlled by the _____.

  Which of the following best completes the sentence above?

  A. Pineal gland
  B. Aorta
  C. Spinal cord
  D. Hypothalamus

13. What is a possible situation in which an autoimmune disease could develop?

  A. The immune system attacks the body's own cells.
  B. A person has a cold or flu.
  C. Antibodies develop against a pathogen.
  D. The spleen functions normally.

14. What is the name of the waterproofing protein developed in the epidermis?

  A. Melanin
  B. Keratin
  C. Dermis
  D. Sebum

15. The _____ plane divides the body into right and left parts.

  Which of the following best completes the sentence above?

  A. Axial
  B. Appendicular
  C. Frontal
  D. Sagittal

Answer Key

1. C		**9.** B	
2. D		**10.** C	
3. A		**11.** B	
4. B		**12.** D	
5. D		**13.** A	
6. C		**14.** B	
7. A		**15.** D	
8. D			

Answers and Explanations

1. (C) The appendicular portion of the body includes the limbs, which are the legs and arms. The cranium, rib cage, and spinal cord are all part of the axial portion of the body.

2. (D) The main function of the nervous system is to coordinate the body's responses to different stimuli. The nervous system acts a regulator for the body by responding to stimuli through receptors. The muscular system regulates the body's movement. The endocrine system maintains homeostasis. The digestive system breaks down the food we eat. Therefore choices A, B, and C are incorrect.

3. (A) Hormones are the chemical messengers produced by the endocrine glands. Hormones are used to regulate many bodily activities. Sperm is produced by the testes for reproduction. White blood cells are used to protect the body against pathogens. Antigens are foreign cells recognized by the immune system.

4. (B) The right atrium receives oxygen-poor blood from the tissues. It is the first of the four chambers to receive blood from the body. After the blood leaves the right atrium, it travels to the right ventricle and to the lungs and so on, until it leaves the heart through systemic circulation and travels through the body.

5. (D) The ovaries are part of the female reproductive system. The trachea, lungs, and bronchial tree are all part of the respiratory system.

6. (C) The gastrointestinal tract is another name for the digestive tract, which extends from the mouth to the anus.

7. (A) One of the functions of the kidneys is to remove metabolic waste. The kidneys also produce urine. The heart pumps blood; the testes produce sperm; and glands in the skin secrete sweat.

8. (D) The skin is the body's first line of defense against pathogens. The skin also helps to maintain body temperature and communicate through sensory receptors about environmental stimuli. The tonsils and the uterus are both inside the body and would not function as the first line of defense. Hair, while protective of the body, does not protect against pathogens.

9. (B) If an egg, or ovum, is not fertilized, then it is discharged during menstruation. If the egg *is* fertilized, it is fused with the sperm and remains in the uterus to develop during pregnancy. The egg does not travel back to the ovaries.

10. (C) The lymphatic system does not control the level of oxygen in blood; that is determined by the circulatory and respiratory systems. The lymphatic system does, however, absorb excess fluid back into the blood, absorb fats from the digestive system, and defend against pathogens.

11. (B) If you are viewing the posterior of a skeleton, then you are looking at the back of it. The term *anterior* describes the front of the skeleton.

12. (D) The hypothalamus controls much of the endocrine system's functions, including maintaining fluid balance, regulating body temperature, influencing sexual behavior, and acting as the link between the nervous and endocrine systems.

13. (A) An autoimmune disease results when the body attacks its own cells. If a person has a cold or flu, the immune system is fighting foreign pathogens. Antibodies developing against a pathogen would be a normal immune response. The spleen filters blood and is not a vital organ.

14. (B) Keratin is the waterproofing protein developed in the epidermis. Melanin is a protein that determines hair and skin color. The dermis is a layer of skin located beneath the epidermis. Sebum is an oily substance secreted by the sebaceous glands.

15. (D) The sagittal plane divides the body into right and left parts. The axial portion of the body consists of the head, neck, and torso. The appendicular portion consists of the limbs. The frontal plane divides the body into anterior and posterior parts.

CHAPTER 23

Nutrition

Nutrition questions on the TEAS test your understanding of nutrients such as protein, fats, carbohydrates, vitamins, minerals, and water. They may also require an understanding of the process through which food is digested and a general knowledge of dietary guidelines.

Protein, Fats, and Carbohydrates

Protein, fats, and carbohydrates are sources of food energy for the body. **Protein** breaks down into amino acids in the body. Of the 20 primary amino acids, only 11 of these can be produced by the body itself. The remaining 9 must be obtained through the diet. These 9 amino acids are known as essential amino acids. They can be found only in protein sources such as meat, eggs, and fish.

9 Essential Amino Acids

Histidine

Isoleucine

Leucine

Lysine

Methionine

Phenylalanine

Threonine

Tryptophan

Valine

Carbohydrates are the body's source of quick fuel. Carbohydrates break down faster in the body than protein and fats. Carbohydrates convert to sugar, or **glucose**, in the body, providing a ready source of fuel. Simple carbohydrates, such as cane sugar, break down fastest when consumed. Complex carbohydrates, such as grains and starchy vegetables, break down more slowly than simple carbohydrates and turn into sugar less quickly in the bloodstream.

Fiber is a component found in carbohydrates that cannot be digested by the body. Because it does not break down into glucose, fiber adds bulk to the diet and improves the process of transporting foods through the digestive system. Adequate fiber intake can also be helpful for controlling blood sugar levels.

Fats are also a source of fuel for the body; once digested, they break down into fatty acids and glycerol. Fats take longer to digest than either protein or carbohydrates, so they provide the body with sustained energy. **Saturated fats** are derived mainly from animal sources and tend to raise cholesterol and increase the risk of heart attack and stroke. **Unsaturated fats**—derived from certain vegetables, fish, and nuts—can lower cholesterol levels, particularly monounsaturated fats, such as those found in avocado and olive oil.

Vitamins and Minerals

Vitamins and minerals are required for the proper functioning of the body. They do not provide fuel sources as foods do, but they are important components of various biochemical processes. Most vitamins and minerals cannot be made within the body and must be consumed through the diet or supplementation.

Certain vitamins and minerals act as **antioxidants**, which protect the cells against damage caused by destructive agents known as **free radicals**. The primary antioxidants are vitamin C, vitamin E, selenium, and beta-carotene, a substance that turns in to vitamin A in the body.

Vitamins	Minerals
Vitamin A (retinol)	Calcium
Vitamin B_1 (thiamine)	Chlorine
Vitamin B_2 (riboflavin)	Chromium
Vitamin B_6	Cobalt
Vitamin B_{12}	Copper
Niacin	Fluorine
Vitamin C	Iodine
Vitamin D	Iron
Vitamin E	Magnesium
Vitamin K	Manganese
Biotin	Molybdenum
Folate (folic acid)	Nickel
Niacin	Phosphorus

Vitamins	Minerals
Pantothenic acid	Potassium
	Selenium
	Sodium
	Sulfur
	Tin
	Vanadium
	Zinc

If certain vitamins or minerals are lacking in a person's diet, the person may experience **deficiency** symptoms, including certain diseases. A table of common deficiency symptoms is provided below.

Symptom	Vitamin or Mineral Deficiency
Anemia	Iron; other vitamins and minerals may also be responsible
Beriberi	Vitamin B_1 (thiamine)
Goiter	Iodine
Hypocalcemia	Calcium
Hypokalemia	Potassium
Hyponatremia	Sodium
Night blindness	Vitamin A
Osteoporosis	Calcium
Pellagra	Niacin; can also be caused by a deficiency of the amino acid tryptophan
Rickets	Vitamin D
Scurvy	Vitamin C

Water

Water is a vital nutrient, but it is different from proteins, fats, and carbohydrates because it is not a food. It performs multiple vital functions in the body. Water:

- Facilitates the digestion of food

- Helps the body to excrete wastes

- Plays a role in transporting nutrients to the cells

- Assists the body in maintaining a stable temperature

- Provides protection for numerous body components

- Keeps the joints lubricated so they can function properly

The Process of Digestion

As we saw in the previous chapter, the process of digestion occurs in the digestive system. It begins in the **mouth**, where the **salivary glands** secrete saliva as food is chewed. Enzymes in the saliva help food to start breaking down even while it is still in the mouth. Swallowed food mixed with saliva then moves through the **esophagus** and into the stomach. Secretions in the **stomach** further help the food to digest, and the digested material passes through the small intestine into the large intestine. Absorption of nutrients occurs primarily in the **small intestine**, where the **gallbladder** secretes bile made in the **liver**, and the **pancreas** secretes additional enzymes essential to digestion. The **large intestine** performs the role of absorbing water from the undigested food matter and creating solid wastes. These wastes then pass through the body via the **rectum** and the **anus**.

The numbered diagram below shows the order in which food passes through different parts of the body in the process of digestion.

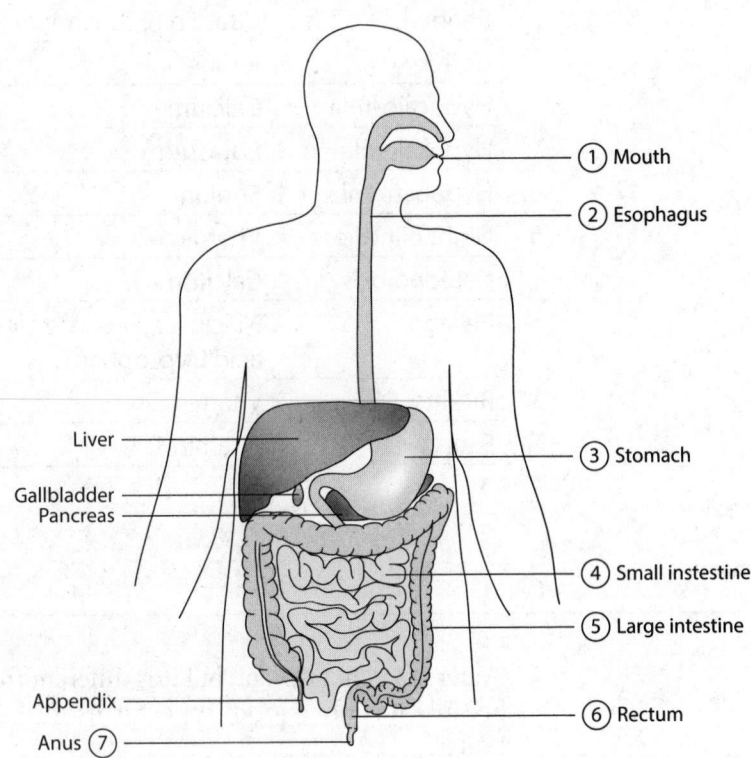

Liver

Gallbladder
Pancreas

Appendix

Anus ⑦

① Mouth

② Esophagus

③ Stomach

④ Small instestine

⑤ Large intestine

⑥ Rectum

Dietary Guidelines

Individuals may be instructed to follow specific dietary guidelines to assist in the management of certain illnesses, such as diabetes and heart disease. **Dietary guidelines for diabetes patients** may include the reduction of carbohydrates in the diet, as carbohydrates convert to glucose in the bloodstream, which can elevate the patient's blood sugar. **Dietary guidelines for patients with heart disease** may include the reduction of saturated fat to help in lowering cholesterol levels and the reduction of sodium to help in lowering blood pressure, among other therapeutic recommendations.

Review Questions

1. In which of the following does the process of digestion start?

   A. Esophagus
   B. Stomach
   C. Mouth
   D. Small intestine

2. Which of the following nutrients is most important for the body?

   A. Water
   B. Protein
   C. Fats
   D. Carbohydrates

3. Which of the following sources of food energy breaks down most slowly in the body?

   A. Protein
   B. Fats
   C. Simple carbohydrates
   D. Complex carbohydrates

4. The primary antioxidants include which of the following?

   A. Chromium
   B. Manganese
   C. Selenium
   D. Tryptophan

5. A patient with rickets is most likely to have a deficiency of which of the following?

   A. Vitamin A
   B. Vitamin B_1
   C. Vitamin C
   D. Vitamin D

6. During digestion, protein breaks down into which of the following?

   A. Amino acids
   B. Glucose
   C. Glycerol
   D. Sucrose

7. Which of the following is responsible for secreting bile into the small intestine in the process of digestion?

   A. Esophagus
   B. Pancreas
   C. Salivary glands
   D. Gallbladder

8. Cholesterol levels can be reduced by dietary intake of which of the following?

   A. Simple carbohydrates
   B. Saturated fats
   C. Trans fats
   D. Monounsaturated fats

9. Which of the following symptoms is most likely to be caused by an iodine deficiency?

   A. Osteoporosis
   B. Scurvy
   C. Goiter
   D. Pellagra

10. A patient with heart failure would most likely be instructed to maintain a low-sodium diet to assist with which of the following?

    A. Reducing insulin levels
    B. Reducing blood pressure
    C. Reducing blood sugar
    D. Increasing caloric intake

Answer Key

1. C	6. A
2. A	7. D
3. B	8. D
4. C	9. C
5. D	10. B

Answers and Explanations

1. (C) The process of digestion begins in the mouth as the food is chewed and continues through the digestive tract.

2. (A) Water is more important to the body than nutrients such as protein, carbohydrates, or fats. An individual can survive without food for longer than he or she could survive without water.

3. (B) Fats break down more slowly in the body than either protein or carbohydrates. Complex carbohydrates break down more slowly than simple carbohydrates, but not as slowly as protein and fats.

4. (C) The mineral selenium is included among the antioxidants, along with vitamin E, vitamin C, and beta-carotene.

5. (D) A patient with rickets is most likely to have a deficiency of vitamin D. A deficiency of vitamin A causes night blindness, whereas a deficiency of vitamin B1 (thiamine) causes beriberi. A deficiency of vitamin C causes scurvy.

6. (A) During digestion, protein breaks down into amino acids. Carbohydrates break down into sugar or glucose, and fats break down into fatty acids and glycerol.

7. (D) The gallbladder is responsible for secreting bile into the small intestine in the process of digestion. Bile is produced in the liver and stored in the gallbladder until it is required for digestion.

8. (D) Cholesterol levels can be reduced by dietary intake of monounsaturated fats, such as those found in avocados and olive oil. B and C are incorrect, because cholesterol levels are increased by both saturated fats and trans fats. Trans fats are created through a process known as hydrogenation, in which hydrogen is added to vegetable oils to help the oils last longer.

9. (C) A goiter is most likely to be caused by an iodine deficiency. Osteoporosis is caused by calcium deficiency; scurvy is caused by a lack of vitamin C, and pellagra is caused by a lack of niacin or the amino acid tryptophan.

10. (B) A patient with heart failure would most likely be instructed to maintain a low-sodium diet to assist with reducing blood pressure. Limiting carbohydrate intake would most likely assist with reducing blood sugar, so choice C is incorrect.

CHAPTER 24

Population Growth and Decline

Population Growth and Decline questions test your knowledge of factors that affect how population growth increases and decreases over time. You may be tested on your understanding of key population terms, as well as the impact of immigration and emigration. You may also encounter questions concerning population studies models and factors affecting birth and death rates.

Key Population Terms

Five important population terms to know are population growth, population decline, zero population growth, crude birth rate, and crude death rate.

At any given time, the population of an area may be in one of three stages: growing, declining, or remaining the same. **Population growth** occurs when the number of people being born or moving into the population outpaces the number of people dying or moving out of the population. **Population decline** occurs when the reverse happens: the number of people dying or moving away is greater than the number of people being born or moving in.

Populations also encounter periods of stability, when there is neither growth nor decline. **Zero population growth** occurs when the number of births plus the number of people moving into the population is roughly equal to the number of deaths combined with the number of people moving out of the population. Under conditions of zero population growth, the size of the population remains about the same.

Estimates of population growth and decline are often based on comparisons of crude birth rates and crude death rates. The **crude birth rate** of a population is the number of births that occur for every 1,000 individuals in a given year. The **crude death rate** is the number of deaths that occur for every 1,000 persons in a year.

Impact of Immigration and Emigration

As we saw in the definitions above, population growth and decline are not influenced only by the numbers of births and deaths in a population. They are also affected by the number of individuals who move into or out of a population in a given time frame. The process of population movement, broadly speaking, is known as **migration**. **Immigration** is the term for the process of individuals moving into a population, and **emigration** is the term for the process of individuals moving out of a population.

Migration levels within a population can be affected by two kinds of factors, known as push and pull factors. **Push factors** are those that cause migration by pushing emigrants out of a certain area. Economic hardship, religious persecution, and political strife are all examples of push factors. **Pull factors**, by contrast, are those that cause migration by pulling emigrants into a certain area. Economic opportunities, religious tolerance, and political freedom are all examples of pull factors.

The Demographic Transition Model

In population studies, societal growth and decline rates may be predicted through the use of the **demographic transition model**. This model postulates that a particular level of growth or decline will occur based on the stage of a country's economic development. The four stages of the demographic transition model are as follows:

Stage One. Societies have little or no technological advances. Birth rates and death rates are both high, so population growth is slow and varied.

Stage Two. Societies begin to advance technologically and economically. Birth rates continue to be high, but death rates fall. Population growth increases.

Stage Three. Societies become economically developed. Birth rates fall, and death rates continue to fall. Population growth slows down.

Stage Four. Societies have been economically developed for some time. Birth rates and death rates fall to low levels. Population growth stops.

Factors Affecting Fertility Rates

Birth rates, or **fertility rates**, can be reduced by the following:

- Birth control

- Education provided to women

- Political recognition of women

- Societal restrictions on family size

- Industrialization and automation

As each of these factors increases, birth rates tend to decrease. Societies become more technologically advanced and have less need to rely on individuals for labor, at the same time as resource concerns cause couples to limit the number of children they have.

Factors Affecting Mortality Rates

Death rates, or **mortality rates**, can be reduced by advances in the following:

- Medical treatment
- Water and sewage sanitation
- Agriculture and food production
- Transportation systems
- Construction technology

As societies experience improvements in each of these areas, mortality rates tend to grow smaller. Societies are better able to treat medical conditions or to prevent them altogether through good hygiene and balanced nutrition. Advances in transportation and construction enable more members of the populace to live in adequate housing, reducing deaths due to natural disasters or extreme climates.

Review Questions

1. Which of the following is true of mortality rates?

   A. They are lower in less-developed countries.
   B. They are higher in more-developed countries.
   C. They are higher in less-developed countries.
   D. They are approximately equal in more-developed and less-developed countries.

2. In which of the following stages of the demographic transition model is a country's population likely to be most stable?

   A. Stage One
   B. Stage Two
   C. Stage Three
   D. Stage Four

3. A country in Stage Three of the demographic transition model is most likely to be characterized by which of the following?

   A. Falling birth rates
   B. Rising birth rates
   C. Rising death rates
   D. Zero population growth

4. Which of the following occurs when the number of births plus the number of immigrants to an area exceeds the number of deaths plus the number of emigrants from the area?

   A. Reverse migration
   B. Zero population growth
   C. Population decline
   D. Population growth

5. Advances in medical treatment are most likely to lead to which of the following?

   A. Reduced mortality rates in less-developed countries
   B. Reduced fertility rates in less-developed countries
   C. Increased immigration to less-developed countries
   D. Increased emigration from more-developed countries

6. A country is beginning to advance both technologically and economically. Its birth rates are high, but its death rates have fallen dramatically, and its population growth has soared as a result. Which stage of the demographic transition model most likely describes this country?

   A. Stage One
   B. Stage Two
   C. Stage Three
   D. Stage Four

7. A population's crude birth rate is based on the number of births that occur for every _____ individuals in a given year.

   Which of the following correctly completes the sentence above?
   A. 1
   B. 10
   C. 100
   D. 1,000

8. An individual who moves to an area to establish permanent residence is knows as which of the following?

   A. Immigrant
   B. Emigrant
   C. Refugee
   D. Expatriate

9. Approximately 2.6 million immigrants of European descent entered the United States during the 1850s, the peak immigration decade in U.S. history. In this decade, the United States most likely experienced which of the following?

A. Fluctuating growth and decline
B. Rapid population decline
C. Rapid population growth
D. Zero population growth

10. Which of the following factors might be most likely to cause a country to experience population decline?

A. Increased fertility rates due to improved nutrition and food production
B. Increased mortality rates due to a widespread illness, such as the plague
C. Reduced infant mortality rates due to the availability of prenatal care
D. Reduced emigration due to the country's refusal to issue travel visas

Answer Key

1. C		**6.** B	
2. D		**7.** D	
3. A		**8.** A	
4. D		**9.** C	
5. A		**10.** B	

Answers and Explanations

1. (C) Mortality rates are higher in less-developed countries, which lack the technological and economic advances necessary to prevent deaths due to hunger, disease, and harsh weather conditions.

2. (D) In Stage Four of the demographic transition model, a country is likely to have zero population growth. Choice A is incorrect because countries in Stage One of the model may see some population growth, albeit very slow.

3. (A) In Stage Three of the demographic transition model, societies become economically developed. Birth rates fall, and death rates continue to fall. Population growth slows down as well.

4. (D) Population growth occurs when the number of people being born or moving into an area (immigrating) outpaces the number of people dying or moving out of the area (emigrating).

5. (A) Advances in medical treatment are most likely to lead to reduced mortality rates in less-developed countries. As medical treatment options improve, individuals are less likely to die from diseases or infection. Birth rates

would be likely to improve in less-developed countries, so choice B is incorrect.

6. (B) Stage Two of the demographic transition model is characterized by initial societal advancement, both technologically and economically. Birth rates continue to be high, but death rates fall. Population growth increases as a result.

7. (D) The crude birth rate of a population is the number of births that occur for every 1,000 individuals in a given year.

8. (A) An individual who moves to an area to establish permanent residence is knows as an *immigrant*. Choice B is incorrect, because *emigrants* are individuals who move away from an area. Choice C is incorrect, because *refugees* are individuals who are forced to leave an area due to violence, persecution, or other unsafe conditions. Choice D is incorrect, because *expatriates* are individuals who leave their native country.

9. (C) The United States experienced rapid population growth in the 1850s due in part to the large wave of European immigrants entering the country at that time.

10. (B) A country with increased mortality rates due to a widespread illness would be most likely to experience a population decline. A country with increased fertility rates would be likely to experience population growth, as would a country with reduced infant mortality rates, so choices A and C are incorrect.

CHAPTER 25

Taxonomy

Taxonomy questions on the TEAS address the structure and hierarchy of the scientific taxonomic classification system.

Taxonomic Classification

All living organisms on Earth are classified. Taxonomy is the classification process by which organisms are named and organized. They are classified in a hierarchy according to their shared features. Scientists use **species** as the basic unit of organization in taxonomy. A **species** can be generally defined as a population that is able to produce offspring; although scientists debate the exact definition of species, the one provided here is the commonly accepted biological definition.

Structure

Rather than use the common names of plants and animals to classify plants and animals, scientists use a two-name Latin system—a binomial (two-word) nomenclature developed by Carl Linnaeus. So, instead of saying *dog*, scientists might use the term *Canis familiaris*. The first name is the **genus**, which is capitalized, and the second name is the **species**, which is not capitalized. Both the genus and the species are either underlined or italicized. There are rules developed and followed for naming in specific scientific communities so that all community members are using the same nomenclature for organisms—this helps to eliminate confusion. There are, however, no hard-and-fast rules for determining classification at each level except that each descending level becomes more specific in grouping organisms according to shared characteristics. For example, a chimpanzee and a human share many similar characteristics and classifications until they are separated at the genus and species level, where they are divided into *Pan troglodytes*, chimpanzees, and *Homo sapiens*, humans.

Hierarchy

Within the classification system, there is a hierarchy as shown in the diagram below. Most organisms can be classified into these seven levels.

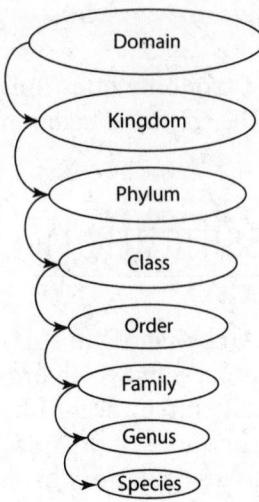

Each of the levels is classified by certain characteristics. The animal or plant is classified as a certain type based on its characteristics and then labeled as such. As each grouping is split, the organisms become more similar. For example:

- The **domain** indicates the characteristics of an organism at the most basic level. This is the broadest classification level and includes only cellular life, not viruses.

- The **kingdom** indicates the cell type, the ability to ingest food, and the number of cells in the body. Originally, there were only two kingdoms: Plant and Animal. Now, however, there are six accepted kingdoms: Plants, Animals, Archaebacteria, Eubacteria, Fungi, and Protists.

- **Phylum** is the division of organisms based on the degree to which they are similar in body plan. For example, in the animal kingdom, organisms are divided into vertebrates and invertebrates. There are 20 different classifications for phyla in the animal kingdom and 10 in the plant kingdom.

- **Class** is another, more specific division based on common traits organisms share.

- **Order** is a further classification based on common traits.

- A **family** is more precise than an order. This classification groups organisms together that have descended from the same ancestor and reflect similar characteristics. Common names are used for family classifications. For example, a particular nut may be part of the walnut family. A family may contain one or more **genus** or **genera**.

- The **genus** makes up the first part of an organism's name. The organisms on this level share similar physical and behavioral characteristics.

- **Species** is the most basic unit of life used for classification and makes up the second part of the organism's name. Members of a species share many common genes; however, they are not identical, as there are variations within the group.

As scientists find and add new information, *sub* or *super* classifications may be added to the order to further identify organisms. Bacteria, for example, have many subspecies that further divide and classify the organisms. Scientists are also using DNA to substantiate current evolutionary relationships and to identify new ones.

The Taxonomy of Humans

Domain	Eukarya
Kingdom	Animalia
Phylum	Chordata
Subphylum	Vertebrata
Superclass	Tetrapoda
Class	Mammalia
Subclass	Theria
Order	Primates
Family	Hominidae
Genus	*Homo*
Species	*sapiens*

Review Questions

1. What is the purpose of using a specific nomenclature to classify organisms?

    A. It ensures that English will be properly used and understood by all scientists within the field.
    B. It helps to alleviate any confusion in identifying organisms.
    C. Darwin's theory of evolution requires specific names at specific levels in the biological taxonomy.
    D. It creates a coding system so that scientists can be discreet when they have new discoveries.

2. *Lithobates catesbianus*, more commonly known as the bullfrog, belongs to which genus?

   A. *L. catesbianus*
   B. *catesbianus*
   C. *Lithobates*
   D. *L.C.*

3. In the taxonomic ranks, two organisms that are part of the same genus but are *not* part of the same species could be a part of which other level or levels?

   A. Only family and kingdom
   B. Only family
   C. Only genus
   D. All but species

4. What is indicated by adding a *sub* or *super* in front of a classification?

   A. It means that the classification is worse or better than the previous level.
   B. It indicates there has been a defective mutation.
   C. It shows whether the organism is a plant or animal.
   D. It indicates further classification or division within a level.

5. In the taxonomy hierarchy, if the domain is the broadest classification, which of the following is the most specific?

   A. Kingdom
   B. Genus
   C. Species
   D. Family

6. One of the classifications of a chimpanzee is *Hominidae*. Which taxonomic rank does that mean it shares with humans?

   A. Domain
   B. Family
   C. Species
   D. Order

7. Which of the following is a characteristic of an organism that would define it as a species?

   A. Having the ability to produce viable offspring
   B. Being a vertebrate
   C. Having two genera
   D. Having the ability to walk on two legs

8. Determining whether an organism is an animal, plant, or fungus is decided first in which of the following classifications?

    A. Species
    B. Family
    C. Order
    D. Kingdom

9. To both support classifications identified through taxonomy and to determine new classifications, what are scientists now using to determine evolutionary relationships?

    A. An organism's relationship to humans
    B. DNA
    C. The organism's common names
    D. Environmental evidence

10. An organism is classified at the phylum level as *Chordata*. In order to determine the organism's class, one would need to do which of the following?

    A. Determine the kingdom classification
    B. Identify more specific characteristics
    C. Look at the name to identify the genus
    D. Perform genetic testing on the fossil of the organism

Answer Key

1.	B	**6.**	B
2.	C	**7.**	A
3.	D	**8.**	D
4.	D	**9.**	B
5.	C	**10.**	B

Answers and Explanations

1. (B) Using specific nomenclature in Latin creates a uniformity that reduces confusion that may be caused in translation. Scientists do not need to translate into different languages; they can use the Latin nomenclature universally.

2. (C) The genus can be determined by the first name in an organism's Latin nomenclature. The second uncapitalized name indicates the species. The organism's full name is the genus and the species.

3. (D) If organisms are part of the same genus but not the same species, then they share the same characteristics of all of the other levels except species. In order to share the same characteristics at the genus level, the organisms would have to share similar characteristics at higher levels as well.

4. (D) The delineation of *sub* or *super* simply indicates a further distinction within that level of taxonomy.

5. (C) The species is the most basic and smallest unit of classification. The hierarchy begins with the domain, the most general, and at each descending level becomes more specific in its classifications.

6. (B) *Hominidae* indicates the shared family characteristics as shown on the example of the human taxonomy chart. If two organisms are labeled the same at a particular level, such as the family level, they possess similar traits.

7. (A) A species can be defined by the characteristic that the organisms could produce viable offspring. Being a vertebrate, walking on two legs, or having two genera are all more broad characteristics that determine classification higher up in the hierarchy.

8. (D) Being classified as a plant, animal, or fungus is a broad definition and would lie near the top of the hierarchy. The kingdom is one of the first classifications, and organisms are narrowed as the classification descends the taxonomic hierarchy.

9. (B) Modern advances have allowed scientists to use DNA to further support observations that have previously determined the classifications of organisms. The organism's relationship to humans and its common name are irrelevant in its formal classification. The study of the organism's habitat is something that was previously done before modern science.

10. (B) The class is a more specific level of classification than the phylum. To determine the class, one would need to evaluate more specific characteristics.

CHAPTER 26

The Cell

TEAS questions concerning **the cell** test your understanding of the differences between prokaryote and eukaryote cells as well as the various parts of a cell. You may also be tested on your knowledge of cell reproduction, including the processes of mitosis and meiosis.

Cells and Life

Life takes many forms, from the simplicity of bacteria to the complexity of primates. According to **cell theory**, all living things are comprised of cells. Complex life forms have more cells and more complexity to their cell structure. Cell theory goes on to state that cells are the unit of function for organisms. They are responsible for life functions like digestion, circulation, reproduction, and immunity, among others.

The life cycle depends on two different types of organisms, autotrophs and heterotrophs. The word **autotroph** comes from the Greek language and means self-feeder. Autotrophs produce glucose through photosynthesis and feed themselves and other living beings. They are mainly plants. The prefix *hetero-* means different, so **heterotrophs** get their nutrition from outside sources. Animals eat plants and other animals to survive. The cell structures of autotrophs and heterotrophs differ.

Prokaryote and Eukaryote Cells

There are two basic types of cells that form the building blocks of all organisms, prokaryote and eukaryote cells. **Prokaryote** cells, shown in the figure below, are simpler, having no nucleus and lacking some of the complex organelles of eukaryotes. Their DNA is not tightly contained as in a eukaryote nucleus. Prokaryote cells are represented in two types of organisms, **bacteria** and **archaea**. Most organisms in these two groups are just a single cell with a **flagellum** for movement. They replicate themselves through a process called **binary fission** in which they split apart, creating two exact copies of the same cell.

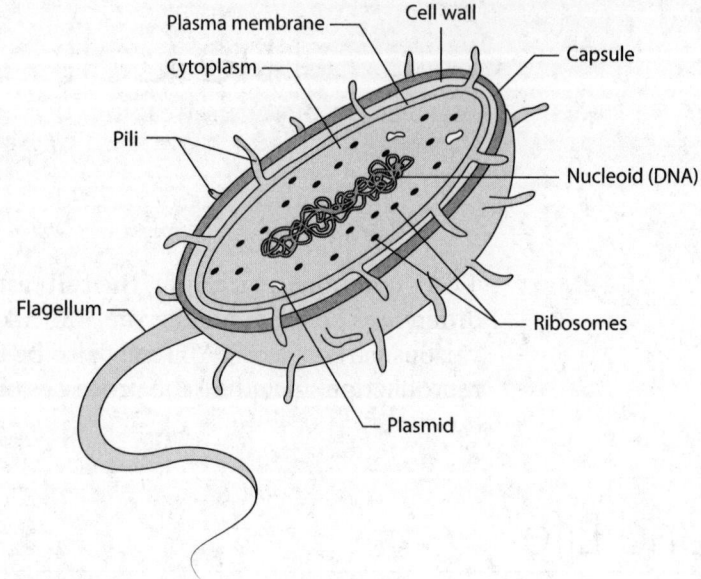

Eukaryote cells are present in almost all of the abundance of life visible to the eye, from plants and animals to fungi and even some bacteria. They have membrane-covered organelles, including a nucleus that holds the cell's DNA. They reproduce through either mitosis or meiosis.

Parts of the Cell

A typical animal cell, shown below, is filled with **cytoplasm** within a **cell membrane**. The cell membrane allows select substances (proteins, enzymes, and chemicals) to pass through while keeping others out. Resting in the cytoplasm are various organelles. Organelles serve to regulate the metabolic functions of the cell.

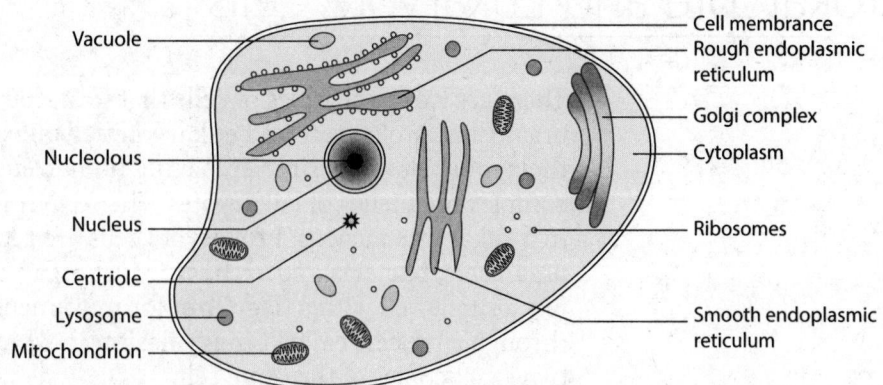

The **nucleus** is the control center of the cell and contains the **nucleolus**. The cell's DNA is contained in the nucleus, and it delivers information to control the metabolic functions of the cell. The nucleolus produces **ribosomes**. Ribosomes are found throughout the cell and synthesize proteins.

The **mitochondrion** is the energy center of the cell where glucose and oxygen are broken down into water and carbon dioxide. As a result of breaking these chemical bonds, energy in the form of adenosine triphosphate (ATP) is produced.

The **endoplasmic reticulum** of a cell is a membrane where proteins, the building blocks of cellular life, are built and stored. **Rough endoplasmic reticulum** has ribosomes attached, whereas **smooth endoplasmic reticulum** has none. Working with the **Golgi complex,** or **Golgi apparatus**, the endoplasmic reticulum assembles proteins and makes structures with those proteins.

Centrioles are organelles that assist in cell reproduction, either mitosis or meiosis.

Lysosomes capture the products of cellular function that the cell cannot use. They break down this cellular waste.

Plant Cells

Plant cells are similar to animal cells in most respects. They have all the same organelles, but they also have a **cell wall** and contain **chloroplasts**. Chloroplasts are organelles that aid in photosynthesis, through which plants use water, carbon dioxide, and the sun's energy to create glucose and oxygen.

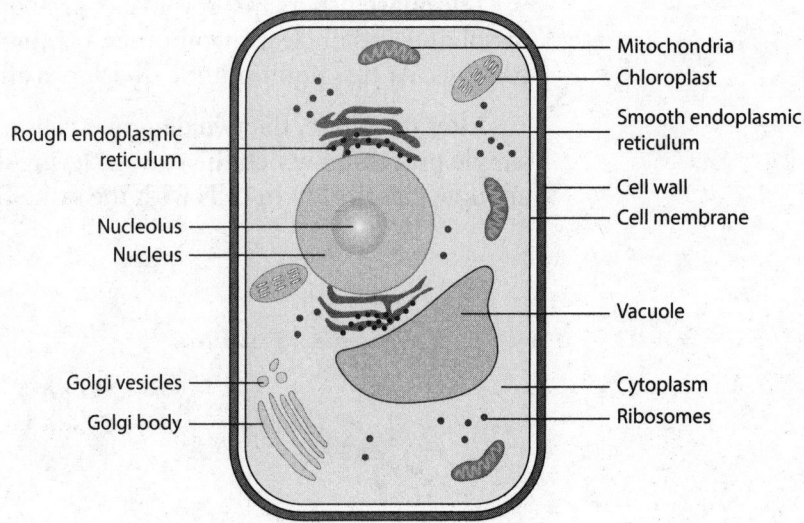

Cell Reproduction

Cells proliferate in two ways, through mitosis or meiosis. **Mitosis** is the way that cells proliferate through asexual reproduction. In mitosis, cells reproduce an exact copy of themselves.

Meiosis is how cells reproduce through sexual reproduction. In this case, each daughter cell has half of the DNA of the original cell. In sexual reproduction, the daughter cells combine with such cells from another individual to form offspring, leading to genetic variation.

Cells that are thriving and conducting metabolic functions are considered to be in **interphase**. During interphase, cells' energy expenditure goes to the function of the organism.

Mitosis

Mitosis, shown in the following figure, occurs when a cell duplicates itself. This can happen in single-cell organisms, like protozoa or bacteria, and is how they reproduce. It also happens in other living organisms when they grow or heal. New cells are created with the same DNA as the original cells.

When more cells are needed or a sexual stimulus is introduced, chromosomes and centrioles are replicated.

Prophase is the first phase of mitosis. In this phase, the nuclear membrane dissolves, allowing the doubled chromosomes to float freely. Spindle fibers congregate around structures known as centrosomes to produce a spindle apparatus, which separates the floating DNA into separate poles.

Metaphase sees an orientation of the spindle apparatus, drawn by the centrosomes, to push the DNA to opposite ends of the cell.

During **anaphase**, spindle fibers retract, again influenced by the centrosomes, pulling apart chromosomes into their v-shaped halves.

Telophase ushers in a reversal of previous processes, with spindle fibers dissolving and nuclear membranes forming around the new chromosome pairings. At this point mitotic division is all but complete.

After telophase, the two daughter cells undergo **cytokinesis.** This is a simple process in which the two nuclei are divided by cell membranes. There are now identical twin cells with the same DNA ready for interphase.

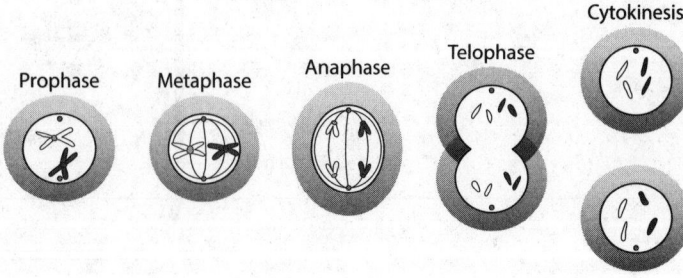

Prophase Metaphase Anaphase Telophase Cytokinesis

Meiosis

Meiosis, shown in the following figure, is a more complex process than mitosis. Cells in meiosis go through two rounds of prophase, metaphase, anaphase, and telophase. These two stages are called **meiosis I** and **meiosis II**.

Prophase I is similar to mitotic prophase in that the nuclear membrane disappears, allowing chromosomes from each parent to mingle. In this case, chromosomes perform a crossing-over in which similar chromosomes from each parent bundle together. An allele from one parent may replace an allele from another, causing genetic variation.

Metaphase I, **anaphase I**, and **telophase I** mimic their mitotic counterparts. The new chromosomal pairings, called **tetrads**, migrate, and cytokinesis begins creating two **diploid** cells containing a full, but unique, complement of mixed DNA (46 chromosomes in humans). These two daughter cells then begin the process of meiosis II.

Prophase II, metaphase II, anaphase II, and telophase II mirror the previous process. Centrosomes and spindle fibers push apart chromosomes. When the spindle fibers retract, chromosomes are pulled apart. When telophase II begins, each daughter nucleus has only one of each pair of chromosomes (23 chromosomes rather than 46 in humans). The result is four **haploid** cells, or **gametes**.

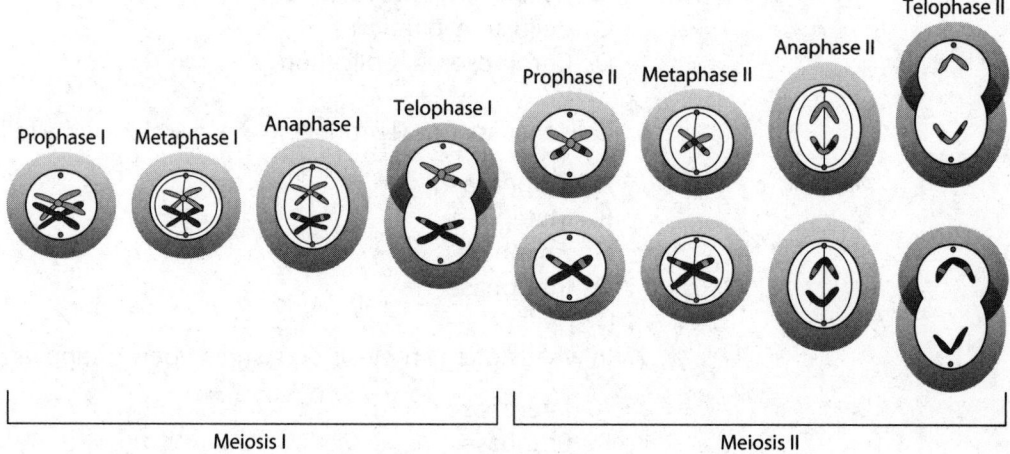

Review Questions

1. A cell reproduces itself through binary fission rather than mitosis or meiosis. What kind of cell is it?

A. Prokaryote

B. Eukaryote

C. Gamete

D. Haploid

2. Which of the following is not contained within the cell membrane of a eukaryote cell?

A. Nucleus
B. Cytoplasm
C. Ribosomes
D. Flagellum

3. Which organelle works in concert with the endoplasmic reticulum to produce other organelles?

A. Centriole
B. Lysosome
C. Golgi complex
D. Cytoplasm

4. What is the function of the nucleolus?

A. Ribosome production
B. Protein storage
C. Cellular respiration
D. Reproduction

5. What is the function of lysosomes?

A. Protein transport
B. Cellular waste breakdown
C. Cellular respiration
D. Chromosome replication

6. Cells that are not reproducing are in which of the following states?

A. Prophase
B. Metaphase
C. Anaphase
D. Interphase

7. In what stage of meiosis do spindle fibers disappear?

A. Interphase
B. Prophase
C. Metaphase
D. Telophase

8. The stages of mitosis are interphase, _____ , metaphase, _____ , and telophase. These are followed by a new interphase.

Which of the following correctly completes the sentence above?

A. Prophase; anaphase
B. Interphase; prophase
C. Anaphase; cytokinesis
D. Cytokinesis; glycolysis

9. At the end of meiosis I, in what state is the original cell?

    A. Two haploid cells
    B. Four haploid cells
    C. Two diploid cells
    D. Four diploid cells

10. In which phase of meiosis does genetic variation take place?

    A. Prophase I
    B. Anaphase I
    C. Metaphase II
    D. Telophase II

Answer Key

1. A	**6.** D
2. D	**7.** D
3. C	**8.** A
4. A	**9.** C
5. B	**10.** A

Answers and Explanations

1. (A) Prokaryote cells lack a nucleus. Both mitosis and meiosis begin with DNA replication in the nucleus. Binary fission is the manner in which prokaryote cells divide into two distinct but identical cells.

2. (D) The flagellum exists outside the cell membrane of single-cell organisms. These are predominately prokaryotes.

3. (C) The Golgi complex, or apparatus, uses the proteins created by the endoplasmic reticulum to build new organelles and other cellular structures.

4. (A) The nucleus contains the DNA of the cell. Within the nucleus, the nucleolus produces ribosomes, which help in protein production.

5. (B) Lysosomes capture and break down the unneeded by-products of metabolic activity, or cellular waste.

6. (D) Interphase is the name of the state that cells occupy when they are performing normal metabolic functions. DNA may be replicating in preparation for cell reproduction, but the cell is not undergoing either mitosis or meiosis.

7. (D) The last stage of meiosis I and meiosis II is telophase. The spindle apparatus has done its job of separating and orienting the chromosomes. It now dissolves to allow the cell to enter interphase and its normal metabolic functions.

8. (A) The four stages of mitosis, in order, are prophase, metaphase, anaphase, and telophase. Cytokinesis happens after the mitotic cycle, while glycolysis takes place during cellular respiration.

9. (C) At the end of meiosis I, the chromosomes have crossed over and then migrated to the poles. Nuclear membranes have formed around the DNA creating two diploid cells, cells with 46 chromosomes.

10. (A) In meiosis, genetic variation happens in the first phase, prophase I. The two sets of chromosomes recombine through crossing over. Homologous alleles match up, creating genetic variation.

CHAPTER 27

Respiration vs. Photosynthesis

Respiration vs. Photosynthesis questions on the TEAS test your ability to distinguish between these two types of processes.

Converting the Energy of the Sun

Photosynthesis and cellular respiration form a complementary system through which plants and animals use the sun's energy to power their own life cycles. In a nutshell, green plants, some algae, and bacteria perform photosynthesis, turning the sun's energy, water, and carbon dioxide into glucose and oxygen. Animals and other organisms convert energy in the opposite direction on the cellular level. They take glucose and oxygen to create carbon dioxide.

Green plants are **autotrophs**, organisms that feed themselves. Photosynthesis allows them to create glucose, and respiration allows them to convert it back to energy. Animals are **heterotrophs**. They must eat food in the form of plants or other animals to get their energy. Animals rely on green plants not only for sustenance but also for the oxygen-rich atmosphere in which they thrive. Conversely, plants benefit from the release of carbon dioxide. Without the sun's energy, neither plants nor animals would have the energy to live.

ATP: Cellular Energy

ATP, or **adenosine triphosphate**, is one of the products of both photosynthesis and cellular respiration. In fact, it could be considered the purpose for these processes. ATP is a molecule that exists in a high-energy state and is essential for all of the processes that keep organisms functioning. Some scientists even call ATP the "currency of life." Like money, it is transferable to any situation. When chemical bonds are broken, through respiration or photosynthesis, excess energy is stored in ATP molecules. These are then used as energy for future processes.

ATP is created through one of three pathways. **Glycolysis**, which occurs in the cytoplasm, breaks down glucose ($C_6H_{12}O_6$) into pyruvic acid ($C_3H_4O_3$) and several waste by-products. In the process, **ADP**, or **adenosine diphosphate**, is transformed into ATP with energy stored in an easily broken phosphate bond. The **Krebs cycle**, occurring in the mitochondria, takes pyruvic acid, which is formed through glycolysis, and breaks it down, further squeezing out more ATP. Finally, the **electron transport chain**, occurring in the mitochondrial membrane, creates even more ATP. Through a process called chemiosmosis, by-products from the Krebs cycle are pushed through the mitochondrial membrane and transformed into more ATP.

Components of Respiration

When we think of respiration, we think of breathing, but that is respiration on a macro scale. Cellular respiration happens on a very small scale—within the cells of a living organism.

Cells receive inputs of glucose and oxygen. In a human, for example, glucose is received when the person eats food. The food is then broken down through digestion into its constituent parts: amino acids, glucose, and fatty acids. These parts can pass through cell membranes to be used by cells for different functions. Glucose is necessary for cellular respiration. Oxygen is the other reactant in respiration. Glucose can also be broken down without oxygen in a process known as **fermentation**.

Respiration on the cellular level takes place in the mitochondria of the cell (see figure). These organelles acts like the stomach of the cell, digesting inputs and sending out energy and by-products. The inputs are oxygen (O_2) and glucose ($C_6H_{12}O_6$). When the chemical bonds of the inputs are broken, the energy stored within is released in the form of ATP. ATP is then available as an energy source for the cell. The by-products are water (H_2O) and carbon dioxide (CO_2), which is breathed out into the air.

$$6O_2 + C_6H_{12}O_6 \rightarrow 6CO_2 + 6H_2O \text{ and ATP}$$

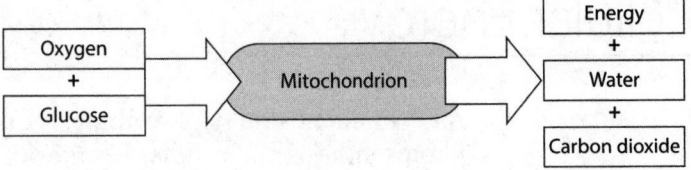

Components of Photosynthesis

Photosynthesis occurs in green plants, some bacteria, and algae. The **chloroplast** is the organelle in plant cells responsible for the process. Inside the chloroplast is **chlorophyll**, a pigment that gives plants their green color.

In fact, chlorophyll reflects light from the green part of the light spectrum. That means that light from the blue and red parts of the spectrum are absorbed and are more effective in photosynthesis.

Chlorophyll is responsible for capturing the sun's energy (see figure). When the cell also has sufficient water and carbon dioxide as reactants, it has the building blocks of glucose. While the cell catches energy in the chemical bonds of the glucose, oxygen is created as a by-product. Both oxygen and glucose are used in cellular respiration to unlock the energy held within.

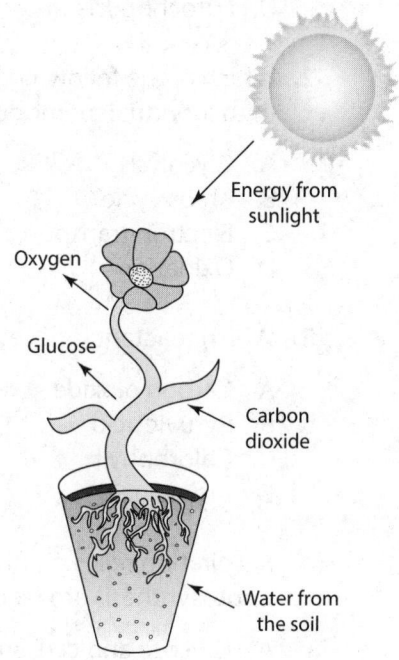

Energy from sunlight

Oxygen

Glucose

Carbon dioxide

Water from the soil

Differences Between Respiration and Photosynthesis

Respiration and photosynthesis sound similar, but they have several important differences. Photosynthesis occurs only in green plants, certain bacteria, and algae. This is because chlorophyll is necessary for photosynthesis and is present in such cells. Cellular respiration occurs in the cells of all living things, including plants. In photosynthesis, **light photons** fuel the process. In respiration, the energy comes from the breaking of chemical bonds. Photosynthesis traps energy, whereas respiration releases it. The by-products of each process are necessary for the functioning of the other. All in all, these two processes form a simple but elegant system.

Review Questions

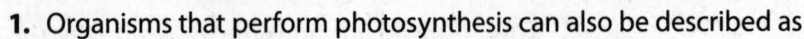

1. Organisms that perform photosynthesis can also be described as
   _____.

   Which of the following correctly completes the sentence above?

   A. Autotrophs
   B. Heterotrophs
   C. Animals
   D. Mitochondria

2. Which of the following substages of ATP production occurs in the
   mitochondrial membrane?

   A. Glycolysis
   B. Krebs cycle
   C. Electron transport chain
   D. Oxidation

3. Which reactant is necessary for the production of ATP in the Krebs cycle?

   A. Carbon dioxide
   B. Pyruvic acid
   C. Chlorophyll
   D. Amino acid

4. Respiration relies on photosynthesis for its inputs. Which by-products of
   photosynthesis are reactants in cellular respiration?

   A. Glucose and carbon dioxide
   B. Water and sugar
   C. Oxygen and sugar
   D. Chlorophyll and nitrogen

5. What is the end result of the chemical process of $6O_2 + C_6H_{12}O_6$ other than
   the production of ATP?

   A. $3O_2 + 3H_2O + 3CO_2$
   B. $6CO_2 + 6H_2O$
   C. $C_6H_{12}O_{12} + 3O_2$
   D. $6H_2O + C_6$

6. The organelle responsible for photosynthesis is the _____.

   Which of the following correctly completes the sentence above?

   A. Chloroplast
   B. Chlorophyll
   C. Mitochondrion
   D. Cytoplasm

7. The mitochondrion is the organelle responsible for _____.

Which of the following correctly completes the sentence above?

A. Protein production
B. Fermentation
C. Photosynthesis
D. Cellular respiration

8. In photosynthesis, light photons provide energy to the cell. Where does the energy come from in cellular respiration?

A. Fermentation
B. Carbon dioxide
C. Light from the blue spectrum
D. The breaking of chemical bonds

9. Cellular respiration differs from photosynthesis in that it occurs in _____.

Which of the following correctly completes the sentence above?

A. Heterotrophs only
B. Green plants and algae only
C. Chloroplasts
D. All living things

10. Green plants appear green because _____ reflects _____ from the color spectrum.

Which of the following correctly completes the sentence above?

A. A mitochondrion; red and blue light
B. Chlorophyll; green light
C. Cellulose; ATP
D. H_2O; a photon of light

Answer Key

1. A

2. C

3. B

4. C

5. B

6. A

7. D

8. D

9. D

10. B

Answers and Explanations

1. (A) Autotrophs, such as green plants, bacteria, and algae, perform photosynthesis to create their own sugars. They can then retrieve the energy through cellular respiration and feed themselves in this way.

2. (C) The three substages of ATP production are glycolysis, the Krebs cycle, and the electron transport chain. Glycolysis occurs in cytoplasm, the Krebs cycle occurs within the mitochondrion itself, and the electron transport chain occurs in the mitochondrial membrane.

3. (B) The Krebs cycle, which occurs in the mitochondria, takes pyruvic acid and transforms it into ATP and by-products.

4. (C) The main by-products of photosynthesis are glucose, or sugar, and oxygen. Both inputs are needed for cellular respiration to take place.

5. (B) $C_6H_{12}O_6$ is glucose. O_2 is oxygen. These are the inputs for cellular respiration. The by-products, other than ATP, are water (H_2O) and carbon dioxide (CO_2). Six molecules of oxygen are needed for each molecule of glucose to produce six molecules of water and six of carbon dioxide.

6. (A) The chloroplast is the organelle in which photosynthesis happens. Chlorophyll is the pigment in the chloroplasts that captures the sun's photons.

7. (D) Cellular respiration occurs in the mitochondria of the cell. This is where glucose and oxygen are broken down to extract ATP. The by-products are water and carbon dioxide.

8. (D) In photosynthesis, the sun's energy is stored in chemical bonds in glucose molecules. Cellular respiration breaks the chemical bonds to release the energy in the form of ATP. The ATP is then used for metabolic functions.

9. (D) All living things, including both autotrophs and heterotrophs, produce energy through cellular respiration. Autotrophs get their energy from cellular respiration. Heterotrophs differ in that they capture the sun's energy. They must also release it to use it for their own functions.

10. (B) Chlorophyll is a pigment in a plant cell. As with anything visible, it reflects the color of the spectrum that creates its own hue. So, chlorophyll reflects the green part of the color spectrum.

CHAPTER 28

DNA and RNA

TEAS questions concerning **DNA and RNA** cover topics including the components of DNA and RNA, nitrogenous bases, and base pairs. You may also see questions concerning transcription and translation.

Functions

Every living organism has instructions for growth in the form of **DNA** and **RNA**. DNA stands for **deoxyribonucleic acid**. RNA stands for **ribonucleic acid**. RNA comes in different forms, such as **mRNA** (messenger RNA), **tRNA** (transfer RNA), and **rRNA** (ribosomal RNA). DNA, the larger molecule, stores genetic information for the organism as a whole. It contains the code for creating new cells and is essential for the creation of new organisms during reproduction. RNA is smaller. In fact, it is created from the nucleic acids in DNA. Its function is to help in the creation of proteins and amino acids, and it is found in ribosomes. It also acts as a messenger carrying genetic information around a cell and beyond.

Chromosomes, Amino Acids, and Proteins

Chromosomes are strands of DNA and related proteins that reside in the nuclei of living cells. They carry the genetic information needed to create new cells and organisms. **Amino acids** are the building blocks of organic material. They are produced by RNA as the building materials for **proteins**, which in turn are the content of cells and cellular organs. Proteins make up enzymes, which carry out the work of cellular life, like metabolic functions. Proteins also make up polymerases, which transcribe and transfer genetic material.

Nucleic Acids

Complex compounds that are present in all organic cells, **nucleic acids** are the core units of life. Both DNA and RNA are nucleic acids. A nucleic acid is composed of **nucleotides**. Nucleotides are **nucleosides** together with a phosphate group. Nucleosides are sugars (ribose or deoxyribose) combined with either a **purine** or a **pyrimidine**.

Nitrogenous Bases

The five nitrogenous bases, **adenine (A)**, **guanine (G)**, **cytosine (C)**, **thymine (T)**, and **uracil (U)**, are needed to make nucleotides. The sequence in which they appear allows genetic information to be stored in DNA and RNA. This information comes in three nucleotide groupings called **codons**. They are written as three letters, for example CAG, to show which nitrogenous bases they are composed of. With four nitrogenous bases, this leads to a possible 64 combinations of three letters in different orders.

Purines and Pyrimidines

Purine bases, adenine and guanine, are bicyclic. Pyrimidine bases, cytosine and thymine, are monocyclic. Uracil is a form of thymine that replaces this pyrimidine in RNA. They form **hydrogen bonds** in a complementary fashion, meaning that a purine always pairs with a pyrimidine.

Base Pairs

Purines and pyrimidines have different structures that allow them to form hydrogen bonds, crucial for the formation of DNA. One purine, guanine, bonds with a pyrimidine, cytosine. This is one of the **base pairs** discovered by Watson and Crick. The other is adenine and thymine. These base pairs are held together by hydrogen bonds. Cytosine bonds with guanine using three hydrogen bonds, while adenine and thymine require only two hydrogen bonds. These bonds connect the **double helix** of DNA. These codons contain instruction for building amino acids, necessary for building organic structures.

Differences Between DNA and RNA

There are many minor differences between DNA and RNA. The major difference is their function. DNA stores and transmits genetic information for use on a cellular and organismic level. RNA transcribes and translates the genetic information into physical structures. DNA relies on four nitrogenous bases—(A) adenine, (G) guanine, (C) cytosine, and (T) thymine—whereas in RNA, (T) is replaced by (U) uracil. DNA has two strands of nucleic acid, referred to as a double helix due to its physical shape. This doubling of genetic information plays a crucial role in genetic diversity during reproduction. RNA has a single strand.

DNA comes in different forms. Mitochondrial DNA, for example, is only inherited from the mother. RNA also has different forms, such as mRNA (messenger RNA), tRNA (transfer RNA), and rRNA (ribosomal RNA).

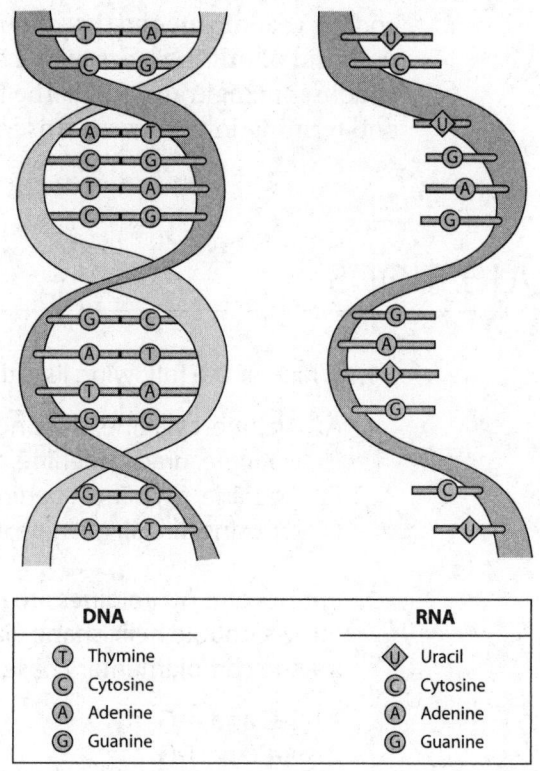

DNA		RNA	
T	Thymine	U	Uracil
C	Cytosine	C	Cytosine
A	Adenine	A	Adenine
G	Guanine	G	Guanine

Transcription

DNA contains all of the genetic information necessary to create living cells and organisms. **Transcription** is the process through which this genetic information is copied to make RNA (see figure). RNA polymerase, an enzyme created from a strand of RNA, binds with a DNA sequence during the initiation phase. This binding loosens the hydrogen bonds holding the double helix together. The bound section elongates with the addition of nucleotides. Proteins called **transcription factors** provide the needed material. The process terminates with a genetic duplicate strand of mRNA being released into the cell.

Translation

At some point, genes must do their work. They contain the instructions for building amino acids and proteins and larger cellular bodies. **Translation** is the process through which that information is put into reality. Translation means making a protein. The first step in translation is transcription. After the cell's genetic code is transcribed to an mRNA molecule, the information within is unlocked in the **ribosomes**. Ribosomes are situated in the cytoplasm of a cell or in the endoplasmic reticulum and are the cell's factories for producing proteins. The mRNA carries the three base pair codons that dictate the type of amino acid needed for a particular protein. A strand of mRNA pairs with a strand of tRNA, carrying complementary codons, during translation. The three-phase process of initiation, elongation, and termination mirrors transcription, but it produces an amino acid.

Review Questions

1. Which of the following lists the four nitrogenous bases found in RNA?

   A. Alanine, cysteine, threonine, glycine (A, C, T, G)
   B. Guanine, uracil, adenine, cytosine (G, U, A, C)
   C. Adenine, thymine, guanine, cytosine (A, T, G, C)
   D. Cytosine, uracil, guanine, thymine (C, U, G, T)

2. Purines and pyrimidines are nitrogenous bases that allow DNA to form into its double helix shape via hydrogen bonding. Which of the following are the complementary base pairs that form DNA?

   A. T-C and A-G
   B. A-C and T-G
   C. G-C and A-T
   D. A-U and G-C

3. DNA is composed of which of the following substances?

   A. Nucleotides
   B. Cells
   C. Neurons
   D. Proteins

4. Which of the following is used during the transcription phase of protein synthesis?

   A. Snippets
   B. tRNA
   C. rRNA
   D. mRNA

5. During which of the following processes is tRNA active?

   A. Translation
   B. Transcription
   C. Meiosis
   D. Mitosis

6. Which of the following is inherited only from the mother?

   A. Phenotype
   B. Genotype
   C. Lysosomal DNA
   D. Mitochondrial DNA

7. Amino acids are the building blocks of which of the following?

   A. Blood
   B. Neurons
   C. Proteins
   D. Cell walls

8. DNA and RNA share almost identical nitrogenous bases. Which nitrogenous base is found only in RNA?

   A. Thymine
   B. Adenine
   C. Uracil
   D. Cytosine

9. DNA uses hydrogen bonds to hold the purines and pyrimidines together. How many hydrogen bonds are there between cytosine and guanine?

   A. 1
   B. 2
   C. 3
   D. 4

10. TAC-GGT-GTA-ACT Gene

    ? - ? - ? - ? mRNA

    During transcription, messenger RNA carries the code from the genes to the ribosomes. To do this, the RNA polymerase must add matching RNA nucleotides to the complementary DNA sequence. Looking at the gene sequence above, which of the following reflects the correct mRNA sequence?

    A. ATG-CCA-CAT-TGA
    B. CGU-AAC-ACG-GUC
    C. GUC-AAG-AGU-UCG
    D. AUG-CCA-CAU-UGA

Answer Key

1. B		**6.** D	
2. C		**7.** C	
3. A		**8.** C	
4. D		**9.** C	
5. A		**10.** D	

Answers and Explanations

1. **(B)** When RNA transcribes a codon from DNA during transcription, thymine is replaced with uracil. Thymine is less prone to mutation, which makes it a good storage vehicle for DNA. Uracil is more flexible, which makes it more suited to its temporary role in RNA. The other three nitrogenous bases, adenine, guanine, and cytosine, are used in both DNA and RNA.

2. **(C)** Base pairs combine in only a few ways because of the unique nature of the hydrogen bonds that hold them together. Cytosine bonds with guanine using three hydrogen bonds. Adenine and thymine require only two hydrogen bonds as do adenine and uracil in RNA. These base pairs are typically written using their letter symbols, G-C and A-T.

3. **(A)** Understanding the role of DNA is important in answering questions about it. DNA stores the genetic information necessary to create living matter and beings. Choices B, C, and D are all created by DNA and RNA. DNA itself is composed of nucleotides.

4. **(D)** Messenger RNA, called mRNA, is created during transcription. Its function is to carry the genetic code to the ribosomes for protein formation. It holds the genetic information in three base pair sequences, called codons.

5. **(A)** Transfer RNA, called tRNA, is needed during translation. It recognizes the specific codon in mRNA needed to create a specific amino acid. There are 64 different possible codons and 20 amino acids, so only the appropriate tRNA will unlock the code and create proteins.

6. **(D)** Mitochondrial DNA is inherited only from the mother in almost all organisms that reproduce through sexual reproduction. Sperm cells contain mitochondrial DNA, but the egg cell's processes destroy it.

7. **(C)** Proteins are the engines of cellular, and thus life, function. In the form of enzymes they manage the cell's metabolic processes. DNA and RNA, through transcription and translation, build the amino acids necessary to create proteins. Without proteins, the other aspects of living material—blood, neurons, and cell walls—would not exist.

8. **(C)** While DNA uses thymine as a pyrimidine to bond with adenine, RNA uses uracil. Thymine is less prone to mutation, which makes it a good storage vehicle for DNA. Uracil is more flexible, which makes it more suited to its temporary role in RNA. The other three nitrogenous bases, adenine, guanine, and cytosine, are used in both DNA and RNA.

9. **(C)** There are only a certain number of possibilities of base pairs due to the unique nature of the hydrogen bonds that hold them together. Cytosine bonds with guanine using three hydrogen bonds. Adenine and thymine require only two hydrogen bonds, as do adenine and uracil in RNA.

10. (D) The discovery of base pairs by Watson and Crick proved that there were only certain combinations of nitrogenous bases possible. This is the meaning of the term *complementary* in the question. For example, guanine always bonds with cytosine. The three possible bonds are G-C, A-T, or A-U. In the example, the first codon is TAC, meaning that the complementary codon *must* be AUG. For the rest of the sequence, GGT-GTA-ACT, the complementary nitrogenous bases are CCA-CAU-UGA.

CHAPTER 29

Genetics

TEAS **Genetics questions** cover topics including chromosomes, genes, alleles, phenotypes, and genotypes. Some questions may also test your knowledge of the use of Punnett squares.

Genetics is the discipline in biology wherein scientists focus on heredity. Whereas biology deals with individuals and groups, genetics deals with the heredity information carried in DNA.

Chromosomes and Genes

The **chromosome** is the fundamental unit of genetics. Contained in the nucleus of plant and animal cells, a chromosome is a linear strand that caries the hereditary information of the individual. It is composed of DNA and related proteins. Humans, for example, have 46 chromosomes, 23 each from their mother (through the egg cell) and from the father (carried in the sperm). All organisms that procreate through sexual reproduction are **diploid**, meaning they carry two sets of chromosomes. The two strands, connected by a single **centromere**, are referred to as **chromatids** (see figure). The number of chromosomes differs between species, and there is no correlation between the number of chromosomes in a species and the number of genes.

The **gene** is a core unit of genetics. It contains the heredity information that, singularly or through a particular grouping of genes, leads to a characteristic. A **characteristic**, or trait, may be physical, like eye color or left-handedness. It can also be behavioral or psychological, such as a predisposition to addictive behaviors. Genes are located in a particular position on a chromosome. They are the loci of mutation, which leads to genetic variation. Mutations occur randomly or through environmental agency.

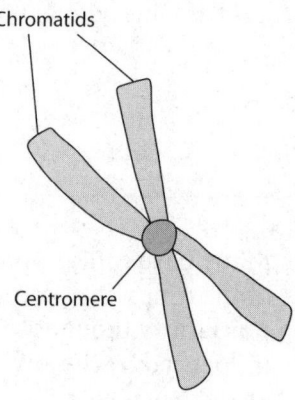

Chromatids

Centromere

Alleles

An **allele** is a version of a gene. A gene can be composed of a pair of alleles that call for a different distinct trait. In diploid organisms there are two alleles, one from each parent. The alleles meet at a **locus**. For any pairing of alleles we can talk about an individual's genes being **homozygous** or **heterozygous**. If the alleles are identical, the gene is homozygous. The characteristic that the gene produces will be the same as in the two parents. When the allele from each parent is different, the gene is heterozygous. Some traits are dominant, and some are recessive. The dominant trait is the one that will be expressed in the offspring.

Phenotypes and Genotypes

Genetic variation takes place at the cellular level, but it can be seen on the surface in individuals. We can view an individual's hair color, height, and hear his or her tone of voice. These observable characteristics are known as **phenotypes**. Some traits, like blood type, are not observable to the naked eye, but they are measurable, so they fall under the phenotype rubric. This includes those traits selected through heredity and influenced by environment. An individual's height, for instance, is a product of its genes, but growing up in a poor environment with a lack of nutrition can lead to a stunting of growth. The observable height of the adult individual is part of its phenotype.

The **genotype** of an individual refers to the genetic makeup in its chromosomes. An individual may carry a recessive gene for a trait that does not appear in its phenotype but is still present and can be handed down to its genetic heirs. Although an individual's height may be inhibited by its environment, its heirs still carry the genotype for a range of height. This is not to be confused with a **genome**. A genome refers to the entire genetic material of an individual—in a human's case, all 46 chromosomes together. Genotype can refer to a specific allele. We can talk about an individual's genotype carrying DNA for both blue and brown eyes. At the phenotype level, the individual has brown eyes because the trait is dominant.

Mendel

Many have called Gregor Mendel, a German monk who lived in the middle of the nineteenth century, the father of genetics. At the time, evolution was largely thought to work along Lamarckian lines, with traits being influenced by the environment. Mendel, through careful observation and experimentation, proved that heredity was instead at work. On the individual level, traits depended solely on the genes of the mother and the father. His work with pea plants led him to notice a mathematical distribution in traits among offspring allowing him to codify the laws of inheritance.

He discovered that some traits are recessive, while others are dominant. He showed this by crossbreeding pea plants that varied in certain characteristics from height to color to seed shape. By tracking the appearance of phenotypic traits in the offspring, he came across the distribution of traits predicted in a Punnett square.

Punnett Squares

The English geneticist Reginald Punnett created a diagram for predicting the outcomes when crossbreeding genotypes. The Punnett square is used to show how the genes of parents (the genes of which are already known) might combine in their offspring. It is a simple box of four squares. The alleles of one parent are placed across the top, and the alleles of the other are placed along the side. The four boxes show all the possible distributions of alleles in offspring (first filial generation, or F1) of the two homozygous parents (parental generation, or P).

	H	H
h	Hh	Hh
h	Hh	Hh

H = tall (dominant); h = short (recessive)

In the Punnett square above, there is a 100% chance that the offspring will exhibit the dominant gene, becoming a tall pea plant.

In the following Punnett square, between two heterozygous parents with one dominant and one recessive allele, the offspring are shown to have a 25% chance of exhibiting the recessive gene.

	H	h
H	HH	Hh
h	Hh	hh

H = tall (dominant); h = short (recessive)

When a homozygous parent with two recessive alleles and a parent with heterozygous alleles are crossed, the results are as shown below:

	H	h
h	Hh	hh
h	Hh	hh

H = tall (dominant); h = short (recessive)

Even though the recessive alleles represent 75% of the genetic material, the dominant gene will be represented in the phenotype 50% of the time. This demonstrates the difference between an organism's genotype and phenotype.

Review Questions

1. Which of the following reflects the genetic makeup of an organism?

    A. Mitochondrion
    B. Protein
    C. Phenotype
    D. Genotype

2. Which of the following reflects the outward observable expression of an organism's genetic makeup?

    A. Phenotype
    B. Allele
    C. Genotype
    D. Codon

3. Diploid organisms contain alleles that code for a specific gene. Which of the following terms describes two identical alleles at the same locus?

    A. Heterozygous
    B. Recessive
    C. Homozygous
    D. Dominant

4. Which of the following terms describes two different alleles at the same locus?

    A. Heterozygous
    B. Homozygous
    C. Recessive
    D. Dominant

5. A homozygous individual (RR) procreates with an individual who is heterozygous for a recessive trait (Rr). Which of the following is the correct percentage of offspring who will be carriers of the recessive trait?

    A. 0%
    B. 25%
    C. 50%
    D. 100%

6. A homozygous individual (NN) procreates with an individual who is heterozygous for a recessive trait (Nn). Which of the following is the correct percentage of offspring who will express the recessive trait?

A. 0%
B. 25%
C. 50%
D. 100%

7. A specific disease is carried on allele (s), which is recessive to the general condition of (S). If a heterozygous male (Ss) procreates with a female who is also heterozygous for the recessive trait (Ss), which of the following is the correct percentage of offspring who will have the disease?

A. 0%
B. 25%
C. 50%
D. 100%

8. A specific disease is carried on allele (X), which is dominant to the normal condition of (x). If a heterozygous male (Xx) procreates with a female who is normal homozygous (xx), which of the following is the correct percentage of offspring who will have the disease?

A. 0%
B. 25%
C. 50%
D. 100%

9. The Punnett square assists in the identification of which of the following?

A. Offspring with genes expressing incomplete dominance
B. Offspring with genes expressing complete dominance
C. Offspring with genes expressing shared dominance
D. All genotypes possible in offspring

10. An individual's genome is composed of which of the following?

A. Only sex chromosomes
B. Only mitochondrial DNA
C. All of the DNA
D. All of the RNA polymerase

Answer Key

1. D		6. A	
2. A		7. B	
3. C		8. C	
4. A		9. D	
5. C		10. C	

Answers and Explanations

1. (D) The question forms a general definition of the term *genotype*. It is the genetic material of the organism whether or not those genes have been expressed in the phenotype, choice C. These genes are available to be passed on to offspring. The mitochondrion, choice A, is the organelle in the cell that converts sugar into usable energy. Protein, choice B, is the building block of cellular life.

2. (A) The phenotype is the observable traits of an organism. A person may have brown hair. This is a phenotypic description. The person's genotype might have alleles for blond hair and brown hair. The dominant gene shows up in the phenotype, but the person's offspring may get the allele for blond hair. A codon is a grouping of DNA that correlates with an amino acid.

3. (C) When two alleles at the same locus are identical, we call this gene homozygous. Heterozygous means that the alleles are different. One allele will be dominant, which means that it will override the other, recessive, allele in the phenotype of the individual. In a homozygous gene, both alleles are the same, so the trait will exhibit itself phenotypically in the individual.

4. (A) A diploid organism has two sets of chromosomes, one from each parent. The genes from each match up at a place called the locus. The allele from one parent will meet its paired allele from the other parent at the locus. If the two alleles are identical, the gene is homozygous. When they are different, they

are heterozygous. One allele is dominant, meaning it will exhibit its characteristics over the recessive trait.

5. (C) For this answer we can use a Punnett square to show the probability being sought.

	R	R
R	RR	RR
r	Rr	Rr

R = dominant; r = recessive

Half of the possible offspring of the two parents are Rr, meaning they carry the recessive allele r. Phenotypically, they will show the dominant trait, no disease, but their offspring might exhibit it. According to the Punnett square, 50% will be carriers of the trait.

6. (A) This answer basically uses the same Punnett square as the answer before. The only change is that the letters referring to the traits are different, and the question is asking about the phenotype, not the genotype.

	N	N
N	NN	NN
n	Nn	Nn

N = dominant; n = recessive

Just as in the last question, half of the possible offspring of the two parents are heterozygous, meaning they carry the recessive allele n. None of them show the recessive trait phenotypically, though. According to the Punnett square, 0% will exhibit the disease phenotypically.

7. (B) This answer also can be achieved through the use of a Punnett square.

	S	**s**
S	SS	Ss
s	Ss	ss

S = disease (dominant); s = no disease (recessive)

The Punnett square shows that only the ss, which is one in four offspring, or 25%, will exhibit the disease phenotypically. Three in four offspring or 75%, Ss and ss, will be carriers, while SS, 25%, won't have any trace of the disease. The question asks what percentage will have the disease, rather than what percentage will be carriers of the disease. According to the Punnett square, 25% will have the disease.

8. (C) This answer, as well, can be solved by turning to a Punnett square.

	X	**x**
x	Xx	xx
x	Xx	xx

X = disease (dominant); x = no disease (recessive)

Half of the offspring of these two individuals have the dominant, disease-carrying allele. These offspring will exhibit the disease phenotypically. According to the Punnett square, 50% will have the disease.

9. (D) The purpose of using the Punnett square is to show the possibility of genetic variation among all offspring. It is probabilistic in nature. Mendel had to crossbreed pea plants over and over to produce accurate results. The Punnett square shows all of the possible combinations of alleles in the offspring genotypes.

10. (C) The term *genome* refers to the complete set of genetic material available to an individual or a group. The important unit of genetic material as it pertains to both genotype and phenotype is DNA. An individual's genome is all of its DNA.

CHAPTER 30

Evolutionary Biology

TEAS questions on **Evolutionary Biology** test your understanding of the biological theory of evolution. Questions may address concepts including natural selection, adaptation, mutation, and genetic drift.

Evolutionary processes are processes by which organisms have evolved from a common ancestor. Through natural selection, mutations, adaptation, and genetic drift, certain genes are passed on, changed, or eliminated. Evolution is a change in species over time; this change is caused by the variant frequency of an allele or alleles in a population. The changes in these genes have created diverse species—and sometimes altogether new species. The processes mentioned previously foster these changes.

The Theory of Evolution

Charles Darwin was a nineteenth-century British scientist who is often considered the father of evolution. He spent many years conducting a comparative study between fossils and live species in South America and on the Galapagos Islands, just off the South American coast. Darwin conducted his studies well before the discovery of DNA; however, many of his observations on evolution and natural selection continue to hold true.

Darwin could only base his theory on phenotypes, the traits that were physically expressed by an organism. He observed that organisms that no longer lived together displayed similar characteristics. He continued to study their similarities but also their differences. Their differences indicated ways in which the organisms had developed over time.

Darwin noted that each population produced more offspring than were required. As a result, many of those in the population died either being caught by predators or through disease or starvation. Such a large population naturally breeds competition among members of the population. Therefore, those organisms with the skill set to survive pass down those survival traits to their progeny. This process is called **natural selection.**

Natural Selection

Natural selection is often coined "survival of the fittest" because those organisms within a species that have the necessary traits to survive predators and disease are the strongest of their population. Within each species population, there are differences in genetic makeup. These differences in traits can result in organisms within the same species varying in color, size, or behavior. In the process of natural selection, the organisms with the traits that are most conducive to survival live to pass on those traits. The demands on a population to provide enough resources dictate that not all members of the population will survive. A species evolves, therefore, through its "fittest" members.

Mutation

Mutations are changes in the genetics of an organism. In order to be passed on through reproduction, mutations must occur in the gametes, or sex cells, of the organism. Normally, as genes are shuffled around during meiosis (the production of cells), some DNA is exchanged—this process is called recombination. Recombination is responsible for many of the variances within a species and the inheritance of certain traits. Mutations can also cause variances because they involve a change in the DNA as well. Mutations, however, are caused by radiation, poisonous substances, or a copying error during meiosis.

Mutations that are favorable to a species are passed down to the offspring and gradually increase the presence of the mutated trait in the species. Beneficial mutations are relatively uncommon in natural selection, however; usually mutations that occur in the gametes are harmful to a species. Harmful mutations can impede survival rates within a population. There are some neutral mutations as well: these occur in non-sex cells and are not passed down. Neutral mutations do not affect evolution.

Adaptation

Adaptation is another process by which evolution occurs. Adaptation occurs when an animal experiences a change in traits as a result of a change in environment. For example, Darwin studied finches, which he observed had beaks of different shapes based on the type of food the finches ate. Although the finches shared similar traits, the type of food a finch ate determined the type of beak it had. The finches had to adapt to the environment for survival. Eventually scientists discovered through analyzing DNA that a particular gene or group of genes controlled the type of beak that was presented and that the favorable beak gene was passed down.

Genetic Drift

Genetic drift is a process of adaptation by which some members of a species are forcibly separated. For example, if members of a species were to be separated by a storm—some members staying at the original location and other members being washed to a new island—through evolution, a new species might be formed. The individuals on the new island would need to adapt to their new environment; those who were better able to do so would survive and pass down their traits. This process would inevitably create variance within the species. If the original and new species were reunited but were unable to produce viable offspring, then a new species would have been formed. This process can also be called reproductive isolation.

Review Questions

1. A certain type of moth exists in two forms: a dark-colored version and a light-colored one. The dark version is prevalent when pollution is more concentrated because it can better camouflage itself. However, when there is less pollution, the light-colored moths are in abundance. The population alters itself based on the landscape of its environment. This would be an example of which of the following?

   A. Genetic drift
   B. Mutation
   C. Adaptation
   D. DNA

2. Sometimes during the evolutionary process, a new species is created. But, since there are many variations of an organism within the same species, how can a scientist tell if a completely new species has developed?

   A. If one set has lived apart from the other for more than five years, scientists consider it a new species.
   B. Any time a mutation occurs, a new species is created.
   C. When the fittest of a species survives, these survivors are considered to be the new species.
   D. If no viable offspring can be produced between the two species, scientists determine that a new species has been created.

3. Which of the following are two significant processes during evolution that account for gene variance on a cellular level in a given species?

   A. Mutation and recombination
   B. Mutation and genetic drift
   C. Natural selection and extinction
   D. Reproductive isolation and recombination

4. Darwin's theory of evolution is based on which of the following concepts?

   A. DNA replication
   B. Natural selection
   C. Reproductive isolation
   D. Recombination

5. As the father of evolution, what was Darwin's main methodology of study?

   A. Comparing DNA
   B. Making observations of various traits of species
   C. Conducting clinical test trials
   D. Dissecting earthworms

6. Which of the following is true about natural selection?

   A. It can be caused by radiation or chemicals.
   B. It occurs only when a species is separated forcibly.
   C. It is the only biological process that causes variance during cell production.
   D. It dictates that those who have the most favorable traits within a species will survive.

7. Mutations that are inherited must occur in _____.

   Which of the following correctly completes the sentence above?

   A. Gametes
   B. The process of reproductive isolation
   C. Phenotypes
   D. The process of natural selection

8. After baby sea turtles hatch from their eggs and dig out of the sand, they head for the ocean. Although the ocean is not far, there are many perils along the way. Often the slowest baby turtles are caught by predators. This is an example of which of the following?

   A. Recombination
   B. Mutation
   C. Natural selection
   D. Meiosis

9. Genetic drift is a type of adaptation. Which of the following describes what happens when a species undergoes genetic drift?

   A. The species becomes extinct due to harmful mutations.
   B. The species is forcibly split apart, and some of its members must adapt to a new environment.
   C. The species moves from being a land animal to becoming a type of fish.
   D. The species is always rendered sterile.

10. In natural selection, competition for _____ is won by the species with the most favorable traits.

    Which of the following correctly completes the sentence above?

    A. Resources
    B. Genetic material
    C. Basic needs
    D. Climate changes

Answer Key

1. C

2. D

3. A

4. B

5. B

6. D

7. A

8. C

9. B

10. A

Answers and Explanations

1. (C) When a change in environment causes a population to change for survival, this process is called adaptation. In the case of the moth, to create better camouflage, the population changed from having more light-colored moths to having more dark-colored moths as the environment changed.

2. (D) There is no specific time frame for how long it takes for a new species to be created, so choice A can be eliminated. However, it is crucial that no viable offspring can be produced in order to indicate that a new species has been created. Only when a species can no longer interbreed can scientists say that a new species has been formed.

3. (A) Although during evolution there are many variables that can cause changes, the only two processes listed that can cause genetic variation on a cellular level are mutation and recombination. These processes occur during cell division.

4. (B) Darwin observed that a species tended to have more offspring than needed. As a result, there was a strain on resources available to the population, and only those whose traits were favorable to securing those resources were able to survive. Therefore, Darwin theorized that evolution occurs by natural selection.

5. (B) DNA had not been discovered during the time that Darwin was making his observations, so choice A is incorrect. The tools Darwin had available to him were his own observations of the similarities and differences in species at various locations.

6. (D) Choices A and C refer to evolution on a cellular level and are therefore incorrect. The theory of natural selection states that only those who inherit the most favorable traits within a population will survive.

7. (A) Mutations occur during cell production. They can occur in any cell, but only gametes carry the genes that will be passed down. Therefore, in order for a mutation to be inherited, it must occur in a gamete.

8. (C) Choices A, B, and D all occur on the cellular level. A baby sea turtle that is slow exhibits a trait that is unfavorable to survival and thus falls to the fate of natural selection.

9. (B) Both genetic drift and adaptation deal with changes in the environment that can cause organisms to change on a cellular level. In genetic drift, the species is subjected to a forced change in environment that separates members of the species. As a result, the separated members must adapt to their new environment.

10. (A) In natural selection, there are often more offspring than there are resources to provide for those offspring. As a result, only the offspring that exhibit favorable traits for survival will be able to compete successfully for those resources.

CHAPTER 31

Earth Science and Astronomy

Earth Science and Astronomy questions on the TEAS focus on our understanding of the Earth and the dynamics of celestial bodies. These questions may cover subjects including Earth's structure, geology, meteorology, and space science.

Earth's Structure

The interior of the Earth is composed of four layers: the crust, the mantle, the outer core, and the inner core (see figure). The **crust** is the outermost layer, and the **inner core** is the innermost layer, as shown in the figure below:

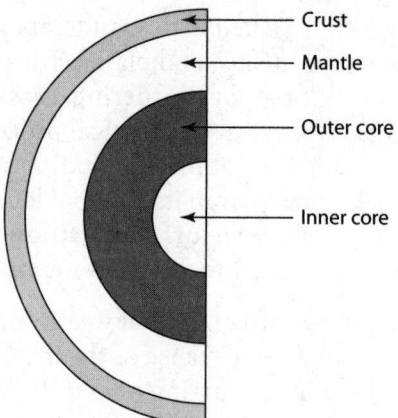

Figure not drawn to scale.

The mantle is made up of viscous magma, and the outer core is believed to be a liquid layer, whereas the other two layers are solid.

Extending out beyond the Earth's surface is the Earth's atmosphere. The **atmosphere** is also composed of four layers, as shown in the figure:

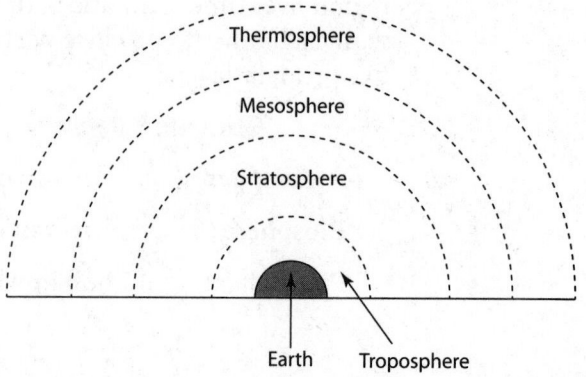

Figure not drawn to scale.

Geology

The Earth's crust is made up of three types of rock: igneous, sedimentary, and metamorphic. **Igneous rocks** are rocks that are formed from magma, or molten rock that has cooled. **Sedimentary rocks** are formed by weathering on the surface of the Earth. **Metamorphic rocks** are formed when igneous and sedimentary rocks are placed under extreme amounts of pressure within the Earth itself.

Rock Type	Formation Process
Igneous	Cooled magma
Sedimentary	Weathering
Metamorphic	Extreme pressure

Rocks in turn are made up of **minerals**, which provide the primary building blocks of the Earth's crust. Minerals can be identified based on specific properties, such as how easy they are to scratch, called hardness, and how smoothly they break apart, called cleavage or fracture.

The Earth's landscapes consist of three primary regions: mountains, plateaus, and plains. These landscapes develop in part due to the combined forces of weathering, erosion, and deposition. **Weathering** occurs when physical or chemical processes cause rock to break down and form smaller pieces of rock, including soil. **Erosion** occurs when weathered rock is moved away from its original location with the help of gravity, water, wind, and other factors. **Deposition** involves the process through which weathered, eroded rock is now deposited in a new place.

The forces of weathering, erosion, and deposition are themselves brought about because of the impact of the water cycle. The **water cycle** consists of five recurring phases, listed in order as follows: evaporation, condensation, precipitation, infiltration, and runoff.

Meteorology

Climate is used to refer to the typical weather patterns experienced by a region over time. Climatic patterns are influenced by factors that interact with each other to produce particular effects. These factors can arise from five primary layers:

Climatic Factors	
Atmosphere	Air surrounding the Earth
Biosphere	Layer of living things on the surface of the Earth
Pedosphere	Soil in which living things grow

| **Lithosphere** | Rocks and minerals that make up the Earth's crust |
| **Hydrosphere** | Water on the Earth's surface, including oceans |

Space Science

The Earth is part of a **solar system** that contains eight planets and a number of dwarf planets. In order of their distance from the sun, the planets are: Mercury, Venus, Earth, Mars, Jupiter, Saturn, Uranus, and Neptune. Pluto, which was formerly called a planet but is now considered a dwarf planet, is beyond Neptune. With a diameter of about 12,756 kilometers at its equator, the Earth is larger in size than Mercury, Venus, Mars, and Pluto and smaller than the other four planets. The sun, by contrast, is over 100 times larger than the Earth, at about 1,392,000 kilometers in diameter.

The sun gives off energy that is transmitted to the Earth as **electromagnetic waves**. These waves lie on a spectrum of longer to shorter wavelengths, as indicated in the following figure.

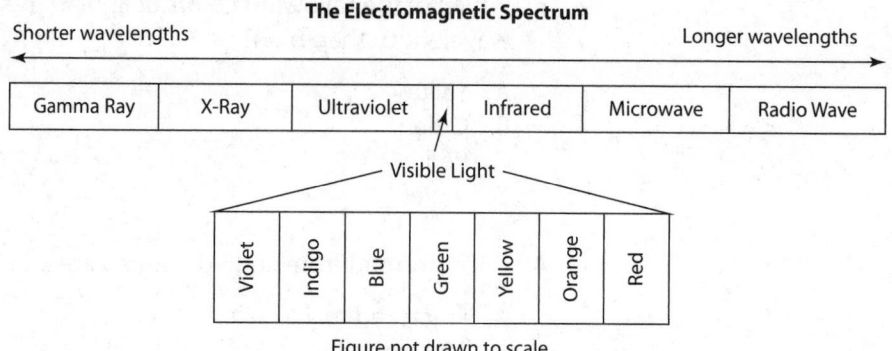

The Electromagnetic Spectrum

Shorter wavelengths — Longer wavelengths

| Gamma Ray | X-Ray | Ultraviolet | Infrared | Microwave | Radio Wave |

Visible Light

| Violet | Indigo | Blue | Green | Yellow | Orange | Red |

Figure not drawn to scale.

Visible light makes up only a small portion of the spectrum. The colors of visible light are foregrounded in the figure, with violet representing the shortest wavelength and red representing the longest.

Review Questions

1. The rocks and minerals that make up the Earth's crust are known as which of the following?

A. Atmosphere
B. Lithosphere
C. Biosphere
D. Hydrosphere

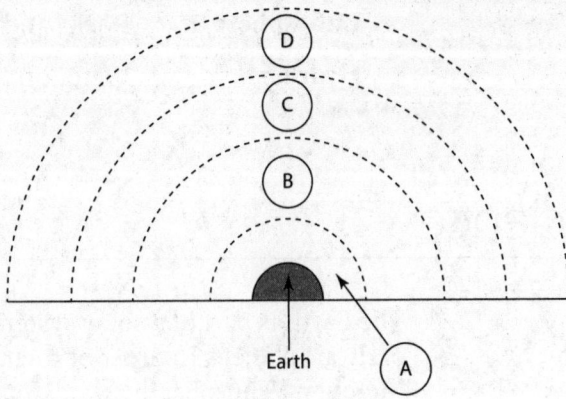

Earth

Figure not drawn to scale.

2. In the figure of the Earth's atmosphere shown above, which of the following layers is the stratosphere?

   A. Layer A
   B. Layer B
   C. Layer C
   D. Layer D

3. Which of the following colors of light in the visible spectrum has a shorter wavelength than blue?

   A. Yellow
   B. Green
   C. Red
   D. Violet

4. Rocks formed from cooled magma are known as which of the following?

   A. Fractured rocks
   B. Metamorphic rocks
   C. Igneous rocks
   D. Sedimentary rocks

5.

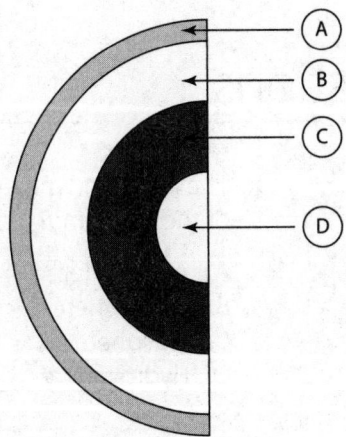

Figure not drawn to scale.

Which of the following layers in the figure shown represents the outer core of the Earth?

A. Layer A
B. Layer B
C. Layer C
D. Layer D

6. The _____ of a mineral indicates how easy it is to scratch.

Which of the following correctly completes the sentence above?

A. Hardness
B. Cleavage
C. Fracture
D. Deposition

7. Which of the following occurs when physical or chemical processes cause rock to break down and form smaller pieces of rock?

A. Precipitation
B. Deposition
C. Weathering
D. Erosion

8. Which of the following layers of the Earth's atmosphere is farthest away from the Earth?

A. Thermosphere
B. Troposphere
C. Mesosphere
D. Stratosphere

9. Which of the following reflects the correct order of the water cycle?

A. Evaporation, runoff, precipitation
B. Condensation, evaporation, runoff
C. Precipitation, runoff, condensation
D. Evaporation, condensation, precipitation

10.

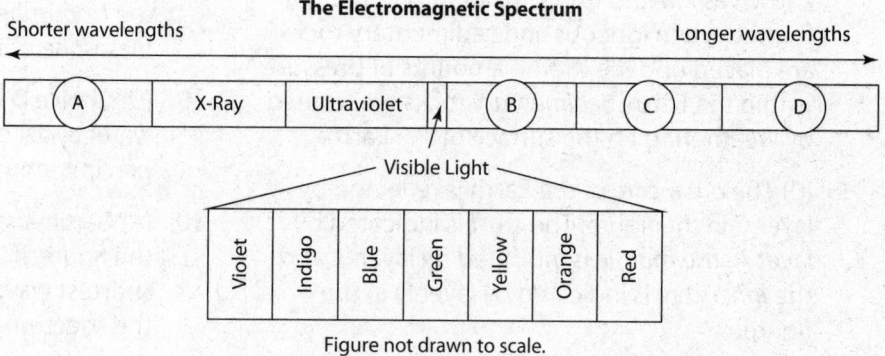

Figure not drawn to scale.

Which of the following indicates the location of gamma rays in the figure above?

A. Location A
B. Location B
C. Location C
D. Location D

Answer Key

1. B
2. B
3. D
4. C
5. C

6. A
7. C
8. A
9. D
10. A

Answers and Explanations

1. **(B)** The rocks and minerals that make up the Earth's crust are known as the *lithosphere*. The *atmosphere* is the air surrounding the Earth, while the *biosphere* is the layer of living things on the Earth's surface. The *hydrosphere* is the water on or near the Earth's surface.

2. **(B)** The *stratosphere* is shown in layer B of the figure. The *troposphere* is indicated by layer A, the *mesosphere* is indicated by layer C, and the *thermosphere* is indicated by layer D of the figure.

3. **(D)** Of the colors mentioned, only violet has a shorter wavelength than blue. Yellow, green, and red all have longer wavelengths than blue light.

4. **(C)** Rocks formed from cooled magma are known as *igneous* rocks. *Metamorphic* rocks are formed when igneous and sedimentary rocks are placed under extreme amounts of pressure within the Earth. *Sedimentary* rocks are formed by weathering on the surface of the Earth.

5. **(C)** The *outer core* of the Earth is reflected by layer C in the figure. The *crust* is indicated by layer A, the *mantle* is indicated by layer B, and the *inner core* is indicated by layer D in the figure.

6. **(A)** The *hardness* of a mineral indicates how easy it is to scratch. *Cleavage* and *fracture* are indicators of how smoothly or jaggedly a mineral breaks apart.

7. **(C)** *Weathering* is the phenomenon that occurs when physical or chemical processes cause rock to break down and form smaller pieces of rock. *Deposition* involves the process through which weathered, eroded rock is deposited in a new place. *Erosion* occurs when weathered rock is moved away from its original location with the help of gravity, water, wind, and other factors.

8. **(A)** The *thermosphere* is the layer of the Earth's atmosphere that is farthest away from the Earth. The first three layers of the Earth are the *troposphere*, the *stratosphere*, and the *mesosphere*, in order from nearest to farthest.

9. **(D)** Choice D reflects the correct order of the water cycle: evaporation, condensation, and precipitation occur in that order.

10. **(A)** Gamma rays are located on the far left of the figure, in location A. Gamma rays have the shortest wavelengths of the waves shown on the spectrum.

CHAPTER 32

The Atom

Atoms questions on the TEAS test your understanding of the components of an atom. You may also be asked to identify parts of atoms based on their atomic number and mass number, and you may be asked to calculate an atom's overall mass. You may see questions regarding isotopes and the overall charge of an atom as well.

Atomic Components

An atom is the smallest unit of an element that still possesses all of the properties of that element. Atoms contain three component parts: protons, neutrons, and electrons. **Protons** are positively charged particles located in the **nucleus**, or center, of the atom. **Neutrons** are also located in the nucleus of the atom along with the protons, but neutrons have a neutral electrical charge.

Electrons are negatively charged particles that orbit around the nucleus of the atom. The figure below shows the four main components of an atom:

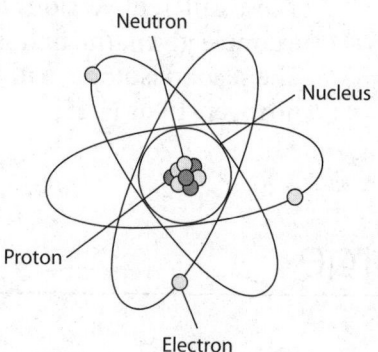

In terms of size, protons and neutrons are roughly the same size, and they are much larger than electrons.

Atomic Number and Mass Number

The **atomic number** of an element is an identifying number that indicates the number of protons found in atoms of that element. An atom of an element with an atomic number of 8 would have 8 protons in its nucleus; an atom with an atomic number of 14 has 14 protons. The atomic number is equivalent to the number of protons.

The **mass number** of an element is an identifying number that indicates the number of protons plus the number of neutrons found in atoms of that element. An atom with an atomic number of 8 and a mass number of 17 would have 8 protons and 9 neutrons. To calculate the number of neutrons that an atom possesses, subtract the number of protons from the mass number:

$$\text{Mass number} - \text{number of protons} = \text{number of neutrons}$$

An atom with 12 protons and a mass number of 24 would have 24 − 12, or 12, neutrons.

Protons and neutrons each have a mass of 1 **atomic mass unit** (AMU). To determine the approximate overall mass of an atom in AMUs, we add the number of protons and neutrons. Electrons are left out of this equation because the mass of electrons is so small relative to that of protons and neutrons.

Isotopes

Atoms of a given element always have the same number of protons, but the number of neutrons may vary. One atom of nitrogen may have 7 protons and 7 neutrons, while another atom may have 7 protons and 8 neutrons. These different versions of atoms are called **isotopes**. In the nitrogen example given, the first isotope would be referred to as nitrogen-14 or N-14. The second isotope, with a mass number of 15, would be referred to as nitrogen-15 or N-15.

Atomic Charge

The charge of an atom can be either positive, negative, or neutral. The **atomic charge** is affected by the numbers of protons and electrons in the atom; neutrons do not affect the charge, as they have no charge themselves. A **neutral atom** has the same number of protons and electrons. The protons are positively charged, and the electrons are negatively charged, so when they are present in equal numbers, they balance each other out.

An atom can give off or gain electrons, which causes its charge to shift from neutral to positive or negative. An atom that has an electrical charge is known as an **ion**. If an atom gives off electrons, it will have fewer electrons than protons, and its charge will be positive. If an atom gains electrons, it will have more electrons than protons, so its charge will be negative.

A neutral isotope of nitrogen-14 would have 7 protons, 7 neutrons, and 7 electrons. The atomic number of nitrogen is 7, so we know that it has 7 protons, and the mass number of the nitrogen-14 isotope is 14. This means the number of neutrons is 14 − 7, or 7. The isotope is neutral, so it must have the same number of electrons as protons.

A negatively charged isotope of nitrogen-14 would have more electrons than protons. If the charge was −1, the isotope would have 7 protons, 7 neutrons, and 8 electrons. The −1 charge tells us that this isotope contains 1 more electron than the number of protons. In shorthand, this −1 charge would be written as N⁻. An ion with a positive charge of +1 would be written as N⁺.

Review Questions

1. Which of the following indicates the number of protons and neutrons in an atom with an atomic number of 6 and a mass number of 14?

   A. 6 protons and 6 neutrons
   B. 6 protons and 8 neutrons
   C. 8 protons and 6 neutrons
   D. 12 protons and 14 neutrons

2. The mass and electrical charge of a neutron can best be described by which of the following statements?

   A. A neutron has the same mass as a proton and a negative charge.
   B. A neutron has the same mass as a proton and a neutral charge.
   C. A neutron has the same mass as an electron and a neutral charge.
   D. A neutron has the same mass as an electron and a positive charge.

3.

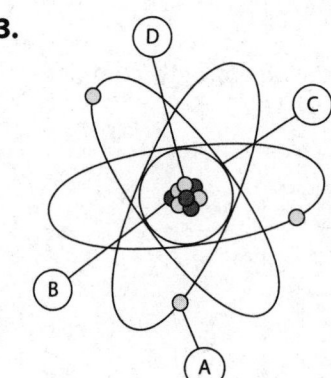

   In the model of the atom shown, label A indicates which of the following?

   A. Nucleus
   B. Neutron
   C. Electron
   D. Proton

4. Which of the following reflects the overall charge of an atom with 10 protons, 12 neutrons, and 11 electrons?

    A. −2
    B. −1
    C. +1
    D. +2

5. What is the approximate overall mass of an atom with 19 protons and 23 neutrons?

    A. 19 AMU
    B. 23 AMU
    C. 38 AMU
    D. 42 AMU

6. Which of the following indicates the number of protons in an atom with an atomic number of 21 and a mass number of 55?

    A. 21
    B. 23
    C. 24
    D. 27

7. What are the overall charge and mass number of an atom with 6 protons, 8 neutrons, and 7 electrons?

    A. Charge −1; mass number 14
    B. Charge −1; mass number 21
    C. Charge +1; mass number 14
    D. Charge +1; mass number 21

8. An atom has 47 protons, 48 neutrons, and 49 electrons. This atom has an overall charge of _____ and an overall mass of approximately _____ AMU.

    Which of the following correctly completes the sentence above?

    A. +2; 96
    B. +2; 95
    C. −2; 96
    D. −2; 95

9.

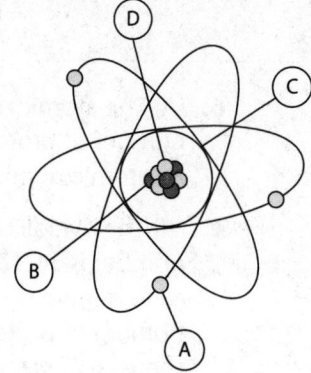

In the model of an atom shown, label B reflects which of the following if it is a positively charged atomic particle?

A. Neutron
B. Proton
C. Nucleus
D. Electron

10. A neutral atom isotope has an atomic number of 16 and a mass number of 34. How many protons, neutrons, and electrons does the atom have?

A. 16 protons, 16 neutrons, and 16 electrons
B. 16 protons, 16 neutrons, and 18 electrons
C. 16 protons, 18 neutrons, and 16 electrons
D. 18 protons, 16 neutrons, and 18 electrons

Answer Key

1. B		**6.** A	
2. B		**7.** A	
3. C		**8.** D	
4. B		**9.** B	
5. D		**10.** C	

Answers and Explanations

1. (B) The atomic number reflects the number of protons in the atom. So, an atom with an atomic number of 6 would have 6 protons. The mass number reflects the number of protons and neutrons added together. So, an atom with 6 protons and a mass number of 14 would have 14 − 6, or 8, neutrons.

2. (B) Protons and neutrons have approximately the same mass, and neutrons have a neutral charge. Electrons are much smaller in mass than protons and neutrons.

3. (C) In the model of the atom, label A indicates an electron. Electrons orbit around the nucleus of the atom.

4. (B) In an atom, protons are positively charged, and electrons are negatively charged. When an atom has an equal number of protons and electrons, its overall charge will be neutral. When the atom has more electrons than protons, its overall charge will be negative. This atom has 11 electrons and 10 protons, so its overall charge is negative. The number of electrons exceeds the number of protons by 1, so the overall charge is −1.

5. (D) The approximate overall mass of an atom, in AMU, is equal to the number of protons plus the number of neutrons. The approximate overall mass of this atom is 19 + 23, or 42, AMU.

6. (A) The atomic number of an atom reflects the number of protons in the atom. This atom has an atomic number of 21, so it has 21 protons.

7. (A) The overall charge is −1, and the mass number is 14. The charge is calculated by determining the difference between the number of protons and electrons. In this case, there are 7 electrons and 6 protons, which means that the atom has 1 more electron than the number of protons. The overall charge is therefore −1. The mass number is the number of protons plus the number of neutrons: in this case, 6 + 8 = 14.

8. (D) This atom has more electrons than protons. It therefore has a negative charge, which eliminates choices A and B. The mass in AMU is determined by adding the number of protons and neutrons: 47 + 48 = 95.

9. (B) Protons are positively charged atomic particles. In the model shown, label B indicates a proton.

10. (C) The atom has an atomic number of 16, so it has 16 protons. The atom has a mass number of 34, so it has 34 − 16, or 18, neutrons. The isotope is neutrally charged, so it has the same number of electrons as protons, or 16 electrons.

CHAPTER 33

The Periodic Table

Periodic Table questions test your understanding of how to read the periodic table of the elements. You may also be tested on various properties shared by different groups of elements. Other questions may address atomic radii, ionization potential, and electronegativity, based on an element's location on the periodic table.

Reading the Periodic Table

The **periodic table** is a table of chemical elements arranged by atomic number. Here is an example:

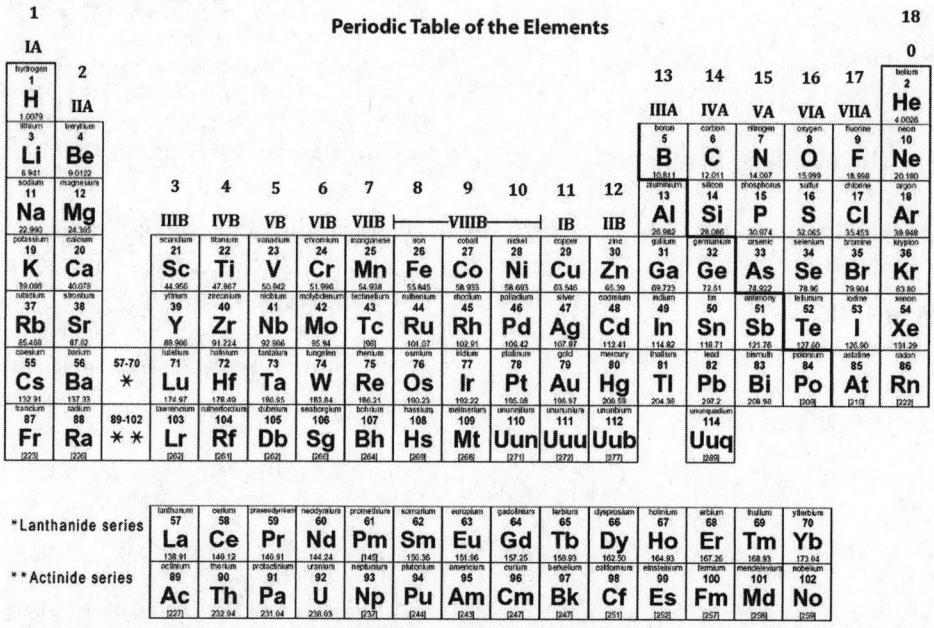

The elements on the periodic table are listed in order of their atomic number. Some periodic tables provide the atomic mass of the element as well:

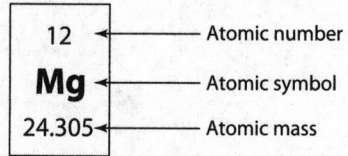

From the periodic table, by reading the atomic number, you can determine the number of protons and electrons in a neutral atom of an element. The number of neutrons can also be determined if the mass number of the atom is known.

Periods and Groups

Elements of the periodic table are arranged in periods and in groups. **Periods** of the periodic table are organized horizontally across the table in rows. In the table shown, the shaded row represents a period:

Periodic Table of the Elements

Groups in the periodic table are organized vertically down the table in columns. (Groups may also be referred to as families.) In the table shown, the shaded column represents a group:

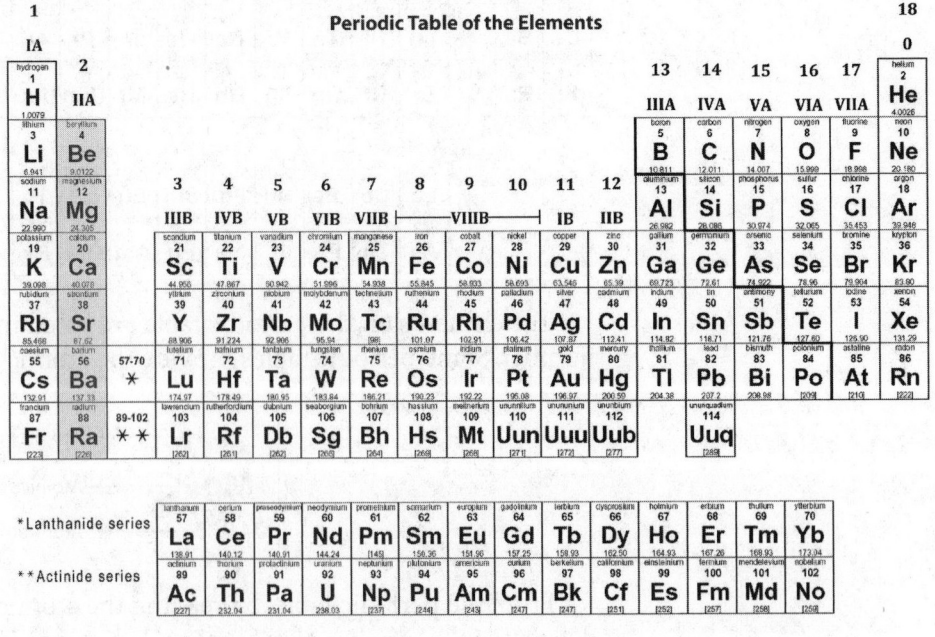

Elements in different groups share certain properties. The **alkali metals** in group 1 are shiny, soft, and highly reactive. The **alkaline earth metals** in group 2 are fairly soft and fairly reactive. The **transition metals** in groups

3 to 12 are hard and have low to negligible reactivity. The **halogens** in group 17 are extremely reactive, whereas the **noble gases** in group 18 are extremely stable. Metals overall tend to be malleable and highly conductive of heat and electricity, whereas nonmetals break easily and are generally poor conductors. **Metalloids**, such as boron, silicon, and germanium, have properties between those of metals and nonmetals.

Atomic Radii

The **atomic radius** of an atom is the measure of the distance from the center of the atom to its outermost orbital shell. Atoms with greater numbers of orbital shells have larger atomic radii because the outermost electrons are farther away from the nucleus. The length of the atomic radii decreases as you move from left to right across a period (row) of the table. The length of the atomic radii increases as you move down a group (column) of the table.

Ionization Potential and Electronegativity

The term **ionization energy** is used to refer to the amount of energy required for the removal of one electron from an atom. The ionization energy of an atom increases as the atomic radius of the atom decreases. This means that ionization energy increases as you move from left to right across a period (row) of the table. It also decreases as you move down a group (column) of the table.

The term **electronegativity** is used to refer to the tendency of an atom to want to bond with other atoms by taking electrons from those atoms. Like ionization energy, the electronegativity of an atom increases as the atomic radius of the atom decreases. This means that electronegativity increases as you move from left to right across a period (row) as atomic radius decreases, and it decreases as you move down a group (column) of the table as the atomic radius increases.

Review Questions

1. Which of the following elements is most highly reactive?

    A. Argon (Ar)
    B. Neon (Ne)
    C. Radon (Rn)
    D. Fluorine (F)

2. Which of the following indicates the number of electrons in a neutral atom of zinc (Zn)?

   A. 16
   B. 20
   C. 30
   D. 40

3. Which of the following elements is the best heat conductor?

   A. Iron (Fe)
   B. Phosphorus (P)
   C. Sulfur (S)
   D. Selenium (Se)

4. Which of the following atoms has a larger atomic radius than copper (Cu)?

   A. Zinc (Zn)
   B. Gold (Au)
   C. Arsenic (As)
   D. Bromine (Br)

5. Tungsten (W) has greater electronegativity than which of the following?

   A. Tin (Sn)
   B. Chromium (Cr)
   C. Hafnium (Hf)
   D. Molybdenum (Mo)

6. The greatest number of protons is found in an atom of which of the following elements?

   A. Chromium (Cr)
   B. Cobalt (Co)
   C. Lithium (Li)
   D. Carbon (C)

7. Atoms of which of the following elements have the highest ionization energy?

   A. Potassium (K)
   B. Nickel (Ni)
   C. Calcium (Ca)
   D. Manganese (Mn)

8. Which of the following statements is true about the relationship between mercury (Hg) and lead (Pb)?

   A. Mercury atoms have fewer protons and a larger atomic radius than lead atoms.
   B. Mercury atoms have more protons and a smaller atomic radius than lead atoms.
   C. Mercury atoms have fewer protons and a higher ionization energy than lead atoms.
   D. Mercury atoms have a smaller atomic radius and a higher ionization energy than lead atoms.

9. Which of the following atoms has the smallest atomic radius?

   A. Rubidium (Rb)
   B. Radium (Ra)
   C. Strontium (Sr)
   D. Barium (Ba)

10. Which of the following lists elements ordered in terms of lowest to highest electronegativity?

   A. Iron (Fe), cobalt (Co), rhodium (Rh)
   B. Nickel (Ni), palladium (Pd), platinum (Pt)
   C. Titanium (Ti), vanadium (V), manganese (Mn)
   D. Zinc (Zn), copper (Cu), nickel (Ni)

Answer Key

1. D		**6.** B	
2. C		**7.** B	
3. A		**8.** A	
4. B		**9.** C	
5. C		**10.** C	

Answers and Explanations

1. **(D)** Fluorine is a member of the halogen group, whose elements are highly reactive. Argon, neon, and radon are members of the noble gases group, whose elements are extremely stable.

2. **(C)** Zinc is found in the fourth row of the periodic table with an atomic number of 30. Its atoms therefore have 30 protons. A neutral atom of zinc would have the same number of electrons as protons, or 30 electrons.

3. **(A)** Metals are better conductors of heat and electricity than are nonmetals. Iron is the only metal among the answer choices. Phosphorus, sulfur, and selenium are all nonmetals.

4. **(B)** The length of the atomic radius decreases as you move from left to right across a period (row) of the table. Zinc, arsenic, and bromine are all located to the right of copper on the fourth row of the table, so atoms of these elements would all have smaller atomic radii than copper. The length of the atomic radius increases as you move down a group (column) of the table, however, so gold atoms would have a larger atomic radius than copper atoms.

5. **(C)** Tungsten is located on the sixth row of the periodic table, and it has an atomic number of 74. Electronegativity increases as you move

from left to right across a period (row) of the table, and it decreases as you move down a group (column) of the table. Hafnium is located to the left of tungsten on the sixth row, so it has a lower electronegativity value.

6. (B) Cobalt has an atomic number of 27, so it contains 27 protons. Chromium has 24 protons, lithium has 3 protons, and carbon has 6 protons.

7. (B) Ionization energy increases as you move from left to right across a period (row) of the table. Nickel is the element located the farthest to the right of the four elements mentioned, which all lie on the fourth row of the periodic table. Nickel therefore has the highest ionization energy.

8. (A) Mercury has an atomic number of 80, while lead has an atomic number of 82, so mercury has fewer protons than lead. Mercury is located to the left of lead on the sixth row of the table, so its atoms have a larger atomic radius than lead atoms.

9. (C) The length of the atomic radius decreases as you move from left to right across a period (row) of the table, and it increases as you move down a group (column) of the table. Strontium is located to the right of rubidium on the fifth row and above barium and radium in the second column, so its atoms have the smallest atomic radii.

10. (C) Electronegativity increases as you move from left to right across a period (row) of the table, and it decreases as you move down a group (column) of the table. Titanium, vanadium, and manganese are listed in order of their positions from left to right on the fourth row of the table, so they are listed in order of least to greatest electronegativity.

CHAPTER 34

Chemistry

Chemistry questions on the TEAS test your knowledge of chemical properties and processes. You may be asked questions about states of matter, properties of matter, phase changes, chemical bonds, chemical solutions, chemical reactions, and acids and bases. You may also be asked to balance chemical equations.

States of Matter

Matter is made up of microscopic particles that move at different speeds depending on the energy they are exposed to. We measure this energy as temperature. The molecules can move either quickly and randomly or hardly at all. When the energy is high, matter takes the form of a **gas**, in which molecules are moving about quickly and are far apart. Lower temperatures result in a **liquid**, in which molecules cohere but are fluid. Coherence means that the molecules remain close together, but they can change position by sliding over one another. When the temperature is low, matter takes the form of a **solid**, in which molecules are packed closely together and retain their positions. A somewhat unusual state of matter is **plasma**, which is similar to a gas in many of its properties but carries an electric charge.

Properties of Matter

Gases have no fixed form. Molecules are free to move at random past each other, and they tend to fill any container that holds them. If a gas is not contained, its molecules will disperse. In liquids, molecules move less freely than in a gaseous state, sliding past one another. They have a fixed volume but will flow freely unless they fill a portion of a container. Solid matter is rigid, and molecules retain a uniform spacing. A solid has a defined form, which is brittle. It can be broken into pieces but has a tendency to stay together.

Phase Changes

States of matter are not constant. They depend on the energy, measured in temperature, applied to that matter. A solid, when heated enough, will go through a **phase change**, becoming a liquid. The molecules that compose the matter begin to move more quickly. If more heat or pressure is applied, the matter will go through another phase change, from liquid to gas. The process works in reverse as molecules slow down when energy inputs are reduced. It is possible for matter to skip a phase, moving from a solid directly into a gas in a process known as **sublimation**. **Deposition** is when a gas directly becomes a solid.

Chemical Bonds

A **chemical compound** is created when two or more atoms join to form a **chemical bond** that leaves the atoms in a less excited state than they were in before the bond. Such bonds form in two ways.

A **covalent bond** occurs when atoms share electrons between them. This type of bond is common between two atoms of the same element, as in hydrogen (H_2) or in similar elements. When a molecule shares a pair of electrons in a stable state, it has formed a covalent bond. Alkanes, for example, share a single bond. In some compounds, one atom takes the shared electron for more time, due to its structure, forming a **polar covalent bond**. This molecule is partly negatively charged and partly positively charged. Some molecules form a **double bond**, sharing four electrons as opposed to two. These bonds are commonly represented in the alkenes, hydrocarbons with twice as many hydrogen molecules as carbon molecules. It is possible to form triple bonds as seen in a group of hydrocarbons called alkynes.

An **ionic bond** is created between atoms when one atom gives an electron to the other. These bonds typically take place between metals and nonmetals due to the unique electron configuration of metals, with the metal giving an electron to the nonmetal. This transfer creates a positive charge and a negative charge at the ends of the compound. The positive charge, or **cation**, is created by the giver of an electron. The negative charge, or **anion**, is located at the receiving end of the electron. The **net charge** of the compound remains balanced at zero.

Chemical Solutions

A chemical solution is a group of chemical compounds evenly distributed in a state of matter. The solution is a **homogenous mixture** where one chemical compound is completely dissolved in the others. This is most easily achieved in a liquid state. There are mixtures that are not solutions. A **heterogeneous mixture** maintains separation between two substances, like oil and water.

The **solute** is the compound dissolved in the **solvent**. Liquids make excellent solvents. The **solubility** of a solvent depends on the nature of the liquid as well as external factors like temperature. The **concentration** of the solution is the amount of solute in the solution. The **mole** is the unit of measurement for chemical reactions and refers to a compound's molecular mass.

Chemical Reactions

To create a new chemical compound from other elements and compounds, a **chemical reaction** is needed. Two or more reactants are added together, often with an input of energy, creating one or more products and by-products. Photosynthesis occurs, for instance, when a plant cell combines carbon dioxide and water. The sun's rays provide the energy. The chemical reaction produces sugar and oxygen.

Chemical reactions occur in nature and in the laboratory. A **catalyst** will speed up the reaction by lowering the amount of energy needed to start the reaction. **Enzymes** act as catalysts in cellular processes. They quicken the chemical reaction, turning a molecule, known as a **substrate**, into a product without being altered themselves.

Acids and Bases

Many acids and bases can be understood from the perspective of the theory developed by Arrhenius, a Swedish scientist. In this view, an **acid** is a substance that gives off hydrogen (H^+) ions when it is dissolved in water. A **base**, or alkaline substance, is a substance that gives off hydroxide (OH^-) ions when it is dissolved in water. Acidic solutions have higher concentrations of hydrogen ions, whereas alkaline solutions have lower concentrations of hydrogen ions.

The presence of acids and bases can be tested using tools known as **indicators**. One indicator in common use is litmus paper. **Litmus paper** turns red in the presence of an acid and blue in the presence of a base.

Here are some examples of acids and their chemical formulas:

Acid	Chemical Formula
Acetic acid	$HC_2H_3O_2$
Phosphoric acid	H_3PO_4
Citric acid	$H_3C_6H_5O_7$
Hydrochloric acid	HCl
Sulfuric acid	H_2SO_4

Here are some examples of bases:

Base	Chemical Formula
Ammonium hydroxide	NH_4OH
Lithium hydroxide	$LiOH$
Magnesium hydroxide	$Mg(OH)_2$
Potassium hydroxide	KOH
Sodium hydroxide	$NaOH$

The acidity or alkalinity of a solution is measured using a scale known as the **pH scale**. The figure below shows examples of substances and lists where they fall on the pH scale:

Strongly Acidic	−1	Hydrochloric Acid
	0	Lead Acid Battery
	1	Sulfuric Acid
	2	Gastric Acid/Lemon Juice
	3	Vinegar/Orange Juice
Weakly Acidic	4	Tomato Juice
	5	Coffee/Beer
	6	Urine/Milk
pH Neutral	7	Pure Water
Weakly Alkali	8	Ocean Water/Eggs
	9	Baking Soda
	10	Hand Soap/Milk of Magnesia
Strongly Alkali	11	Ammonia
	12	Bleach
	13	Oven Cleaner
	14	Sodium Hydroxide

Each step of the pH scale has 10 times the difference in concentration of hydrogen (H^+) ions as the step before or after it. So, a solution with a pH of 7 will have 10 times more hydrogen ions than a solution with a pH of 8 and 10 times fewer hydrogen ions than a solution with a pH of 6.

Balancing Chemical Equations

The TEAS Science section may contain questions that ask you to balance chemical equations. We will outline the steps in this process later in this chapter.

One of the most important chemical equations for humans is the one that represents photosynthesis. Without the following equation, there would be no life on Earth:

$$CO_2 + H_2O \rightarrow C_6H_{12}O_6 + O_2$$

This equation shows how green plant cells, with the help of the sun's energy, convert carbon dioxide (CO_2) and water (H_2O) into glucose and oxygen (O_2). The two **reactants**, carbon dioxide and water, are on the left side of the arrow. The arrow shows the direction of production. The two **products**, sugar and oxygen, are on the right side of the arrow.

According to the **Law of the Conservation of Mass**, in a chemical reaction, no energy is lost, but neither is mass destroyed. The amount of reactant must match the amount of products that are made, even if those products escape as a gas or a liquid.

In the photosynthesis equation, there is a difference in the number of atoms on the right and left sides:

Element	Reactants	Products
C	1	6
H	2	12
O	3	8

To produce sugar and oxygen requires more reactants than we have on the left side. The solution is to balance the two sides.

We can multiply any molecule with a number, called a **coefficient**. We cannot change the subscript, however, without changing the nature of the molecule. By adding coefficients to the reactants and products, we can balance the equation in a few simple steps.

The best way to do this is by balancing each element in turn. Start with the carbon. The right side has 6 carbon atoms, so the left side needs 6:

$$\underline{6}CO_2 + H_2O \rightarrow C_6H_{12}O_6 + O_2$$

Here we have multiplied the CO_2 by 6 to result in 6 carbon atoms on the left side. When we multiply CO_2 by 6, this also changes the number of oxygen atoms on the left side from 3 to 13. There are now 12 oxygen atoms in the CO_2 molecule, plus 1 in the H_2O molecule, for a total of 13. The changed numbers are shown underlined in the following table.

Element	Reactants	Products
C	**6**	6
H	2	12
O	**13**	8

Now the carbon is equal, but the hydrogen remains unequal, and the oxygen has changed in number. Next, fix the hydrogen:

$$\underline{6}CO_2 + \underline{6}H_2O \rightarrow C_6H_{12}O_6 + O_2$$

Here we multiplied the H_2O molecule by 6 to result in 12 hydrogen atoms on the left side. When we multiply H_2O by 6, this further changes the number of oxygen atoms on the left side from 13 to 18. There are now 12 oxygen atoms in the CO_2 molecule, plus 6 in the H_2O molecule, for a total of 18.

Element	Reactants	Products
C	**6**	6
H	**12**	12
O	**18**	8

The last remaining imbalance rests with the oxygen. At this point, there is plenty of oxygen in the reactants. We can balance the equation by producing more O_2.

$$\underline{6}CO_2 + \underline{6}H_2O \rightarrow C_6H_{12}O_6 + \underline{6}O_2$$

In this step, the O_2 molecule on the right side was multiplied by 6. This resulted in 18 oxygen atoms on the right side. The equation is now balanced. Each element has the same number of atoms on the left and right sides.

Element	Reactants	Products
C	**6**	6
H	**12**	12
O	**18**	**18**

Review Questions

1. A solution with a pH of 13 is considered to be which of the following?

   A. Weak acid
   B. Strong acid
   C. Weak base
   D. Strong base

2. A molecule that is acted upon by an enzyme is called a _____.

   Which of the following correctly completes the sentence above?

   A. Solvent
   B. Solution
   C. Substrate
   D. Sievert

3. A hydrocarbon with one triple bond is called an _____.

   Which of the following correctly completes the sentence above?

   A. Alkyne
   B. Alkane
   C. Alkene
   D. Anion

4. ___Mg + ___HNO$_3$ → ___H$_2$ + ___Mg(NO$_3$)$_2$

   Which of the following correctly balances the equation above?

   A. $2Mg + HNO_3 \rightarrow H_2 + Mg(NO_3)_2$
   B. $Mg + 2HNO_3 \rightarrow H_2 + Mg(NO_3)_2$
   C. $Mg + 2HNO_3 \rightarrow 2H_2 + Mg(NO_3)_2$
   D. $2Mg + HNO_3 \rightarrow H_2 + 2Mg(NO_3)_2$

5. Which of the following is the chemical formula for pentane?

    A. C_6H_{12}
    B. C_8H_{12}
    C. C_5H_{12}
    D. C_7H_{12}

6. Which of the following represents an example of ionic bonding?

    A. The bonding of nonmetal atoms
    B. The sharing of electrons
    C. The transfer of electrons
    D. The bonding of metal atoms

7. Which of the following describes the phase change of sublimation?

    A. Solid to liquid
    B. Liquid to gas
    C. Solid to gas
    D. Liquid to solid

8. Which of the following hydrocarbons contains double bonds?

    A. C_2H_8
    B. C_6H_8
    C. C_8H_6
    D. $C_{12}H_{24}$

9. A solid item (X) with the density of 0.917 g/cm³ is placed in a beaker containing an aqueous substance (Y) with the density of 1.0000 g/cm³. Which of the following things do you expect to happen?

    A. X will float on surface.
    B. X will sink halfway down the beaker.
    C. X will sink to the bottom of the beaker.
    D. X and Y have such close density that X will move around freely within Y.

10. Which of the following is a function of enzymes?

    A. Stop a reaction
    B. Speed up the reaction rate
    C. Slow down the reaction rate
    D. Reduce the number of reactions

11. ___H_3PO_4 + ___$LiOH$ → ___H_2O + ___Li_3PO_4

Which of the following correctly balances the acid-base reaction above?

    A. $H_3PO_4 + LiOH \rightarrow 3H_2O + 2Li_3PO_4$
    B. $H_3PO_4 + 3LiOH \rightarrow 2H_2O + Li_3PO_4$
    C. $2H_3PO_4 + LiOH \rightarrow 3H_2O + Li_3PO_4$
    D. $H_3PO_4 + 3LiOH \rightarrow 3H_2O + Li_3PO_4$

12. Liquids have the capability of flowing. Which of the following statements below explains this phenomenon?

A. The spacing of the particles is close together
B. The spacing of the particles is far apart
C. The particles can glide over one another
D. The particles are attracted to one another

13. $\_\_C_2H_6 + \_\_O_2 \rightarrow \_\_CO_2 + \_\_H_2O$

Which of the following correctly balances the combustion reaction above?

A. $2C_2H_6 + 8O_2 \rightarrow 4CO_2 + 4H_2O$
B. $2C_2H_6 + 7O_2 \rightarrow 4CO_2 + 6H_2O$
C. $6C_2H_6 + 5O_2 \rightarrow 3CO_2 + 2H_2O$
D. $6C_2H_6 + 7O_2 \rightarrow 4CO_2 + 2H_2O$

14. In which of the following states of matter are molecules located closest together?

A. Gas
B. Liquid
C. Plasma
D. Solid

15. Acids provide H^+ ions in water, while bases provide OH^- ions. Which of the following is a pair of bases?

A. HCl, HNO_3
B. H_2SO_4, HNO_3
C. $NaOH$, KOH
D. $Ba(OH)_2$, H_3PO_4

Answer Key

1. D		**9.** A	
2. C		**10.** B	
3. A		**11.** D	
4. B		**12.** C	
5. C		**13.** B	
6. C		**14.** D	
7. C		**15.** C	
8. D			

Answers and Explanations

1. **(D)** A solution with a pH of 13 is a strong base. Household bleach and oven cleaner are two examples of strong bases.

2. **(C)** Enzymes are proteins that act as catalysts. They speed up chemical processes. Without them, these reactions would take longer. Enzymes act upon a molecule known as a substrate.

3. **(A)** An alkane has a single bond. An alkene has a double bond. Alkynes are characterized by a triple bond. An anion refers to the negatively charged end of an ionic bond.

4. **(B)** To balance the equation, we must make the left side have the same number of elements as the right:

$$\_\_Mg + \_\_HNO_3 \rightarrow \_\_H_2 + \_\_Mg(NO_3)_2$$

The elements in this example number as follows:

Element	Reactants	Products
Mg	1	1
H	1	2
N	1	2
O	3	6

The Mg (magnesium) is already balanced. We move on to the next element, H (hydrogen). We double it in the reactants and look at the result:

$$\_\_Mg + \underline{\mathbf{2}}HNO_3 \rightarrow \_\_H_2 + \_\_Mg(NO_3)_2$$

Element	Reactants	Products
Mg	1	1
H	**2**	2
N	**2**	2
O	**6**	6

The two sides are balanced by adding the coefficient 2 to the second reactant.

5. **(C)** The chemical formula for pentane is C_5H_{12}. A member of the alkane family, it has five carbon atoms, giving it its name.

6. **(C)** Ionic bonds differ from covalent bonds in that they transfer an electron from one compound to another rather than sharing electrons. They occur between metals and nonmetals in conjunction.

7. **(C)** Sublimation is the process in which a solid skips the liquid state and becomes a gas immediately. This somewhat rare phase change is seen in special compounds like dry ice, which goes from a solid to steam at room temperature. Choice A, solid to liquid, is known as melting. Choice B, liquid to gas, can be characterized as vaporization, evaporation, or even boiling, depending on the energy input. Choice D, liquid to solid, is typically known as freezing.

8. **(D)** Hydrogen bonds come in different forms. Double bonds form among hydrocarbons in different ways, as well, but the ratio is always one carbon atom for every two hydrogen atoms. The basic form is C_1H_2. $C_{12}H_{24}$ is the only example given that fits this 2-to-1 ratio.

9. **(A)** The relative densities of solids and liquids are important for determining how they will react. A solid that is denser than a liquid will sink when placed in it. A solid that is less dense will float.

10. **(B)** Enzymes serve as catalysts in chemical reactions. They speed up reaction times by lowering the energy required to activate a reaction. They change the environment in which a reaction takes place without being altered by the reaction themselves.

11. **(D)** To balance the equation, we must make the left side have the same number of elements as the right:

$$\_\_H_3PO_4 + \_\_LiOH \rightarrow \_\_H_2O + \_\_Li_3PO_4$$

The elements in this example number as follows:

Element	Reactants	Products
H	4	2
P	1	1
O	5	5
Li	1	3

The Li (lithium) stands out as being unbalanced. Adding a coefficient of 3 to the reactant gets us this distribution:

$$\_\_H_3PO_4 + \underline{\textbf{3}}LiOH \rightarrow \_\_H_2O + \_\_Li_3PO_4$$

Element	Reactants	Products
H	**6**	2
P	1	1
O	**7**	5
Li	**3**	3

Since the Li is balanced, we want to change the other molecule in the product, like this:

$$\_\_H_3PO_4 + 3LiOH \rightarrow \underline{\textbf{3}}H_2O + \_\_Li_3PO_4$$

The elements in this example number:

Element	Reactants	Products
H	6	**6**
P	1	1
O	7	**7**
Li	3	3

The two sides are balanced by adding the coefficient 3 to the product.

12. (C) Choice A could apply to both liquids and solids. Choice B could apply relatively to both gases and liquids. Choice D could apply to solids as well as liquids. The ability of particles to move fluidly is what describes the viscosity of liquids.

13. (B) To balance the equation, we must make the left side have the same number of elements as the right:

$$\_\_C_2H_6 + \_\_O_2 \rightarrow \_\_CO_2 + \_\_H_2O$$

The elements in this example number as follows:

Element	Reactants	Products
C	2	1
H	6	2
O	2	3

Let's start by balancing H (hydrogen):

$$\_\_C_2H_6 + \_\_O_2 \rightarrow \_\_CO_2 + \underline{\textbf{3}}H_2O$$

That gives us the following distribution:

Element	Reactants	Products
C	2	1
H	6	**6**
O	2	**5**

Now, C (carbon):

$$\_\_C_2H_6 + \_\_O_2 \rightarrow \underline{\textbf{2}}CO_2 + 3H_2O$$

That gives us the following distribution:

Element	Reactants	Products
C	2	**2**
H	6	6
O	2	**7**

To balance O (oxygen), we would need to multiply the reactant by 3.5. Coefficients must be whole numbers. We can double everything to fix the problem:

$$\underline{\textbf{2}}C_2H_6 + \underline{\textbf{7}}O_2 \rightarrow \underline{\textbf{4}}CO_2 + \underline{\textbf{6}}H_2O$$

That gives us the following distribution:

Element	Reactants	Products
C	**4**	**4**
H	**12**	**12**
O	**14**	**14**

The answer is:

$$2C_2H_6 + 7O_2 \rightarrow 4CO_2 + 6H_2O$$

14. (D) The differences between the three main states of matter is the distance between molecules and their motion. These are caused by the energy put into the system. Lower energy means less movement and smaller distances between molecules, which describes solids. Plasma is closer to a gas than any other state.

15. (C) Sodium hydroxide (NaOH) and potassium hydroxide (KOH) are both bases. Barium hydroxide (Ba(OH)$_2$) is also a base, but it is paired with phosphoric acid (H$_3$PO$_4$), so choice D is incorrect. Choice A contains hydrochloric acid (HCl) and nitric acid (HNO$_3$), while choice B contains sulphuric acid (H$_2$SO$_4$) and nitric acid (HNO$_3$).

CHAPTER 35

Mechanics

Mechanics questions on the TEAS may test your understanding of Newtonian physics concepts including velocity, speed, force, acceleration, momentum, and gravity. Newton's first, second, and third laws may also be addressed.

Mechanics is the science of motion. It is often broken down into two subfields: kinematics and dynamics. **Kinematics** focuses on how something moves, drawing a mathematical picture of motion. **Dynamics** explores what causes movement.

Velocity and Speed

Mechanics relies on two kinds of measurements: vectors and scalars. Vector measurements have direction, but scalar measurements do not. To understand the difference between vectors and scalars, one need only look at the difference between speed and velocity. In English, we often use these terms interchangeably, but in physics, they have distinct meanings.

Speed can be understood in terms of instantaneous speed and average speed, without regard to direction. When you are driving and a policeman pulls you over because his radar gun shows you going 85 mph, he has captured your **instantaneous speed**. This is the speed of your car at the instant it registered on the radar gun. On a long car trip, your **average speed** is equal to the total distance traveled divided by the total time it takes to make the trip. If you drive 500 miles and it takes you 10 hours, your average speed is 50 mph:

$$v = \frac{d}{t}$$

$$\frac{500 \text{ miles}}{10 \text{ hours}} = 50 \text{ mph}$$

Velocity is a vector measurement. In the radar gun case above, your instantaneous speed is 85 mph. Your **instantaneous velocity** is also 85 mph, but it has a direction, heading east on the highway.

Average velocity differs from average speed, however. Whereas speed is directly related to distance, velocity is directly related to displacement. When you look at a pendulum swinging, it goes back and forth, speeding up and slowing down. Its average speed is relative to the distance it covers. It moves back and forth over the same space, though. It moves a meter to the right, then back to the middle, then a meter to the left, and back. Its average velocity is zero, because over time its displacement is zero.

Force

Force is a vector measurement, which represents the effect of one object on another. When a billiard ball strikes another it provides a force to the second. It has a momentum. In the process, both objects have their momentum changed by the interaction. They change velocities and directions.

We measure force using a figure called a Newton (N). This is the amount of force required to accelerate a 1-kilogram object at 1 meter per second squared on a flat surface.

Acceleration

Acceleration is one of the more important vector measurements in physics. It shows the change in movement of an object. A car driving at a steady rate of 55 mph is not accelerating. When you step on the gas pedal or the brake pedal, that's when acceleration can be measured. It is a measure of the object's change in velocity when it encounters a force.

If you're driving at 100 meters per second (about 45 miles per hour) and you slam on the brakes because of an obstacle in the road, it will take some time for your car to stop. If it takes 10 seconds to come to a complete stop, you can figure out your **average acceleration** (where a stands for acceleration):

$$a = \frac{\text{final velocity} - \text{initial velocity}}{\text{time}}$$

$$a = \frac{\text{change in velocity}}{\text{time}}$$

$$a = \frac{\Delta v}{t}$$

$$a = \frac{0 \text{ m/s} - 100 \text{ m/s}}{10 \text{ seconds}}$$

Your acceleration is −10 meters per second per second, or **−10 m/s²**.

Momentum

Another way of describing the movement of an object through space is through its momentum. **Momentum** takes into account not only the velocity of an object but also its mass.

Imagine a child learning to roller skate on a flat road. He is traveling at 1 meter per second. You might stand in his way without fear to catch him if he falls. Now imagine a teenager learning to drive. Even if the car is traveling at 1 m/s, there is no way you will stand in its way. Why? The answer is momentum. Momentum includes both the speed, 1 meter per second, and the direction of the object, and also accounts for the mass of the object in a significant way.

In physics, lowercase *p* stand for momentum. Momentum equals mass times velocity. Here is the formula:

$$p = m \times v$$

Since momentum is the product of mass and velocity, this explains why a large object has much more momentum than a small one and is harder to stop. Let's imagine that the car in the example weighs 1,000 kg while the child weighs 20 kg.

The child's momentum: 20 kg × 1 m/s = 20 kg • m/s

The car's momentum: 1,000 kg × 1 m/s = 1,000 kg • m/s

The car's momentum is 500 times higher than the child's. It would require that much more of a force to counter it.

Gravity

Gravity is a universal force of attraction that exists between all masses. We are all in thrall to the Earth's gravity because its mass is so great and we are so close to it. When you throw a ball up in the air, the ball comes back down because the force of the Earth's gravity is so great. The acceleration caused by the Earth's gravity on the surface is denoted as:

$$g = 9.8 \text{ m/s}^2$$

Newton's Laws

Isaac Newton contributed a great deal to explaining the rules of motion in the physical world. Newton's Laws remain valid centuries later:

* **Newton's First Law** states that an object at rest will stay at rest, while an object that is moving will continue moving at a steady pace. This idea is also called **inertia**. The only caveat is that if a force is applied to the object, inertia will be broken.

* **Newton's Second Law** concerns what happens when force is applied to an object. It states that the acceleration of an object when a force is applied depends on two variables. It depends directly on the amount of force applied and inversely on the mass of the object.

* **Newton's Third Law** states simply that for every action, there is an equal and opposite reaction. There must be two objects that interact when a force is applied. When that interaction takes place, both objects are affected by a force of equal size in a vector of the opposite direction.

Review Questions

1. When a car hits a brick wall, what force is applied to the car?

   A. Half the force of the car's momentum
   B. Twice the force of the car's momentum
   C. The same force as the car's momentum
   D. The force cannot be determined.

2. How is velocity different than speed?

   A. Velocity is a vector measurement.
   B. Velocity is a scalar measurement.
   C. Speed includes a direction.
   D. Speed accounts for an object's mass.

3. Which of the following has the greatest momentum?

   A. A 200-kg gorilla running at 12 m/s
   B. A 75-kg impala running at 35 m/s
   C. A 60-kg human running at 15 m/s
   D. A 25-kg hyena running at 20 m/s

4. A car traveling at 50 m/s takes 5 seconds to reach a complete stop. What is its average acceleration?

   A. -5 m/s^2
   B. -10 m/s^2
   C. -50 m/s^2
   D. -250 m/s^2

5. How fast would a 75-kg person need to run to match the momentum of a 100-kg person running at 12 m/s?

   A. 8 m/s
   B. 12 m/s
   C. 16 m/s
   D. 24 m/s

6. To find the momentum of an object, which of the following would you *not* need to know?

   A. Speed
   B. Mass
   C. Velocity
   D. Time

7. Which of the following would be enough to calculate a horse's average speed around a racetrack?

   A. The horse's mass and the length of the course
   B. The length of the course and the amount of time the horse took
   C. The amount of time the horse took and the mass of the jockey
   D. The length of the course and the velocity of the horse out of the gate

8. A shopping cart full of groceries weighs 24 kg and is being pushed down the aisle at 1.5 m/s. What is its momentum?

   A. 16 kg • m/s
   B. 24 kg • m/s
   C. 36 kg • m/s
   D. There is not enough information to calculate the momentum.

9. Which of Newton's laws explains why a parked car doesn't move?

   A. First Law
   B. Second Law
   C. Third Law
   D. None of Newton's laws explains why a parked car doesn't move.

10. A bowling ball weighing 6 kg is rolled toward a billiard ball weighing 1 kg. The two balls strike each other. According to Newton's Third Law, which force is greater, the force on the bowling ball or the force on the billiard ball?

    A. The force on the bowling ball
    B. The force on the billiard ball
    C. The forces are equal.
    D. The forces cannot be determined.

Answer Key

1. C		**6.** D
2. A		**7.** B
3. B		**8.** C
4. B		**9.** A
5. C		**10.** C

Answers and Explanations

1. (C) Newton's Third Law states that every action is met with an equal and opposite reaction. If the car hits the wall with a momentum of 10,000 kg • m/s, the wall will respond with an equal force in the opposite direction.

2. (A) Velocity is related to speed, but it is a vector measurement, whereas speed is a scalar measurement. Velocity includes a direction and measures displacement rather than distance traveled.

3. (B) Momentum is velocity times mass. The impala weighs 75 kg and travels at 35 m/s making its momentum 2,625 kilogram meters per second. The gorilla's momentum is 2,400 kg • m/s, the human 900 kg • m/s, and the hyena 500 kg • m/s.

4. (B) The equation for acceleration is $\frac{\Delta v}{t}$, where Δv is the change in velocity. In the scenario given, the change in velocity is 0 m/s –50 m/s, or –50 m/s. The change of –50 m/s divided by 5 seconds equals –10m/s².

5. (C) The 100-kg person running at 12 m/s has a momentum of 1,200 kg • m/s. To achieve the same momentum, we divide 1,200 kg • m/s by 75 kg, which results in a speed of 16 m/s. The smaller person will have to run faster, but proportionately so.

6. (D) Momentum is calculated using velocity, which has speed as a component. The mass of an object is also required. No time component is needed to calculate momentum.

7. (B) Average speed is the distance covered and the time elapsed. No other measurements are necessary to calculate it.

8. (C) To calculate momentum, you use mass and velocity. Both are provided here. Multiplying 24 kg by 1.5 m/s results in 36 kilogram meters per second.

9. (A) Newton's First Law explains the idea of inertia. An object at rest will stay at rest unless a force is applied. A parked car is at rest.

10. (C) Newton's Third Law states that for every action there is an equal but opposite reaction. When the balls collide, they will experience the same force in opposite directions.

CHAPTER 36

Energy

TEAS **Energy questions** test concepts including kinetic energy, potential energy, mechanical energy, heat energy, and chemical energy. You may be asked to differentiate between these concepts and to solve physics problems involving them.

Energy comes in many forms. It is contained in motion, in gravity, and in chemical bonds. Energy can be transferred from one object to another, and it can be converted from one form to another.

Kinetic Energy

Kinetic energy is a measure of the energy in a moving object. A moving object has an energy directly related to its mass and velocity. The formula for kinetic energy (*KE*) is as follows:

$$KE = \frac{1}{2}mv^2$$

When a cue ball in billiards is struck, it carries kinetic energy to the next ball it strikes. That energy is a measure of the amount of work it can do. Kinetic energy tells us how far and how fast the cue ball can move the next ball. Objects with a larger mass carry more kinetic energy than smaller objects. Objects moving quickly carry more energy than those moving slowly. The **joule** is the measure for kinetic energy.

Potential Energy

When an object is in a position that would allow it to move in the future, it has **potential energy**. If a boulder is held in place at the top of a hill by a stick, its potential energy can be measured. The boulder has **gravitational potential energy**, wherein the height of the position of the boulder and the Earth's gravitational constant affect the equation. How much energy will be released when the stick is removed and the boulder rolls down the hill? Potential energy is a product of the mass of the object, *m*, its height above the ground, *h*, and the gravitational constant of the Earth, *g* (9.8 m/s²):

$$PE_g = m \times g \times h$$

A slingshot that has been pulled back has measurable potential energy. The energy is not related to gravity or height, however. It has to do with the elasticity of the slingshot's band. The energy of the slingshot band is stored as **elastic potential energy**. In this equation, we use a constant (k) that measures the elastic potential of the slingshot band, or spring, or whatever material is being manipulated:

$$PE_e = \frac{1}{2} kx^2$$

In this equation, x represents the measure of how much the slingshot band or other material is being compressed or stretched.

Mechanical Energy

Mechanical energy is the measure of an object's ability to do work. It includes both the kinetic energy of an object and its potential energy. A diver, for example, has the kinetic energy gained from leaping from the diving board as well as the energy that gravity provides for pulling her downward toward the pool. Total mechanical energy equals an object's kinetic energy plus its gravitational potential energy plus its elastic potential energy:

$$ME = KE + PE_g + PE_e$$

This is a measure of the work that an object can do. It is also measured in joules.

Heat Energy

Heat energy is a representation of energy being transferred from one object to another. Boiling water will eventually cool down to room temperature. Conversely, an iced drink will eventually warm up to room temperature. This flow of energy from a warm object to a colder object is known as heat energy. When the two objects have reached the same temperature (the cold beverage is the same temperature as the room's air), they have achieved **thermal equilibrium**.

Chemical Energy

Energy that is stored in the bonds connecting molecules is known as **chemical energy**. Photosynthesis stores the sun's energy in the chemical bonds of glucose. When an animal eats a plant, its body's metabolic processes unlock the chemical energy in those bonds for the animal's use.

Similarly, chemical energy can be released through combustion or some other chemical reaction.

Measuring Energy

Kinetic energy is measured in joules. Since the joule is a measure of both mass and velocity, it equals one kilogram per meter squared per second squared:

$$1 \text{ joule} = 1 \text{ kg} \cdot \left(\frac{m}{s}\right)^2$$

Chemical energy is measured in moles. A **mole** is the amount of chemical energy stored in one gram of hydrogen atoms.

Power is work over time. The standard measure of power is the watt. A **watt** is a joule per second. Large engines sometimes are measured in horsepower. One horsepower is about 750 watts.

Law of Conservation of Energy

The Law of Conservation of Energy states that energy can never be destroyed. Instead, it is transferred from one object to another, such as when a billiard ball strikes another, causing it to move. It can also be transformed from one kind into another. A windmill uses the wind to turn, but it eventually converts that energy into electricity. Energy is dissipated as waste products like heat, light, or sound, but the total amount of energy in a system is constant.

Review Questions

1. What kinds of energy can be measured in a ball rolling down a hill?

   A. Potential and heat
   B. Potential and kinetic
   C. Chemical and heat
   D. Chemical and kinetic

2. What is the kinetic energy (*KE*) of a 4-kg bowling ball rolling down a lane at 2 meters/second?

   A. 2 joules
   B. 4 joules
   C. 8 joules
   D. 12 joules

3. A skier makes two ski runs down a hill. During the first run, his velocity is 10 miles per hour. During the second run, his velocity is doubled. Which of the following statements correctly compares the energy of the skier during his two runs?

   A. The kinetic energy of the second run is twice that of the first run.
   B. The kinetic energy of the second run is four times that of the first run.
   C. The kinetic energy of the second run is half that of the first run.
   D. The kinetic energy of the second run is equal to that of the first run.

4. When a cup of hot tea is left cooling on a countertop, what is happening to the energy in the cup?

   A. Heat energy is being transferred from the tea to the surrounding air.
   B. Heat energy is being transferred from the surrounding air to the tea.
   C. Chemical energy is being converted into kinetic energy.
   D. Kinetic energy is being converted into chemical energy.

5. Mechanical energy is a measure of how much work an object can do. Which of the following kinds of energy does it include?

   A. Chemical energy
   B. Heat energy
   C. Nuclear energy
   D. Elastic potential energy

6. A cat and a mouse are sitting on a desk. They are about to leap off. Which of the following statements is true?

   A. The cat has more potential energy than the mouse.
   B. The mouse has more potential energy than the cat.
   C. The cat and the mouse have an equal amount of potential energy.
   D. Neither the cat nor the mouse has potential energy.

7. The gravitational potential energy of an object does *not* depend on which of the following measurements?

   A. Mass
   B. Gravity
   C. Height
   D. Time

8. What happens to the gravitational potential energy of an object whose mass is halved?

   A. It is halved.
   B. It remains the same.
   C. It is doubled.
   D. It rises by a factor of four.

9. What does a mole measure?

A. Kinetic energy
B. Potential energy
C. Chemical energy
D. Nuclear energy

10. According to the Law of Conservation of Energy, which of the following *cannot* happen during an interaction between two objects?

A. Energy is transferred from one object to another.
B. Energy is converted from one form to another.
C. Energy is turned into a by-product, like heat energy.
D. Energy is lost to the system forever.

Answer Key

1. B

2. C

3. B

4. A

5. D

6. A

7. D

8. A

9. C

10. D

Answers and Explanations

1. (B) The ball rolling down a hill is using kinetic energy. It also has gravitational potential energy stored up in it while it still has some height left in its roll.

2. (C) The equation for determining kinetic energy is: $KE = \frac{1}{2}mv^2$. Here is the math:

$$KE = \frac{1}{2}mv^2$$

$$= \frac{1}{2}(4\text{ kg})(2\text{ m/s})^2$$

$$= \frac{1}{2}\,4 \times 4$$

$$= 8\text{ kg} \bullet \left(\frac{\text{m}}{\text{s}}\right)^2$$

$$= 8\text{ joules}$$

3. (B) The equation for determining kinetic energy is: $KE = \frac{1}{2}mv^2$. The value for any velocity is multiplied by itself. A run that is twice as fast has four times as much kinetic energy.

4. (A) Heat energy is transferred directionally until the object reaches thermal equilibrium with its environment. The cooling of the tea involves such a transfer.

5. (D) To measure mechanical energy, add up the kinetic energy and the two types of potential energy of an object: its gravitational potential energy and its elastic potential energy.

6. (A) The potential energy of an object is $PE_g = m \times g \times h$. If they are sitting on the desk together, their height off the ground is the same, and g, the gravitational force, is a constant. The mass of the cat is much greater, however, so it has more potential energy.

7. (D) The equation for determining an object's gravitational potential energy is its mass times its height above ground times the gravitational constant of the Earth. Time is not a factor in its energy potential.

8. (A) The gravitational potential energy of an object is directly related to its mass. If you double the mass, you double its PE_g. If you halve its mass, you halve the PE_g.

9. (C) A mole is the amount of chemical energy stored in one gram of hydrogen atoms. It measures the energy held in bonds between atoms. Moles are used to measure chemical energy.

10. (D) According to the Law of Conservation of Energy, energy is never destroyed in an interaction. It is always conserved by the system and can only be transferred or converted.

CHAPTER 37

Electricity and Magnetism

TEAS questions about **Electricity and Magnetism** cover the concepts of electric charges, electric currents, electric circuits, and magnetism.

Electric Charges

Electricity begins at the molecular level. In the nucleus of an atom, electrons and protons carry electrical charges. Protons carry a positive charge, while electrons carry a negative charge. On the material level, these charges add up and are measured in a unit called the Coulomb (C). A **coulomb** is the amount of energy in 6.24×10^{18} electrons passing a given point in one second.

Since each charge has either a **positive** or **negative** force, they react differently to each other. Like charges repel, while opposing charges attract. The force of the repulsion or attraction can be measured:

$$F = \frac{k \times Q_1 \times Q_2}{d^2}$$

Q_1 is the charge of the first object, and Q_2 is the charge of the second object. The distance between the two objects is represented by d, and k is a constant depending on the medium holding the two charged objects. This equation shows that the force of repulsion or attraction is directly related to the size of the charge. Larger charges mean more force. The force is inversely related to distance. The closer the charged objects are together, the more force exists between them. As they move farther away from each other, the force between them is diminished.

Electric Currents

An **electric current** is the flow of an electric charge through an electric circuit. The measurement of current takes place at a specific point on the circuit and measures the rate of the charge as it passes that point. The measurement for current (I) is the amount of charge (Q) over time (t).

$$I = \frac{Q}{t}$$

The standard unit for current is the **ampere** or, more simply, the **amp**. An amp is 1 coulomb per second.

Electric currents have a direction. Positive charges move one way, while negative charges move in the opposite direction. The "+" and "−" symbols on a battery show the directionality of the electric circuit. **Alternating current (AC)** is a standard that allows the direction of the current to reverse at times. **Direct current (DC)** is an electrical standard that allows the current to flow in only one direction.

Electric Circuits

An **electric circuit** is created when conducting material forms a properly closed system, allowing a charge to move freely. The conducting material needs to be run through an electrochemical cell, like a battery. The material must be routed through both the negative and positive ends of the cell for the charge to move freely.

Conducting material must be used in a circuit. Metal conducts electricity, while wood does not. Wood by-products are used in insulation because they hamper electrical current.

A circuit also needs an **electric potential** difference. This difference is supplied by the battery or other power source. This difference is measured in volts. A **volt** shows the amount of electric potential difference in a circuit necessary to create one watt of power. One volt can push one amp of current against one ohm of resistance. Batteries are rated by their voltage. Two 12-volt batteries are equal to one 24-volt battery.

When someone flips a light switch on, a circuit is closed, allowing the current to move through the wires. If a switch or light does not work, the circuit may be broken somewhere along its course.

Resistance in a Circuit

Current runs through a wire or other circuit, but not seamlessly. **Resistance** is a measure of the difficulty that current has running through a circuit. Resistance is affected by the length of the circuit, by the width through which the current passes, and by the conductor used in the circuit. Resistance is measured in **ohms** (Ω). Less width means more resistance. Longer distance also means more resistance, as does poor electrical conductivity.

Static Electricity

Not all electricity emanates through a closed circuit. **Static electricity** is found on the surface of objects. It has the same power to attract or repel. It can be seen on some surfaces more easily than others. When two balloons are rubbed together, for example, friction creates static electricity on their surfaces, allowing them to be attached to other surfaces or to repel each other.

Magnetism

Both magnetism and electricity are ruled by a single force, **electromagnetism**. A **magnetic field** acts much like an electric one, attracting and repelling objects at a distance. A magnetic field's force is measured in **teslas**. The measurement for a tesla (B) is volts (V) multiplied by seconds per meter squared:

$$B = \frac{V \times s}{m^2}$$

Magnetism, like electricity and gravity, creates a field of force. It allows objects to act upon each other at a distance. Any object that enters a magnetic object's field of force gets acted upon by that force.

Review Questions

1. Which of the following units are used when measuring electric current?

   A. Amps
   B. Ohms
   C. Teslas
   D. Joules

2. What happens to two positively charged objects when they are brought into close proximity?

   A. They attract each other.
   B. They repel one another.
   C. They cancel out each other's charges.
   D. They have no reaction to each other.

3. What happens to two negatively charged particles as they spread apart?

   A. The force between them grows.
   B. The force between them diminishes.
   C. Their charge polarities reverse.
   D. They increase in mass exponentially.

4. Which of the following is true of direct current and *not* true of alternating current?

   A. It is always a high voltage.
   B. It is always a low voltage.
   C. Current travels in a single direction.
   D. Current travels in both directions.

5. The resistance of a wire depends on its _____, _____, and _____.

   Which of the following correctly completes the sentence above?

   A. Length; material; watts
   B. Width; ohms; joules
   C. Material; positive charge; negative charge
   D. Length; material; width

6. The force between two charged objects is related to the amount of the two charges, _____, and the distance between them.

   Which of the following correctly completes the sentence above?

   A. The temperature of the environment
   B. The medium between the two charges
   C. The polarity of the charges
   D. The time the two objects are exposed to one another

7. How many 12-volt batteries are required to produce 48 volts in an electric circuit?

   A. 1
   B. 2
   C. 4
   D. 8

8. Where does static electricity take place?

   A. In a closed electric circuit
   B. Across an electric potential difference
   C. Through an insulating material
   D. On the surface of an object

9. Which of the following is necessary to create a working electric current?

   A. An electric potential difference and a closed circuit
   B. A closed circuit and a voltage indicator
   C. A conducting material and an insulating material
   D. A conducting material and a power source

10. A magnetic field's force is measured in _____.

    Which of the following correctly completes the sentence above?

    A. Ohms
    B. Amps
    C. Teslas
    D. Volts

Answer Key

1. A   **6.** B

2. B   **7.** C

3. B   **8.** D

4. C   **9.** A

5. D   **10.** C

Answers and Explanations

1. (A) Electric current is measured in amps, also known as amperes. It measures the number of coulombs passing a point on a circuit per second.

2. (B) Objects of like charge repel one another. Objects of opposite charge attract. The strength of the force between them depends on their proximity.

3. (B) The force between two charged objects is inversely related to the distance between the two. This means that the smaller the distance is, the larger the force is. As the distance is increased, the force is decreased.

4. (C) Alternating current is an electrical standard in which the current can travel in both directions. Direct current is an electrical standard in which the current travels in a single direction.

5. (D) Ohms are a measurement of the resistance in a wire or other circuit conductor. Resistance varies depending on the length, width, and material of the conductor.

6. (B) The equation for the force of two charges includes a constant, *k*, which depends on the medium in which the charges are found.

7. (C) The voltage of a battery is independent of the voltage of other batteries. Used in a group on a circuit, four 12-volt batteries will produce 48 volts of current.

8. (D) Static electricity is electric charges occurring on the surface of an object. These charges can attract or repel other charged surfaces.

9. (A) First, a circuit needs to be closed in order for current to pass through it. Second, there needs to be an electric potential difference, like one present in a battery, to provide a current.

10. (C) Teslas are a measurement of a magnetic field's force. They show the relationship between volts, time, and distance.

PART 4

English Language and Usage

The **TEAS English Language and Usage section** tests your understanding of English in three main areas: grammar and word meaning, spelling and punctuation, and sentence structure. The review that follows covers grammatical components you'll need to know, as well as important considerations concerning clarity and style.

CHAPTER 38

Parts of Speech

Parts of Speech questions address the differences between subjects, verbs, nouns, pronouns, adjectives, adverbs, conjunctions, articles, and prepositions. You must identify these parts of speech in a sentence. These questions also test the difference between singular and plural nouns.

In the English language, we use different parts of speech to convey different types of information in sentence form. The parts of speech identify the role that a particular word or words play in a sentence. Essentially, parts of speech are sentence components.

Subjects and Verbs

The most important sentence components are subjects and verbs. **Subjects** convey who or what is performing the action in a sentence. **Verbs** describe the action that is taking place:

> Matt couldn't keep a secret.

In this sentence, the subject of the sentence is *Matt*. The verb is *couldn't*, a contraction for *could not*. Consider this example:

> Sarah's brother couldn't keep a secret.

In this sentence, the subject of the sentence is *Sarah's brother*. The verb is *couldn't*.

> Here's a subject that's slightly more complex:

> Sarah's sincere but talkative little brother couldn't keep a secret.

In this form of the sentence, the subject is *Sarah's sincere but talkative little brother*. The verb is still *couldn't*, as in the previous two examples.

Nouns and Pronouns

A **noun** is a person, place, or thing, and a **pronoun** is a word that refers to a noun:

> Jamie entered the room before she saw Charles.

This sentence contains three nouns: *Jamie*, *the room*, and *Charles*. The word *she* is a pronoun that refers to *Jamie*.

Nouns and pronouns often make up the subjects of sentences, but they aren't always the subjects. Sometimes a form of a verb may be the subject of the sentence:

Laughing is contagious in our household.

In this example, the word *laughing* is a form of the verb *to laugh*. *Laughing* is the subject of the sentence, followed by the verb *is*.

Nouns can be singular or plural. A **singular** noun represents only one person, place, or thing. A **plural** noun represents more than one person, place, or thing being described.

Pronouns can also be singular or plural, depending on the noun they refer to:

Laughing is contagious in our household, especially when we are watching television.

In this example, *household* is a singular noun: it describes only one household. *Television* is also a singular noun, indicating one TV. The pronoun *we* is plural. It indicates more than one person watching TV.

Adjectives and Adverbs

Adjectives and adverbs are descriptive words. In grammatical parlance, we say that **adjectives** modify nouns, and **adverbs** modify verbs. That just means that adjectives describe nouns, and adverbs describe how the action of a verb is taking place.

Adverbs can also modify adjectives and other adverbs:

The beach had massive waves.

In this sentence, the word *massive* is an adjective. It modifies the noun *waves*. Consider this example:

The beach's massive waves immediately caused a scare.

In this sentence, the word *massive* is still an adjective modifying *waves*. The word *immediately* is an adverb, modifying the verb *caused*. *Immediately* is used to describe how the action of causing a scare took place.

Conjunctions, Articles, and Prepositions

Other important parts of speech to know are conjunctions, articles, and prepositions. These components are less central to the meaning of a sentence than are subjects and verbs, but they must be included in order to make the meaning understood. **Conjunctions** are connecting words. They join together the ideas in a sentence. **Articles** are identifiers; they let us know if a noun is specific or general. Finally, **prepositions** indicate relationships between components of a sentence, often showing the location or direction of action. Prepositions are commonly included as parts of prepositional phrases:

> The weather was cool and inviting.

In this sentence, the word *and* is a conjunction. It joins the words *cool* and *inviting*. In the following sentence, the word *a* is an article. It identifies the noun *golf cart*.

> Leonard decided to go shopping for a golf cart.

> Let's consider the following example, which contains the preposition *to*.

> Hayley went to the library.

This preposition is part of the prepositional phrase *to the library*. The phrase indicates where Hayley went, showing the direction of her action.

Review Questions

1. The <u>severe</u> thunderstorm developed <u>later</u> than predicted, so we had time to finish our picnic.

   Which of the following correctly identifies the parts of speech in the underlined portions of the sentence above?

   A. Noun; adverb
   B. Adjective; adverb
   C. Adverb; adjective
   D. Adjective; noun

2. Antibacterial soap should be used to help prevent <u>the</u> spread of germs.

   The underlined word in the sentence above is an example of which of the following parts of speech?

   A. Pronoun
   B. Noun
   C. Adverb
   D. Article

3. Although the plumber repeatedly attempted to fix the drainpipe, it still remains clogged.

   The word *repeatedly* serves as which of the following parts of speech in the sentence above?

   A. Verb
   B. Noun
   C. Adverb
   D. Preposition

4. Which of the following plural nouns is written in the correct form?

    A. Alumni
    B. Mouses
    C. Phenomeni
    D. Syllabuses

5. After the team played its championship game, the coach treated the children to ice cream.

    Which of the following correctly identifies the parts of speech in the underlined portions of the sentence above?

    A. Pronoun; verb
    B. Adjective; adverb
    C. Adverb; noun
    D. Adjective; verb

6. Surveillance videos reveal suspicious activity behind the store around midnight.

    The underlined word in the sentence above is an example of which of the following parts of speech?

    A. Article
    B. Pronoun
    C. Preposition
    D. Verb

7. Dolphins are social creatures and tend to live in pods ranging in size from ten to over one hundred animals.

    The word *social* serves as which of the following parts of speech in the sentence above?

    A. Adjective
    B. Preposition
    C. Verb
    D. Noun

8. Which of the following plural nouns is written in the correct form?

    A. Patioes
    B. Melodies
    C. Geeses
    D. Cactuses

9. When the cruise <u>ship</u> pulled into port, the seaside town was flooded <u>with</u> tourists.

   Which of the following correctly identifies the parts of speech in the underlined portions of the sentence above?

   A. Preposition; adverb
   B. Adjective; verb
   C. Noun; preposition
   D. Preposition; noun

10. Samuel left <u>his</u> riding boots at the stable last week.

    The underlined word in the sentence above is an example of which of the following parts of speech?

    A. Preposition
    B. Noun
    C. Adverb
    D. Pronoun

11. This year's concert series features rock, folk, and country music.

    The word *features* serves as which of the following parts of speech in the sentence above?

    A. Noun
    B. Verb
    C. Adverb
    D. Adjective

12. Which of the following plural nouns is written in the correct form?

    A. Nucleuses
    B. Childs
    C. Criteria
    D. Potatos

13. Each <u>exquisite</u> necklace is <u>meticulously</u> crafted by hand.

    Which of the following correctly identifies the parts of speech in the underlined portions of the sentence above?

    A. Noun; adverb
    B. Adjective; adverb
    C. Adverb; adjective
    D. Adjective; adverb

14. Constructed with sustainable materials, the new music building on campus is powered by <u>an</u> array of solar panels.

The underlined word in the sentence above is an example of which of the following parts of speech?

A. Article
B. Noun
C. Preposition
D. Pronoun

15. Mechanics generally advise motorists to have their cars serviced every 3,000 miles.

The word *motorists* serves as which of the following types of speech in the sentence above?

A. Pronoun
B. Article
C. Preposition
D. Noun

Answer Key

1. B		**9.** C	
2. D		**10.** D	
3. C		**11.** B	
4. A		**12.** C	
5. A		**13.** B	
6. C		**14.** A	
7. A		**15.** D	
8. B			

Answers and Explanations

1. (B) Since the word *severe* modifies the noun *thunderstorm*, it functions as an adjective in this sentence. The word *later* functions as an adverb in this sentence, modifying the verb *developed*.

2. (D) Choice D is correct because the word *the* is an article that modifies the word *spread*.

3. (C) Because the word *repeatedly* modifies the verb *attempted*, it is used as an adverb in this sentence. Therefore, choice C is the correct answer.

4. (A) The word *alumni* is the plural form of the nouns *alumnus* and *alumna*. The other answer choices are incorrect because *mice* is the plural of *mouse*; *phenomena* is the plural of *phenomenon*; and *syllabi* is the plural of *syllabus*.

5. (A) The word *its* refers back to the noun previously introduced in the sentence, *team*, so it is a pronoun. The main action of the sentence is described by the verb *treated*.

6. (C) The word *behind* links the prepositional phrase *behind the store* to the rest of the sentence and therefore acts as a preposition in this sentence.

7. (A) Since the word *social* modifies the noun *dolphins*, it serves as an adjective in this sentence. Therefore, choice A is the correct answer.

8. (B) The word *melodies* is the plural form of the noun *melody*. The other answer choices are incorrect because *patios* is the plural of *patio*; *geese* is the plural of *goose*; and *cacti* is the plural of *cactus*.

9. (C) Because the word *ship* identifies a person, place, or thing, it is a noun. The word *with* links the prepositional phrase *with tourists* to the rest of the sentence.

10. (D) Because the word *his* refers to the noun antecedent *Samuel*, the word *his* functions as a pronoun in this sentence.

11. (B) The word *features* presents the main action in this sentence and therefore serves as a verb, making choice B the correct answer.

12. (C) The word *criteria* is the plural form of the noun *criterion*. The other answer choices are incorrect because *nuclei* is the plural of *nucleus*; *children* is the plural of *child*; and *potatoes* is the plural of *potato*.

13. (B) Since the word *exquisite* modifies the noun *necklace*, it functions as an adjective in this sentence. The word *meticulously* functions as an adverb in this sentence, modifying the verb *crafted*.

14. (A) Choice A is correct because the word *an* is an article that modifies the word *array*.

15. (D) The word *motorists* serves as the direct object of the noun *Mechanics* in this sentence and functions as a noun. Therefore, choice D is the correct answer.

CHAPTER 39

Subject-Verb Agreement

The subject of a sentence must always agree with its verb. This means that the subject and verb must both be either singular or plural. **Subject-Verb Agreement questions** address whether there is a match between single and plural subjects and verbs.

Consider the following sentence:

Her niece was never in the mood to play hopscotch.　✓ CORRECT

The subject of this sentence, *her niece*, is singular. The verb, *was*, is also singular. This sentence has subject-verb agreement because the subject and verb are both singular. Now look at this sentence:

Her nieces was never in the mood to play hopscotch.　✗ INCORRECT

In this case, the subject is plural: *her nieces* refers to more than one niece. This sentence therefore requires the plural verb *were*:

Her nieces were never in the mood to play hopscotch.　✓ CORRECT

The singular verb *was* in the incorrect sentence has been replaced by the plural verb *were*. Now the subject and the verb are both plural, so the subject and verb agree. Here's another example:

Why doesn't your grandfather like to fish?　✓ CORRECT

The subject here, *grandfather*, is singular. The verb, *doesn't like*, is also singular. This sentence has subject-verb agreement.

This sentence, on the other hand, is incorrect:

Why doesn't your grandfather and grandmother like to fish?　✗ INCORRECT

Whenever a subject contains two nouns joined by the word *and*, this makes the subject plural. Since the subject of the sentence is now plural, the sentence needs a plural verb:

Why don't your grandfather and grandmother like to fish?　✓ CORRECT

The singular verb *doesn't like* from the sentence above has been replaced with the plural verb *don't like*. The subject and the verb are both in plural form, so they now agree.

Review Questions

1. Which of the following sentences has correct subject-verb agreement?

   A. After a heavy rainfall, the dry creek beds often overflows.
   B. The barns surrounding the farmhouse were painted shades of red and brown.
   C. Many trees in this orchard produces a variety of delicious apples.
   D. Freezing temperatures last winter is blamed for the lackluster harvest.

2. Which of the following sentences contains subject-verb agreement?

   A. Both Jenna and Patrick is interested in playing soccer this year.
   B. Brian and Eileen expects to hear their favorite song at the dance tonight.
   C. The dog and the cat is both due for their annual veterinary visits.
   D. My aunt and my uncle plan to visit our family over the holidays.

3. Which of the following sentences provides an example of correct subject-verb agreement?

   A. The herd of elephants are being driven from their natural habitat.
   B. The flock of baby ducks search for bread crumbs near the edge of the pond.
   C. The pride of lions is traveling across the plains in search of fresh water.
   D. The pack of hungry wolves follow their prey until the early morning hours.

4. Which of the following sentences contains a correct example of subject-verb agreement?

   A. Neither Howard nor Phillip likes to play board games.
   B. Either the host or hostess greet guests when they arrive at the restaurant.
   C. Sally or Brenda volunteer at the hospital nearly every weekend.
   D. Hiking or jogging provide excellent cardiovascular exercise.

5. Which of the following sentences contains an example of correct subject-verb agreement?

   A. Both of the children prefer pink lemonade instead of iced tea.
   B. Everyone attend orientation meetings before the start of the semester.
   C. Somebody mow the grass regularly even though the house is vacant.
   D. All of the students enjoys the school trip at the end of the year.

6. Which of the following sentences has correct subject-verb agreement?

   A. Topics included in the manual ranges from welding to pipefitting.
   B. Captains of the ship rotates their time on and off duty.
   C. Dates for each club meeting is posted by the door.
   D. Numbers for current program enrollment indicate a high degree of interest.

7. Which of the following sentences contains subject-verb agreement?

    A. After practice this Saturday, the team play its season opener.
    B. Before the pool opens for the season, the waterpark staff provides lifeguard training.
    C. As classical music enthusiasts, the audience tend to favor works by Baroque composers.
    D. In addition to geometry and algebra, the class study calculus this year.

8. Which of the following sentences provides an example of correct subject-verb agreement?

    A. The list of standing committees is in the folder.
    B. One reason for college visits are to help students narrow down the many choices available.
    C. Peter's collection of model airplanes were started by gifts from his grandfather.
    D. A rare volume of classic folktales were donated to the library.

9. Which of the following sentences provides an example of correct subject-verb agreement?

    A. Street signs depicting small children at play is visible all over the neighborhood.
    B. Students pursuing degrees in healthcare take anatomy and physiology courses.
    C. Vendors selling food at the state fair undergoes regular safety inspections.
    D. Politicians running for office in this town frequently visits with local residents.

10. Which of the following sentences contains an example of correct subject-verb agreement?

    A. Julia and David performs solo pieces in this evening's choral concert.
    B. Brian or Alice plan to assist at the school science fair next week.
    C. Mary and her sisters browse antique stores for unique gift items.
    D. Donald or his brother stop at the grocery store on Fridays to pick up milk and bread.

11. Which of the following sentences has correct subject-verb agreement?

    A. Visitors who toured the botanical garden was impressed with its lush beauty.
    B. Members of the honor society are chosen based on academic achievement.
    C. Archaeologists working at the excavation site has discovered evidence of ancient civilizations.
    D. Lawyers at the firm serves as mentors to law student interns.

12. Which of the following sentences contains subject-verb agreement?

    A. Charles and Katherine, veteran news reporters, interview the mayoral candidate.
    B. Charles and Katherine, veteran news reporters, interviews the mayoral candidate.
    C. Several veteran news reporters interviews the mayoral candidate.
    D. Veteran news reporters, Charles and Katherine, interviews the mayoral candidate.

13. Which of the following sentences provides an example of correct subject-verb agreement?

    A. The damaged wiper blades on the truck is being replaced.
    B. The two mailboxes in front of the house overflows with newspapers.
    C. The bright rays of the sun are strongest between 10 a.m. and 2 p.m.
    D. The many pickets of the backyard fence is painted white.

14. Which of the following sentences contains a correct example of subject-verb agreement?

    A. Everyone who hears that song comment on its catchy rhythm.
    B. Anyone who cares about the environment recycles plastic water bottles.
    C. Somebody who listens to that radio station call in every morning.
    D. Both professors who are on sabbatical intends to write a book this year.

15. Which of the following sentences contains an example of correct subject-verb agreement?

    A. Because of the excellent school district, houses for sale in this area sells quickly.
    B. Since there are many clouds this evening, stars in the night sky is not visible.
    C. With the excellent park system, visitors to the area enjoys many recreational activities.
    D. Despite the disappointing stock report, investors in the company remain optimistic.

Answer Key

1. B		9. B	
2. D		10. C	
3. C		11. B	
4. A		12. A	
5. A		13. C	
6. D		14. B	
7. B		15. D	
8. A			

Answers and Explanations

1. (B) Since the subjects of these sentences are plural, the accompanying verbs must also be plural. Choices A, C, and D present plural subjects with singular nouns, making these answer choices incorrect.

2. (D) Choice D provides an example of a sentence containing subject-verb agreement since the compound subject, *aunt and uncle*, is considered a plural subject. Therefore, the verb must also be plural, as is the case with the verb *plan*.

3. (C) These sentences' subjects are collective nouns that indicate group unity and are singular in number. Only choice C pairs its singular subject with a singular verb.

4. (A) Compound subjects with multiple nouns are still considered singular if they are joined with words like *or* or *nor*. Therefore, choice A is correct because it links a singular subject, *Howard nor Phillip*, with the singular verb *likes*.

5. (A) Indefinite pronouns that are singular, such as *everyone* and *somebody*, require a singular verb; indefinite pronouns that are plural, including *both* and *all*, need a plural verb. Choice A's plural subject, *Both*, agrees with its plural verb, *prefer*.

6. (D) Choice D contains correct subject-verb agreement since the subject *Numbers* is plural, and the verb *indicate* is also plural. The other answer choices present plural subjects with singular verbs and are therefore incorrect.

7. (B) Each of these sentences contains a collective noun that indicates group unity. Since this type of noun is considered a singular noun, the proceeding verb must also be singular.

8. (A) Choice A correctly conjugates the singular subject *list* with the singular verb *is*; the other answer choices incorrectly link plural verbs to plural nouns in the preceding prepositional phrases rather than to the singular subjects of these sentences.

9. (B) Each of these sentences contains a plural subject that requires a plural verb. Only choice B correctly pairs the plural subject *Students* with the plural verb *take*; the other sentences all use plural subjects with singular verbs.

10. (C) Compound subjects joined by the word *and* are considered plural and require plural verbs; compound subjects linked with the word *or* are considered singular and must be followed by singular verbs. Therefore, only choice C is correct.

11. (B) Choice B contains correct subject-verb agreement since the subject *Members* is plural, and the verb *are chosen* is also plural. The other answer choices present plural subjects with singular verbs and are therefore incorrect.

12. (A) Choice A is the only sentence that correctly uses a plural subject, *Charles and Katherine*, with a plural verb, *interview*. The other answer choices connect plural subjects with singular verbs.

13. (C) Choice C's plural subject *rays* is correctly paired with the plural verb *are*. Since choices A, B, and D use plural subjects along with singular verbs, they are incorrect.

14. (B) Choice B is correct because the singular verb *cares* is paired with its singular subject, *Anyone*. Most indefinite pronouns are singular and require singular verbs, except for certain pronouns, such as *both* and *all*.

15. (D) Choices A, B, and C are examples of incorrect subject-verb agreement in which plural subjects, separated from verbs with prepositional phrases, are incorrectly paired with singular verbs. Choice D correctly links a plural subject with a plural verb.

CHAPTER 40

Verb Tenses

Verb tenses are used to show when the action is taking place in the sentence. The most common verb tenses are past, present, and future. If the action of the sentence is taking place in the past, the verbs showing that action should be in the past tense. If the action of the sentence is taking place in the present, the verbs showing that action should be in the present tense, and so on.

Verb Tenses questions address the correct use of verb tenses and whether a verb phrase matches the tense used in the rest of the sentence.

The following example is written in the past tense. It contains the past tense phrase *yesterday*:

Andrew received his class award yesterday.　✓ CORRECT

The verb *received* correctly indicates that the action of the sentence took place in the past.

The following example is incorrect because the past tense verb *received* does not make sense in the context of the sentence. Here we have a future tense phrase, *tomorrow*:

Andrew received his class award tomorrow.　✗ INCORRECT

The correct verb for this sentence is *will receive*, to place this sentence in the future tense:

Andrew will receive his class award tomorrow.　✓ CORRECT

The following sentence also contains a reference to show that the action took place in the past. The phrase *before the movie* shows that some action took place prior to the movie. That action therefore needs a past tense verb.

Before the movie, the group went out to dinner.　✓ CORRECT

This sentence is correct as written. The past tense verb *went* shows that the group had dinner before seeing the film.

Here's a sentence that correctly shows its action taking place in the present. It contains the present tense phrase *today*, and it uses the present tense verb *is choosing*:

She is choosing between her top two colleges today.　✓ CORRECT

The following example also contains the present tense verb phrase *is choosing*. However, the phrase *last week* indicates that the action of the sentence took place in the past. This sentence, as written, is therefore incorrect:

She is choosing between her top two colleges last week.　✗ INCORRECT

The sentence should read that she *chose* between her top two colleges last week, to show clearly that the action took place in the past:

She chose between her top two colleges last week. ✓ CORRECT

Review Questions

1. Because of the frost warning issued yesterday, Henry _____ to take his houseplants off the back porch and bring them indoors last night.

   Which of the following verbs correctly completes the sentence above?

   A. has decided
   B. decide
   C. decided
   D. will decide

2. For the family reunion next weekend, Elizabeth and her sisters _____ apple, cherry, and blueberry pies the morning of the event.

   Which of the following verbs correctly completes the sentence above?

   A. will bake
   B. bake
   C. baked
   D. have baked

3. Students who register for classes today may _____ their class schedules online.

   Which of the following verbs correctly completes the sentence above?

   A. will view
   B. view
   C. viewed
   D. have viewed

4. When Judy arrives at the station later this evening, she _____ the late train to Washington, D.C.

   Which of the following verbs correctly completes the sentence above?

   A. boarding
   B. board
   C. boarded
   D. will board

5. Despite the large crowds at the zoo last Friday, Matthew and his mother _____ to see the new snow leopard cubs.

   Which of the following verbs correctly completes the sentence above?

   A. manage
   B. managed
   C. will manage
   D. have managed

6. Although Pluto was formerly considered the ninth planet from the sun, astronomers now _____ Pluto as one of several dwarf planets orbiting the outer Solar System.

   Which of the following verbs correctly completes the sentence above?

   A. consider
   B. will consider
   C. had considered
   D. considered

7. Katie's parents _____ her school supplies after updated supply lists are posted next week.

   Which of the following verbs correctly completes the sentence above?

   A. had purchased
   B. purchase
   C. purchased
   D. will purchase

8. Typically, student council meetings are held the first Wednesday of the month, and the foreign language club _____ twice a month on Fridays.

   Which of the following verbs correctly completes the sentence above?

   A. had met
   B. meets
   C. met
   D. will have met

9. It is estimated that within the next decade, temperatures _____ to escalate, and coastal areas will be more vulnerable to rising waters.

   Which of the following verbs correctly completes the sentence above?

   A. continued
   B. continue
   C. will continue
   D. had continued

10. With the addition of a third highway lane a few months ago, traffic congestion between the two cities was significantly _____.

    Which of the following verbs correctly completes the sentence above?

    A. reduced
    B. reduce
    C. will reduce
    D. reducing

11. Even though Janice has a gym membership, she _____ to take long walks outside when the weather is so pleasant.

    Which of the following verbs correctly completes the sentence above?

    A. preferred
    B. will prefer
    C. prefers
    D. had preferred

12. The upcoming school trip to the natural history museum _____ an excellent opportunity for students to learn more about many dinosaur species.

    Which of the following verbs correctly completes the sentence above?

    A. had provided
    B. will provide
    C. provided
    D. provide

13. Jacob _____ piano very well; in fact, he is currently mastering one of Bach's Two-Part Inventions.

    Which of the following verbs correctly completes the sentence above?

    A. playing
    B. will play
    C. played
    D. plays

14. Since the company's annual report was due on Thursday, Francis _____ extra hours last week to ensure it was completed.

    Which of the following verbs correctly completes the sentence above?

    A. worked
    B. work
    C. is working
    D. will work

15. In anticipation of increased demand, the local food bank _____ its stock of nonperishable goods at its annual canned food drive next month.

Which of the following verbs correctly completes the sentence above?

A. had replenished
B. replenished
C. will replenish
D. replenish

Answer Key

1. C

2. A

3. B

4. D

5. B

6. A

7. D

8. B

9. C

10. A

11. C

12. B

13. D

14. A

15. C

Answers and Explanations

1. (C) This sentence is written in the past tense, as indicated by the word *yesterday* and the phrase *last night*. Therefore, the correct answer must also be in the past tense.

2. (A) Because this sentence describes an action that will take place in the future, as indicated by the phrases *next weekend* and *morning of the event*, a verb in the future tense is required.

3. (B) The content of this sentence, which includes the word *today*, pertains to the present tense, so choice B is correct. Choice D is not correct since the verb is in the present perfect tense, indicating an action that happened at some unspecified time before the present.

4. (D) Because the time frame indicated by this sentence is revealed by the phrase *later this evening*, the correct answer must be a verb in the

future tense. Therefore, choice D is the correct answer.

5. (B) The phrase *last Friday* places the action in this sentence in the past tense. Therefore, choice B is the best answer since a verb in the past tense is needed.

6. (A) Words such as *now* and the present tense verb *orbiting* indicate that this sentence is written in the present tense. Therefore, choice A is the best answer.

7. (D) The time frame suggested in this sentence is in the future, as shown by the word *after* and the phrase *next week*. Choice D contains a verb in the future tense and is the correct answer.

8. (B) This sentence describes an action that is continuing, so verbs must be written in the present tense. The correct answer, choice B, is a present tense verb.

9. (C) Phases such as *within the next decade* and *will be more vulnerable* place this sentence's time frame in the future. Therefore, a verb written in the future tense is required.

10. (A) This sentence pertains to an action completed in the past, as indicated by the phrase *a few months ago*. Choice A, a verb in the past tense, is the best answer.

11. (C) This sentence is written in the present tense, as indicated by the present tense verbs in the sentence, *has* and *is*. Therefore, the correct answer must also be in the present tense.

12. (B) Because the museum trip mentioned in this sentence is described as *upcoming*, the event must take place in the future. Choice B presents a verb written in the future tense.

13. (D) This sentence is written in the present tense, as revealed by the phrase *is currently mastering*. Therefore, the correct answer must also be in the present tense.

14. (A) Phrases like *was due* and *last week* clearly place the action of this sentence in the past tense, so choice A is the best answer.

15. (C) Since the action of this sentence will take place in the future, as suggested by the phrases *In anticipation* and *next month*, the correct answer must be a verb written in the future tense.

CHAPTER 41

Pronouns

Pronouns are words used to refer to nouns. Usually a pronoun will be used after a noun has already been given in the sentence or paragraph. The noun that the pronoun refers to is called the **antecedent**.

<u>Sasha</u> is a vegetarian, so <u>she</u> will order a nonmeat entrée.

In this example, the pronoun *she* is used to refer to Sasha. *Sasha* is the antecedent of the pronoun.

Similarly, in the following sentence, the pronoun *him* is used to refer to Jorge. *Jorge* is the antecedent of the pronoun:

<u>Jorge</u> loves all the gifts that the bowling team gave <u>him</u>.

In the following example, the pronoun *their* is used to refer to the Rudolphs. *The Rudolphs* is the antecedent in this sentence.

<u>The Rudolphs</u> have an apple tree in <u>their</u> backyard.

Pronoun Forms

When a pronoun is used, it must be in the correct form. Pronouns can act as **subjects** doing the action. They can also act as **objects** receiving the action, and they can show **possession**.

In the following sentence, the pronoun *she* is used as a subject. *She* is completing the action of ordering, so the subjective form of the pronoun is used correctly.

<u>Sasha</u> is a vegetarian, so <u>she</u> will order a nonmeat entrée.   ✓ CORRECT

It wouldn't sound right to use an object form of the pronoun in this sentence:

<u>Sasha</u> is a vegetarian, so <u>her</u> will order a nonmeat
entrée.   ✗ INCORRECT

Instead, the object form should be used when the pronoun is receiving the action of the verb, as in this example:

<u>Sasha</u> is a vegetarian, so the waiter brought <u>her</u> a
nonmeat entrée.   ✓ CORRECT

Here is a list of subjective, objective, and possessive forms of pronouns.

	Subjective	**Objective**	**Possessive**
First Person	I	me	my, mine
	we	us	our, ours
Second Person	you	you	your, yours
Third Person	he	him	his
	she	her	her
	it	it	its
	they	them	their, theirs

These forms of pronouns are also called **cases**.

Gender and Number

Pronouns can show both gender and number. In other words, they can be masculine or feminine, and they can be singular or plural. Pronouns should match their antecedent in both respects. If a noun is singular feminine, the pronoun should be singular feminine as well. If a noun is plural neutral, the pronoun should be plural neutral as well, and so on.

Jorge loves all the gifts that the bowling team gave him.

In this sentence, the antecedent *Jorge* is masculine and singular. The pronoun *him* is also masculine and singular.

In the following example, the antecedent *The Rudolphs* is plural. The pronoun *their* is also plural.

The Rudolphs have an apple tree in their backyard.

Finally, the following sentence shows an example of a gender-neutral antecedent, *the table*. The table has no gender, so it is referenced using the gender-neutral possessive pronoun *its*:

The table was polished to show off the beautiful grain of its wood.

In cases where a single person is being discussed but that person's gender has not been made clear, the singular pronoun phrase *he or she* should be used.

Each camper must make sure that he or she packs
enough warm clothes for the week.   ✓ CORRECT

In this example, *each camper* is the antecedent. This antecedent is singular, but the gender is not clear. The phrase *he or she* is used correctly to refer back to *each camper*.

It may be tempting to use the pronoun *they* when the gender of a singular antecedent is not specified; however, this is incorrect.

The word *they* is a plural pronoun, so it should not be used with singular antecedents.

Each <u>camper</u> must make sure that <u>they</u> pack enough warm clothes for the week.   ✗ INCORRECT

It would be correct to use *they* if the antecedent was also plural, as in the sentence below:

All <u>campers</u> must make sure that <u>they</u> pack enough warm clothes for the week.   ✓ CORRECT

Relative Pronouns

Pronoun questions on the TEAS also test relative pronouns (*who, which,* and *that*) and the correct usage of *who* versus *whom*. Regarding these pronouns, there are two points to keep in mind.

> The relative pronoun *who* is always used to refer to people, whereas *which* and *that* are used to refer to things.

<u>Principal Smith</u> is the one <u>who</u> ordered the extra copies.   ✓ CORRECT

<u>Principal Smith</u> is the one <u>that</u> ordered the extra copies.   ✗ INCORRECT

In these sentences, *Principal Smith* is the antecedent. Since *Principal Smith* is a person, the pronoun *who* should be used.

Here's an example of a relative pronoun that refers back to a thing:

To Kill a Mocking Bird is the book <u>that</u> I told you about.   ✓ CORRECT

To Kill a Mockingbird is the book <u>whom</u> I told you about.   ✗ INCORRECT

> The word *who* is used when the pronoun is the subject completing the action, and the word *whom* is used when the pronoun is a direct object receiving action.

The <u>teacher</u> is a knowledgeable instructor <u>who</u> truly cares about her students.   ✓ CORRECT

The <u>teacher</u> is a knowledgeable instructor <u>whom</u> truly cares about her students.   ✗ INCORRECT

These sentences use relative pronouns to refer back to the noun *the teacher*. In this case, the teacher is performing an action: she truly cares about her students. Because she is performing the action shown by the verb *cares*, the pronoun *who* should be used.

The following examples show a relative pronoun used as the direct object of an action. In this case, the pronoun *whom* should be used. Here, Carol performed the action of speaking. The person to *whom* she spoke was the recipient of her action.

| Carol was not sure to <u>whom</u> she was speaking. | ✓ CORRECT |
| Carol was not sure to <u>who</u> she was speaking. | ✗ INCORRECT |

Review Questions

1. When <u>Joseph</u> arrives at the bookstore, _____ will look for a birthday gift for his niece.

   Which of the following options is the correct pronoun for the sentence above? The antecedent of the pronoun to be added is underlined.

   A. we
   B. he
   C. him
   D. they

2. The high school band will perform _____ new set at the first football game.

   Which of the following is the correct pronoun to complete the sentence above?

   A. their
   B. our
   C. one's
   D. its

3. Steven is a dedicated student _____ always completes his class assignments on time.

   Which of the following correctly completes the sentence above?

   A. whom
   B. which
   C. who
   D. that

4. Since that medical office is so busy, <u>patients</u> often schedule _____ appointments months in advance.

   Which of the following is the correct pronoun for the sentence above? The antecedent of the pronoun to be added is underlined.

   A. their
   B. they're
   C. it's
   D. its

5. Which of the following is an example of a grammatically correct sentence?

   A. Summer courses are offered to students that want to learn more about filmmaking.
   B. Summer courses are offered to students who want to learn more about filmmaking.
   C. Summer courses are offered to students which want to learn more about filmmaking.
   D. Summer courses are offered to students whom want to learn more about filmmaking.

6. After <u>Wendy and Daniel</u> gather their fishing gear,_____ will walk to the pond.

   Which of the following options is the correct pronoun for the sentence above? The antecedent of the pronoun to be added is underlined.

   A. we
   B. she
   C. he
   D. they

7. Many doctors advise _____ patients to get plenty of daily exercise and rest.

   Which of the following is the correct pronoun to complete the sentence above?

   A. their
   B. they're
   C. one's
   D. his

8. After the professor agreed to write a letter of recommendation, she asked to _____ it should be sent.

   Which of the following correctly completes the sentence above?

   A. which
   B. whom
   C. who
   D. that

9. If the <u>team</u> loses tonight's game, _____ chances for playing in the state finals decrease.

   Which of the following is the correct pronoun for the sentence above? The antecedent of the pronoun to be added is underlined.

   A. they're
   B. their
   C. its
   D. it's

10. Which of the following is an example of a grammatically correct sentence?

    A. The store manager forgot whom she issued a refund.
    B. The store manager forgot who she issued a refund to.
    C. The store manager forgot to who she issued a refund.
    D. The store manager forgot to whom she issued a refund.

11. If Maria locks her keys in the car, _____ will have to call a locksmith to open the doors.

Which of the following options is the correct pronoun for the sentence above? The antecedent of the pronoun to be added is underlined.

    A. she
    B. we
    C. her
    D. they

12. Jason and his friends arrived at _____ destination about an hour later than expected.

Which of the following is the correct pronoun to complete the sentence above? The antecedent of the pronoun to be added is underlined.

    A. its
    B. their
    C. they're
    D. his

13. Extra boxed lunches will be given to _____ might want them.

Which of the following correctly completes the sentence above?

    A. whoever
    B. whichever
    C. whatever
    D. whomever

14. Terence and Sonia refused to ride the roller coaster because _____ afraid of heights.

Which of the following is the correct pronoun and verb for the sentence above? The antecedent of the pronoun to be added is underlined.

    A. it's
    B. they're
    C. their
    D. its

15. Which of the following is an example of a grammatically correct sentence?

    A. The pharmacist which filled my prescription gave me information about the medication.

    B. The pharmacist that filled my prescription gave me information about the medication.

    C. The pharmacist who filled my prescription gave me information about the medication.

    D. The pharmacist whom filled my prescription gave me information about the medication.

Answer Key

1. B		**9.** C	
2. D		**10.** D	
3. C		**11.** A	
4. A		**12.** B	
5. B		**13.** D	
6. D		**14.** B	
7. A		**15.** C	
8. B			

Answers and Explanations

1. (B) Since the antecedent, *Joseph*, is singular and masculine, the correct answer must also be singular and masculine. Therefore, choice B, the pronoun *he*, is the correct answer.

2. (D) This sentence has a singular antecedent since the noun *band* refers to one unified body. Therefore, the singular pronoun *its* is needed.

3. (C) In this sentence, the subjective case form *who* is needed since *who* is the subject of the clause *always completes his assignments on time*. The pronouns *that* and *which* refer to things, not people, and *whom* is an objective case pronoun for direct and indirect objects.

4. (A) In this sentence, the antecedent *patients* is a plural noun that requires a plural possessive pronoun before the noun *appointments* to

show ownership. Choice B is incorrect because *they're* is a contraction for *they are* and not a plural possessive pronoun.

5. (B) Choice B is grammatically correct since the subjective case pronoun *who* is needed as the subject of the clause modifying the noun *students*. Choices A and C incorrectly use pronouns that refer to objects, and choice D incorrectly uses the objective case pronoun *whom*.

6. (D) Since the antecedent, *Wendy and Daniel*, is plural, the correct answer must also be plural. Therefore, choice D, the pronoun *they*, is the correct answer.

7. (A) This sentence has a plural antecedent, *doctors*, so it requires a plural pronoun. Therefore, choice A is the best answer.

8. (B) In this sentence, the objective case form *whom* is needed since *whom* serves as the direct object of the sentence. The pronouns *that* and *which* refer to things, not people, and *who* is the subjective case form used for subjects of sentences and clauses.

9. (C) In this sentence, the antecedent *team* is a collective and therefore singular noun that requires a singular possessive pronoun. Choice B is incorrect because it is a plural possessive pronoun. Choices A and D are incorrect since they are contractions for *they are* and *it is* and not relevant to this sentence.

10. (D) Choice D is grammatically correct since the objective case pronoun *whom* is needed as the direct object of the clause modifying the noun *manager*. Choice C uses a subjective case pronoun and is incorrect.

11. (A) Since the antecedent, *Maria*, is singular and feminine, the correct answer must also be singular and feminine. Therefore, choice A, the pronoun *she*, is the correct answer.

12. (B) The antecedent *Jason and his friends* is plural, so the possessive pronoun *their* is needed to complete this sentence. The other options are either singular or do not show possession.

13. (D) An objective case pronoun is needed in this sentence to serve as the direct object, so choice D, *whomever*, is correct. Choice A presents a subjective case pronoun, and choices B and C are pronouns used to refer to things, not people.

14. (B) In this sentence, the antecedent *Terence and Sonia* is a plural noun that requires a plural pronoun and verb, so *they're*, a contraction for *they are*, is correct. Choice C is incorrect because *their* is a plural possessive pronoun used to show ownership and not relevant to this sentence.

15. (C) Choice C is grammatically correct since the subjective case pronoun *who* is needed as the subject of the clause modifying the noun *pharmacist*. Choices A and B incorrectly use pronouns that refer to objects, and choice D incorrectly uses the objective case pronoun *whom*.

CHAPTER 42

Homophones

Homophones are words that sound similar but are spelled differently and have different meanings. Common homophones include the words *it's/its* and *their/there/they're*.

The table below shows homophones found often in English and their definitions.

Homophones	Definitions
Anecdote/antidote	An **anecdote** is a story; an **antidote** is a remedy for an illness or problem.
Blue/blew	**Blue** is a color; **blew** is the past tense of the verb *to blow*.
Capital/capitol	A **capital** letter is a letter written in upper case or the primary political city in a state; a **capitol** is a building or group of buildings used for state governance.
Confident/confidant	**Confident** is an adjective meaning self-assured. A **confidant** is a trusted friend or advisor.
Creek/creak	A **creek** is a small body of water. A **creak** is a sound: the wooden floor *creaked* when she stepped on it.
Edition/addition	An **edition** is a version of text; **addition** is an operation in math.
Effect/affect	The word *effect* is commonly used as a noun. An **effect** is the result produced by some causal factor. The word *affect* is commonly used as a verb. To **affect** something means to have an impact on it.
For/four	**For** is a preposition showing purpose; **four** is a number.
Here/hear	The word **here** indicates location; the word **hear** means to perceive sound.
Insure/ensure	**Insure** is generally used to refer to insurance; when you insure something, you protect it against harm. To **ensure** means to make certain.
Its/it's	The word **its** is a possessive pronoun. The word **it's** is the contraction for *it is*.
Meet/meat	The verb **meet** means to come together; the noun **meat** refers to animal protein.

Homophones	Definitions
Pair/pare/pear	The noun **pair** means two of something: he bought a *pair* of socks. The verb **pare** means to cut away or reduce: he *pared* down his possessions to just the essentials. The noun **pear** is a fruit.
Pale/pail	The word **pale** means light in color; the word **pail** means a bucket.
Peace/piece	The word **peace** indicates harmony or lack of conflict; the word **piece** means a portion.
Peek/peak	**Peek** means to take a look or to spy; **peak** means the top or highest point.
Principal/principle	A **principal** is a person who is the head or leader. A **principle** is a rule or guideline.
Site/cite	The word **site** is a noun meaning location. The word **cite** is a verb meaning to give credit to a source.
Sole/soul	**Sole** is an adjective meaning only. **Soul** is a noun that refers to a person's spiritual nature.
Stationary/stationery	**Stationary** means motionless or fixed in place. **Stationery** is fine paper used for writing.
Their/there/they're	The word **their** is a possessive pronoun: they gave us the address of *their* new home. The word **there** indicates location: we will see you *there*. **They're** is a contraction for *they are*.
Then/than	The word **then** indicates order in a sequence: first this happened, *then* that happened. The word **than** indicates comparison: she is taller *than* him.
Too/two/to	**Too** means also. **Two** refers to the number 2. **To** is a preposition.
Week/weak	The noun **week** is a time interval of seven days. The adjective **weak** means not strong.
Whale/wail	A **whale** is a large sea mammal. To **wail** means to scream or cry.
Which/witch	The word **which** is a relative pronoun: *which* side of the family are you related to? The word **witch** is a noun: she dressed as a *witch* for Halloween.
Whole/hole	**Whole** is an adjective meaning entire. **Hole** is a noun meaning a gap or an opening.
Whose/who's	The word **whose** is a relative pronoun: *whose* side are you on, anyway? The word **who's** is a contraction for *who is*: Sherrie is the one *who's* calling.
Your/you're	**Your** is a possessive pronoun: is that *your* dog? **You're** is a contraction for *you are*.

Review Questions

1. Which of the following underlined words is an example of correct spelling?

   A. Flooding along the <u>creak</u> has caused the embankment to erode.
   B. At the <u>peek</u> of his career, the artist was exhibiting many watercolors.
   C. Seafood will be offered as an alternative to <u>meet</u> dishes at the dinner.
   D. Prior to our trip to England, we will spend a <u>week</u> in Ireland.

2. _____ planning a fall road trip when the leaves start to exhibit _____ fall color.

   Which of the following options correctly completes the sentence above?

   A. They're; their
   B. Their; they're
   C. They're; there
   D. There; they're

3. The class rehearsed for several weeks before _____ annual holiday performance.

   Which of the following correctly completes the sentence above?

   A. they're
   B. their
   C. its
   D. it's

4. Following recent personnel changes, the company decided that _____ time to update _____ website.

   Which of the following sets of words should be used to fill in the blanks in the sentence above?

   A. its; its
   B. it's; its
   C. it's; it's
   D. its; it's

5. At the antiquarian book sale, a signed first _____ of that novel sold for nearly one thousand dollars.

   Which of the following is the correctly spelled word to complete the sentence?

   A. edition
   B. eddition
   C. addition
   D. adition

6. Which of the following underlined words is an example of correct spelling?

    A. Drivers must proceed cautiously in this area because of the large <u>dear</u> population.
    B. Veronica's collection of greeting cards from family members is very <u>deer</u> to her.
    C. At the petting zoo, children may visit with <u>dear</u>, goats, and many other animals.
    D. Although it remains controversial, <u>deer</u> hunting is now legal in this county.

7. If we are going to watch _____ hockey game this evening, we'll need to get _____ before 7 p.m.

    Which of the following options correctly completes the sentence above?

    A. there; they're
    B. they're; their
    C. their; there
    D. they're; there

8. Aerobic exercise is necessary for optimal physical health, but _____ also important to perform weight-bearing exercises.

    Which of the following correctly completes the sentence above?

    A. its
    B. there
    C. their
    D. it's

9. My coffee mug has lost _____ handle, and now _____ starting to chip along the rim.

    Which of the following sets of words should be used to fill in the blanks in the sentence above?

    A. its; it's
    B. it's; its
    C. it's; it's
    D. its; its

10. Although they have only been friends for a few months, Jarrod is Emily's trusted _____ .

    Which of the following is the correctly spelled word to complete the sentence?

    A. confidence
    B. confident
    C. confidant
    D. confidance

11. Which of the following underlined words is an example of correct spelling?

    A. Children should drink plenty of milk to <u>insure</u> healthy bone development.
    B. Jack decided to <u>ensure</u> his valuable painting for the full replacement cost.
    C. Getting enough rest has a positive <u>affect</u> on one's ability to concentrate.
    D. Headaches are a reported side <u>effect</u> of this particular medication.

12. _____ is an ongoing problem with that software that _____ trying to resolve.

    Which of the following options correctly completes the sentence above?

    A. They're; their
    B. Their; they're
    C. There; they're
    D. They're; there

13. Students participating in the science fair should submit _____ project entries by Friday.

    Which of the following correctly completes the sentence above?

    A. they're
    B. their
    C. its
    D. it's

14. Since the levy will be placed on the November ballot, _____ time to recruit volunteers to support _____ passage.

    Which of the following sets of words should be used to fill in the blanks in the sentence above?

    A. it's; its
    B. its; it's
    C. it's; it's
    D. its; its

15. Even though I would like to include that country in my travel itinerary, the current political unrest makes it much _____ dangerous to visit.

    Which of the following is the correctly spelled word to complete the sentence?

    A. to
    B. two
    C. too
    D. tow

Answer Key

1. D
2. A
3. C
4. B
5. A
6. D
7. C
8. D

9. A
10. C
11. D
12. C
13. B
14. A
15. C

Answers and Explanations

1. (D) Choice D is the only sentence with correct usage of the underlined word. Choices A, B, and C provide examples of words that sound like the intended word choices but are incorrect.

2. (A) Choice A is the correct combination of words to complete this sentence. The first part of the sentence requires the contraction *They're* for *They are*, and the second part of the sentence needs the possessive plural pronoun *their* to refer back to the plural antecedent, *leaves*.

3. (C) Because the antecedent *class* is a singular, collective noun, the singular pronoun *its* is the correct answer. Choice B is a plural possessive pronoun, and choice D is the contraction for *it is*, so these choices are incorrect.

4. (B) In the first part of the sentence, the contraction *it's* is needed in place of the words *it is*. The second part of the sentence should be completed with the possessive pronoun *its*, which is not written with an apostrophe.

5. (A) In this sentence, the word *edition* is needed, which is spelled correctly in choice A.

6. (D) Choice D is the only sentence with correct usage of the underlined word. Choices A, B, and C provide examples of homophones that

sound like the intended word choice but are spelled differently and therefore incorrect.

7. (C) Choice C is the correct combination of words to complete this sentence. The first part of the sentence requires the possessive pronoun *their*; the second part of the sentence needs the adverb *there*, which typically indicates placement (in this case, the ice rink or site of the hockey game).

8. (D) In this sentence, the contraction for *it is*, or *it's*, is needed. Choice A presents the singular possessive pronoun *its* and is therefore incorrect in this sentence.

9. (A) The first part of the sentence should be completed with the possessive pronoun *its*, which is not written with an apostrophe. In the second part of the sentence, the contraction *it's* is needed in place of the words *it is*.

10. (C) In this sentence, the word *confidant* is needed, which is spelled correctly in choice C.

11. (D) Choice D is the only sentence with correct usage of the underlined word. Choices A, B, and C provide examples of words that sound like the intended word choice but are incorrect.

12. (C) Choice C is the correct combination of words to complete this sentence. The first part

of the sentence requires the adverb *There*, and the second part of the sentence needs the contraction *they're* for *they are*. The possessive plural pronoun *their* is not needed in this sentence.

13. (B) Because the antecedent *students* is a plural noun, the plural possessive pronoun *their* is the correct answer. Choice A is not a plural possessive pronoun but rather the contraction for *they are*, so this choice is incorrect.

14. (A) In the first part of the sentence, the contraction *it's* is needed in place of the words *it is*. The second part of the sentence should be completed with the possessive pronoun *its*, which is not written with an apostrophe.

15. (C) In this sentence, the adverb *too* is needed, which is spelled correctly in choice C.

CHAPTER 43

Punctuation

Punctuation questions address the correct use of punctuation in regular text and quotations. You must know the appropriate use of periods, question marks, exclamation points, commas, semicolons, colons, apostrophes, hyphens, double quotation marks, and single quotation marks.

Periods, Question Marks, and Exclamation Points

Periods are used at the end of a complete sentence. **Question marks** are used at the end of a question, and **exclamation points** are used to mark the end of a forceful command or a statement that expresses strong emotions.

Amira went skating Sunday.	Period
Did you know Amira went skating Sunday?	Question mark
I'm shocked that Amira went skating Sunday!	Exclamation point

Dependent and Independent Clauses

In order to understand the correct use of commas and semicolons, you must first understand the difference between a dependent and an independent clause. **Clauses** are groups of words that make up sentences. A **dependent clause** can't stand as a complete sentence on its own, whereas an **independent clause** forms a complete sentence and can stand on its own.

She forgot her sunglasses at the library

The clause in this example is an independent clause because it forms a complete sentence. It can stand entirely on its own.

The clause in the following example, by contrast, is a dependent clause. It does not form a complete sentence; we need more information to understand the full meaning being conveyed.

Because she was rushing to get to school

Here are a few more examples of dependent and independent clauses:

After the football game ended	Dependent
The committee voted against the bill	Independent
You really should learn to tie your shoe laces	Independent
Although Laura drove all over town	Dependent

Commas, Semicolons, and Colons

Dependent and independent clauses are important in understanding how and when to use commas and semicolons. A **comma** is a punctuation mark that shows a pause between ideas. Among other uses, commas can be used to separate items in a list and to join parts of sentences.

The following example uses commas correctly to separate three items in a list:

Rashid bought school supplies, water, and a backpack at the store.

Now consider this sentence, which uses commas correctly to join parts of a sentence:

Even though it was cold outside, we went camping anyway.

Notice that here the comma is being used to join a dependent clause—*Even though it was cold outside*—with an independent clause, *we went camping anyway*.

Commas can also be used to join two independent clauses, but the comma must be followed by a connecting word such as *and*, *but*, *for*, or *so*. These connecting words are called **coordinating conjunctions**. There are seven coordinating conjunctions that can be used to join independent clauses:

Coordinating Conjunctions

for

and

nor

but

or

yet

so

Coordinating conjunctions can be remembered by using a memory phrase. The first letter of each conjunction spells out the word *FANBOYS*.

If you use a coordinating conjunction to join two independent clauses, a comma must come directly before the conjunction:

A crowd gathered outside the building, and the protesters began to seem restless.	✓ CORRECT
A crowd gathered outside the building, the protestors began to seem restless.	✗ INCORRECT
A crowd gathered outside the building and the protesters began to seem restless.	✗ INCORRECT

The first example uses the coordinating conjunction *and*, which is correctly preceded by a comma. The second sentence is incorrect because it omits the coordinating conjunction. The last example is incorrect because it omits the comma before the coordinating conjunction.

Semicolons can be used to join two independent clauses without a coordinating conjunction. The second example above could be could be corrected by replacing the comma with a semicolon as follows:

A crowd gathered outside the building; the protesters began to seem restless.	✓ CORRECT

Semicolons are not used to join independent clauses with coordinating conjunctions, but they can be used with transitional words, such as *however*, *nevertheless*, and *therefore*. Whenever a semicolon joins two independent clauses with the help of a transitional word, a comma must follow the transitional word:

The evidence against the defendant was strong; nevertheless, the defendant was acquitted.	✓ CORRECT

In the preceding example, the transitional word *nevertheless* is preceded by a semicolon and followed by a comma. Without both of these punctuation marks, the sentence would be punctuated incorrectly:

The evidence against the defendant was strong; nevertheless the defendant was acquitted.	✗ INCORRECT
The evidence against the defendant was strong nevertheless, the defendant was acquitted.	✗ INCORRECT

Similar to semicolons, **colons** can also be used to join independent clauses. For a colon to be used, the second independent clause must expand upon the ideas in the first independent clause, as in the following sentence:

The evidence against the defendant was strong: the prosecution had gathered testimony from multiple eye witnesses.	✓ CORRECT

Colons can also be used to introduce elements in a list:

Three items should accompany you on every rafting trip: a rain poncho, a waterproof lunch kit, and a sturdy life jacket.	✓ CORRECT

Apostrophes and Hyphens

Apostrophes are used to show possession and to form contractions. To show possession, we normally add an apostrophe followed by an *s*:

Noun Form	Possessive Form	Example
the sun	the sun's	the sun's rays
a dog	a dog's	a dog's toy
our car	our car's	our car's horn

If the noun that is showing possession is a plural that ends in the letter *s*, normally only an apostrophe is used:

Noun Form	Possessive Form	Example
the families	the families'	the families' picnic baskets
the windows	the windows'	the windows' panes
your sneakers	your sneakers'	your sneakers' laces

Hyphens are used to separate some prefixes from the main part of the word, or root word. Hyphens should always be used following the prefixes *all-*, *ex-*, and *self-*. They should also be used after prefixes that precede a proper noun or a proper adjective:

Prefixes	Proper Nouns and Adjectives
all-seeing	trans-Siberian
ex-employer	mid-Atlantic
self-supporting	un-American

Hyphens are also used with compound adjectives that come before the word they modify.

Emma was a strong-willed person.	✓ CORRECT
Treats are an often-used incentive at the vet's office.	✓ CORRECT
Sunday's game was full of record-breaking plays.	✓ CORRECT

Hyphens are not used, however, in compound adjectives that start with adverbs ending in *-ly*:

✗ INCORRECT	✓ CORRECT
a frequently-made error	a frequently made error
a flimsily-built house	a flimsily built house
an awfully-loud noise	an awfully loud noise

In the left column in the table above, the words *frequently*, *flimsily*, and *awfully* are all adverbs ending in *-ly*. Hyphens should not be used following these words, as shown in the column on the right.

Quotation Marks

Quotation marks can come in double or single form, each with its own specific uses. **Double quotation marks** are used to signal direct quotations.

Sarah said, "It's a lovely day to go hiking."

A comma should also follow the direct quotation if the phrase is a statement:

"It's a lovely day to go hiking," Sarah said.

If the quoted phrase is a question, it should end with a question mark:

"Would you like to go on a hike with me?" Sarah asked.

Question marks, periods, commas, and exclamation points should be placed *inside* quotation marks.

The detective asked the witness several times, "Are you sure"?   ✗ INCORRECT

The detective asked the witness several times, "Are you sure?"   ✓ CORRECT

Single quotation marks are used to denote a quotation within a quotation:

Mrs. Juarez replied, "Sam said that he would 'need the car soon,' so don't keep it for too long."

It is not correct to use single quotation marks to show direct quotations. Double quotation marks should always be used for this purpose.

The errand boy told his boss that he was 'just going out for a pizza run.'   ✗ INCORRECT

The errand boy told his boss that he was "just going out for a pizza run."   ✓ CORRECT

Whenever quotation marks are used—either single or double—they should always precede and follow the quoted phrase. Both the beginning and ending quotation marks must be included.

Everyone yelled, "Go team! and cheered the players to victory.   ✗ INCORRECT

Everyone yelled, "Go team!" and cheered the players to victory.   ✓ CORRECT

In this example, the first sentence is missing the quotation marks after *team* that close the quoted phrase. The second example corrects this error by including the opening and closing quotation marks.

Review Questions

1. Which of the following is an example of correctly punctuated direct dialogue in a sentence?

   A. He explained, 'Rain gardens provide attractive landscaping that absorbs stormwater.'
   B. He explained that "Rain gardens provide attractive landscaping that absorbs stormwater."
   C. He explained, Rain gardens provide attractive landscaping that absorbs stormwater.
   D. He explained, "Rain gardens provide attractive landscaping that absorbs stormwater."

2. Which of the following sentences correctly punctuates direct dialogue?

   A. The conductor announced, "Our next selection is 'Spring' from Vivaldi's *Four Seasons*".

   B. The conductor announced, "Our next selection is 'Spring' from Vivaldi's *Four Seasons*."

   C. The conductor announced, "Our next selection is 'Spring' from Vivaldi's *Four Seasons*.'

   D. The conductor announced, 'Our next selection is "Spring" from Vivaldi's *Four Seasons*.'

3. Which of the following sentences correctly applies the rules of punctuation?

   A. In Hemingway's *The Sun Also Rises*, protagonist Jake Barnes explains, "You can't get away from yourself by moving from one place to another."

   B. In Hemingway's *The Sun Also Rises*, protagonist Jake Barnes explains, 'You can't get away from yourself by moving from one place to another.'

   C. In Hemingway's *The Sun Also Rises*, protagonist Jake Barnes explains, 'You can't get away from yourself by moving from one place to another'.

   D. In Hemingway's *The Sun Also Rises*, protagonist Jake Barnes explains, "You can't get away from yourself by moving from one place to another".

4. In addition to perfect form, successful Olympic swimmers possess the following three qualities _____ strength, speed, and stamina.

   Which of the following punctuation marks correctly completes the sentence above?

   A. ;
   B. ,
   C. :
   D. -

5. Which of the following sentences correctly applies the rules of punctuation?

   A. Terence tested out of several first-year classes; therefore he will graduate one semester early.

   B. Terence tested out of several first-year classes; therefore, he will graduate one semester early.

   C. Terence tested out of several first-year classes, therefore, he will graduate one semester early.

   D. Terence tested out of several first-year classes; therefore; he will graduate one semester early.

6. Which of the following is an example of a correctly punctuated sentence?

   A. My friend asked "What are your travel plans this summer?"
   B. My friend asked "What are your travel plans this summer"?
   C. My friend asked, "What are your travel plans this summer"?
   D. My friend asked, "What are your travel plans this summer?"

7. Which of the following sentences is correctly punctuated?

   A. Because of the large number of runners expected at this year's marathon advanced registration is required.
   B. Because of the large number of runners expected at this year's marathon. Advanced registration is required.
   C. Because of the large number of runners expected at this year's marathon, advanced registration is required.
   D. Because of the large number of runners expected at this year's marathon; advanced registration is required.

8. Which of the following is an example of a correctly punctuated sentence?

   A. Anne owns a variety of cookbooks; however, she prefers to search for recipes online.
   B. Anne owns a variety of cookbooks, however, she prefers to search for recipes online.
   C. Anne owns a variety of cookbooks however, she prefers to search for recipes online.
   D. Anne owns a variety of cookbooks; however she prefers to search for recipes online.

9. Which of the following sentences contains the appropriate use of an apostrophe?

   A. The college held it's annual convocation last week.
   B. This season's harvest should be plentiful due to optimal weather.
   C. Students must complete they're capstone projects prior to graduation.
   D. We are joining the Anderson's for a barbecue next Saturday.

10. Which of the following words is written correctly?

   A. un-kind
   B. re-adjust
   C. all-inclusive
   D. non-essential

11. Which of the following sentences is correctly punctuated?

   A. After interviewing several candidates, the hiring committee made its recommendation.
   B. After interviewing several candidates. The hiring committee made its recommendation.
   C. After interviewing several candidates; the hiring committee made its recommendation.
   D. After interviewing several candidates the hiring committee made its recommendation.

12. Which of the following sentences contains the appropriate use of an apostrophe?

    A. Executive Council member's discussed the new initiative at their meeting last month.
    B. Employment rates' in the region are starting to increase as the economy improves.
    C. Signs directing patient's to the registration area are posted throughout the hospital.
    D. Admissions counselors' schedules for next semester are posted in the office.

13. Which of the following sentences correctly applies the rules of punctuation?

    A. Although it costs $11.50 to see the play, discounts are available for senior citizens.
    B. Although it costs $11.50 to see the play. Discounts are available for senior citizens.
    C. Although it costs $11.50 to see the play discounts are available for senior citizens.
    D. Although it costs $11.50 to see the play; discounts are available for senior citizens.

14. Every summer, the Johnsons enjoy participating in the park's popular program, Happy Trails _____ 10 Short Hikes for Families and Children.

    Which of the following punctuation marks correctly completes the sentence above?

    A. ;
    B. ,
    C. :
    D. -

15. Which of the following words is written correctly?

    A. ex-chairperson
    B. un-imaginative
    C. re-apply
    D. non-fiction

Answer Key

1. D   **9.** B
2. B   **10.** C
3. A   **11.** A
4. C   **12.** D
5. B   **13.** A
6. D   **14.** C
7. C   **15.** A
8. A

Answers and Explanations

1. (D) Choice D is an example of direct dialogue with proper use of quotation marks. In choice C, the quotation marks are incorrectly omitted, and choice A incorrectly uses single quotation marks. Choice B, an example of an indirect quote, does not need quotation marks.

2. (B) Choice B is correct because the song title is indicated by single quotation marks, and the entire quote is enclosed by double quotation marks. Choice A places the period at the conclusion of the sentence outside the quotation marks and is therefore incorrect.

3. (A) Choice A provides the only example of a sentence that is punctuated correctly. In this sentence, the direct quote from Jake Barnes is enclosed within double quotation marks, and the ending punctuation, a period, precedes the final quotation marks.

4. (C) Choice C is the correct answer since this sentence requires a colon after the word *qualities*. When a sentence includes a list, a colon should be used after the independent clause preceding the list.

5. (B) To punctuate this sentence properly, the conjunctive adverb *therefore* that connects the two independent clauses must be preceded by a semicolon and followed by a comma. Therefore, only choice B is correct.

6. (D) Choice D provides an example of a direct quote that is punctuated correctly. A comma is used following the introductory phrase to set off the direct quote, and double quotation marks enclose both the quoted material and the final punctuation (in this case, a question mark).

7. (C) The properly punctuated sentence, choice C, separates the dependent clause that begins the sentence from the independent clause in the latter part of the sentence with a comma. The other sentences are incorrect because choice A omits the comma, choice B creates a sentence fragment, and choice D uses a semicolon without two independent clauses.

8. (A) Choice A contains two independent clauses joined by a conjunctive adverb, so the placement of a semicolon before and a comma following the word *however* is correct. Since the other sentences do not follow this required punctuation, they are incorrect.

9. (B) Only choice B provides an example of an apostrophe used correctly, since *season's* shows possession and requires this mark of punctuation. Choices A and C are examples of contractions requiring apostrophes, but they are incorrectly used in place of the pronouns *its* and *their*. Choice D contains an unnecessary apostrophe since the plural form *Andersons* is needed.

10. (C) A hyphen should be used following the prefixes *all-*, *ex-*, and *self-*. The other answer choices do not require hyphenation and should be written as one word.

11. (A) Choice A is an example of a correctly punctuated sentence in which the dependent clause is separated from the independent clause by a comma. Choice B creates a sentence fragment, and choice D incorrectly omits the comma. A semicolon is not necessary in choice C, as the two clauses are not both independent.

12. (D) Only choice D provides an example of an apostrophe used correctly since *counselors'* shows plural possession. Choices A, B, and C are incorrect since these sentences have nouns that are plural, not possessive, and therefore do not require an apostrophe.

13. (A) Choice A is the only correctly punctuated sentence because a comma is needed to separate the dependent and independent clauses. Choice B incorrectly features a period after the dependent clause and a capital *D* to begin a new sentence, while choice C incorrectly has no punctuation after the dependent clause, and choice D has a semicolon after the dependent clause.

14. (C) Choice C is the correct answer since the title and subtitle of the program should be separated by a colon. Subtitles are not distinguished from titles with semicolons, commas, or hyphens, making the other choices incorrect.

15. (A) Since a hyphen should be used following the prefixes *all-*, *ex-*, and *self-*, choice A is the correct answer. Choices B, C, and D incorrectly hyphenate compound nouns that should be written in closed form as one word.

CHAPTER 44

Capitalization

Capitalization questions address capitalization rules involving proper nouns. You must know how to apply capitalization rules to publication titles, individual names, professional titles, names of events, organizations, and geographic locations. Months, days, and holidays may also be tested.

A **proper noun** is the name of a specific person, place, or thing, such as an organization or a landmark. In the English language, proper nouns are always capitalized. Several specific examples of proper noun capitalization are shown in this chapter.

Publication Titles

When referring to a publication, such as a book or magazine, the first word in the title should be capitalized, as should all major words in the title. Minor words, such as *of* and *the*, are not capitalized.

✓ CORRECT	✗ INCORRECT
The Wall Street Journal	*the Wall Street Journal*
A Wrinkle in Time	*A Wrinkle In Time*
The Cat in the Hat	*The Cat In The Hat*

Individual Names

The names of specific people should be capitalized. Words that indicate family titles are capitalized if they are used to refer to a specific person.

✓ CORRECT	✗ INCORRECT
Jim Pearson	Jim pearson
Aunt Sally	aunt Sally
his only living uncle	his only living Uncle

Professional Titles

Professional titles, such as doctor or professor, are capitalized when they are used to refer to the name of a specific individual:

Regina was looking for a good doctor, so I sent her to Dr. Cole.	✓ CORRECT
The professor asked the students to call him Professor Thomas.	✓ CORRECT

Geographic Locations and Event Names

The names of geographic locations are capitalized if they refer to a specific place. This includes national landmarks and historical monuments, such as Lincoln's Memorial. The names of directions—east, west, north, and south—are capitalized if they refer to a specific geographical region or are used as part of a place name. If they are used as adjectives, they should be lowercase.

Capitalize	**Don't Capitalize**
Germany	southern fried chicken
Main Street	east of the city
Hoover Dam	western style
the old West	head north on the highway
South Dakota	

> Formal titles of events should be capitalized. Examples include Macy's Thanksgiving Day Parade, Boston Marathon, and Super Bowl Sunday.

Organizations

The names of organizations should be capitalized. Be sure to capitalize all major words in the title.

The pilot went to work for American Airlines.	✓ CORRECT
The pilot went to work for American airlines.	✗ INCORRECT
Professor Carter graduated from Princeton university.	✗ INCORRECT
Professor Carter graduated from Princeton University.	✓ CORRECT

Months, Days, and Holidays

The full names of months, days, and holidays are all capitalized.

✓ CORRECT	✗ INCORRECT
January	january
Tuesday	tuesday
St. Patrick's Day	St. Patrick's day
New Year's Eve	New Year's eve

The names of seasons—winter, spring, summer, and fall—are not normally capitalized, unless the season is included as part of a proper noun.

Don't Capitalize	Capitalize
spring flowers	Spring Fling
winter snow	Winter Solstice Festival
a summer day	Summer Concert Series
changing fall colors	Autumn Harvest Celebration

Review Questions

1. Which of the following phrases follows the rules of capitalization?

   A. Eastern Michigan
   B. aunt Becky
   C. Sergeant Smith
   D. Labor day

2. Which of the following book titles is correctly capitalized?

   A. *the Little Prince*
   B. *The Catcher In The Rye*
   C. *Anne of green gables*
   D. *Gone with the Wind*

3. Which of the following sentences uses capitalization rules correctly?

   A. I traveled with Aunt Lucy, Uncle Frank, and my Sister to Key West in southern Florida.
   B. I traveled with Aunt Lucy, Uncle Frank, and my sister to Key West in southern Florida.
   C. I traveled with aunt Lucy, uncle Frank, and my sister to Key West in southern Florida.
   D. I traveled with Aunt Lucy, Uncle Frank, and my sister to Key West in Southern Florida.

4. When our train arrived in New York City, Andrew's mother asked the station manager for directions to the Empire State building.

   Which of the following words in the sentence above should be capitalized?

   A. mother
   B. station
   C. manager
   D. building

5. Which of the following phrases follows the rules of capitalization?

   A. Italian bistro
   B. Art class
   C. professor Thomas
   D. Fourth of july

6. To garner support from democrats, each candidate made a campaign stop in the western part of the state.

   Which of the following words in the sentence above should be capitalized?

   A. democrats
   B. candidate
   C. western
   D. state

7. Which of the following phrases follows the rules of capitalization?

   A. their Cousin
   B. your Uncle
   C. my brother John
   D. aunt Barbara

8. Which of the following phrases follows the rules of capitalization?

   A. aunt Jane
   B. Chancellor Jones
   C. Eastern Connecticut
   D. New Year's day

9. Which of the following book titles is correctly capitalized?

   A. *War And Peace*
   B. *The Witch of blackbird pond*
   C. *Mansfield park*
   D. *Tuesdays with Morrie*

10. Which of the following sentences uses capitalization rules correctly?

    A. Last summer, my Family visited Redwood National Park in northern California.

    B. Last summer, my family visited Redwood National Park in Northern California.

    C. Last summer, my family visited Redwood National Park in northern California.

    D. Last summer, my family visited Redwood national park in northern California.

11. As part of their annual Class trip to Washington, DC, students from Jefferson High School visited the Smithsonian National Air and Space Museum.

Which of the following words in the sentence above should *not* be capitalized?

    A. Class
    B. Jefferson
    C. Smithsonian
    D. Museum

12. Which of the following phrases follows the rules of capitalization?

    A. irish heritage
    B. president Cooper
    C. music lessons
    D. Columbus day

13. To provide greater access to a college education, president Benson of Springside University has announced plans to add a satellite campus to the southeastern part of the state.

Which of the following words in the sentence above should be capitalized?

    A. college
    B. president
    C. campus
    D. southeastern

14. Which of the following book titles is correctly capitalized?

    A. *the Millionaire Next Door*
    B. *Last-Minute retirement planning*
    C. *Investing On a Shoestring*
    D. *Personal Finance for Dummies*

15. Which of the following sentences uses capitalization rules correctly?

A. Made up of three large waterfalls, Niagara Falls is located between western new york in the United States and southern Ontario in Canada.

B. Made up of three large waterfalls, Niagara Falls is located between western New York in the United States and southern ontario in Canada.

C. Made up of three large waterfalls, Niagara Falls is located between western New York in the United States and southern Ontario in Canada.

D. Made up of three large waterfalls, niagara falls is located between western New York in the United States and southern Ontario in Canada.

Answer Key

1. C		**9.** D	
2. D		**10.** C	
3. B		**11.** A	
4. D		**12.** C	
5. A		**13.** B	
6. A		**14.** D	
7. C		**15.** C	
8. B			

Answers and Explanations

1. (C) Since a specific title is used with a named person in choice C, it is considered a proper noun and should be capitalized. For choice A, the word *eastern* should not be capitalized since this word is used an as adjective instead of a place name. Choices B and D require capitalization of both words since each is a proper noun.

2. (D) Choice D is the only example of a correctly capitalized book title. Choice A fails to capitalize the first word in the title; choice B capitalizes a preposition and an article in the title, which is unnecessary; and choice C does not capitalize two major words in the title.

3. (B) Choice B correctly capitalizes *Aunt Lucy*, *Uncle Frank*, *Key West*, and *Florida* since these words are used as proper nouns in this

sentence. Choice A incorrectly capitalizes the word *sister*, which is used as a common noun, and choice D incorrectly capitalizes the word *southern*, which is used as an adjective and not a place name in this sentence.

4. (D) Because the word *building* is part of a proper noun describing a specific place, it should be capitalized in this sentence. The other choices are used as common nouns and therefore do not require capitalization.

5. (A) Since nationalities and their languages are capitalized, choice A is correct. Choice B does not require capitalization since it is not a specific course name. Choices C and D are incorrect because professional titles of named individuals and full names of holidays should be capitalized.

6. (A) Since the word *democrats* refers to a specific political party, it should be capitalized. Choices B, C, and D are used as common nouns in this context and therefore do not require capitalization.

7. (C) Words showing family relationships should only be capitalized when they are used as proper nouns. If the name is preceded by a possessive pronoun, the name is capitalized but not the word showing the family relationship: *Callie spoke with her aunt Barbara.*

8. (B) Since a specific title is used in front of a person's name in choice B, it is considered a proper noun and should be capitalized. Choices A and D require capitalization of both words since each is a proper noun. For choice C, the word *eastern* should not be capitalized since this word is used an as adjective instead of a place name.

9. (D) Choice D is the only example of a correctly capitalized book title in which the first word and all other important words are capitalized. Choice A is incorrect since the article *and* is capitalized, and choices B and C fail to capitalize major words in the title.

10. (C) Choice C correctly capitalizes *Redwood National Park* since these words describe a specific place. Choice A incorrectly capitalizes the word *family*, which is not used as a proper noun, and choice B incorrectly capitalizes the word *northern*, which is used as an adjective and not a place name in this sentence.

11. (A) The word *class* does not require capitalization since it is used as a common noun. Choices B, C, and D are all words describing a particular place name, so these proper nouns must all be capitalized.

12. (C) Because choice C is not the name of a specific class, there is no need to capitalize these words. Choices A, B, and D are incorrect because names of languages, professional titles of people, and full names of holidays are always capitalized.

13. (B) The word *president* should be capitalized since it is used as a proper noun referring to a specific person. It is not necessary to capitalize the words *college*, *campus*, or *southeastern* since these words do not name a particular person, place, or thing.

14. (D) Choice D is the only example of a correctly capitalized book title in which the first word and all other important words are capitalized. Choices A and C are incorrect since the article *the* and the preposition *on* are capitalized, and choice B fails to capitalize major words in the title.

15. (C) Choice C correctly capitalizes *Niagara Falls* since these words describe a specific place. Choices A and B are incorrect because the specific geographic place names, *New York* and *Ontario*, should be capitalized.

CHAPTER 45

Sentence Structure

Sentence Structure questions address clarity of expression, subordinating conjunctions, and how to combine sentences into a single sentence. You must also be able to distinguish between simple sentences, complex sentences, compound sentences, and sentence fragments.

Subordinating Conjunctions

In Chapter 43, we reviewed the use of coordinating conjunctions. These are connecting words, such as *and*, *but*, *so*, and *for*, which may be used to join two independent clauses:

> Ezra went to the store, and he bought some milk.

When a coordinating conjunction is used to join two independent clauses, as we saw earlier, the conjunction must always be preceded by a comma:

> Ezra went to the store and he bought some milk.   ✗ INCORRECT

> Ezra went to the store, and he bought some milk.   ✓ CORRECT

Independent clauses are considered independent because they can stand as complete sentences on their own. When we join two independent clauses with a coordinating conjunction, we are joining two clauses of equal weight. Neither is dependent on the other.

Dependent clauses, on the other hand, do not form complete sentences on their own. They start with connecting words known as subordinating conjunctions:

Dependent Clauses

Because she left early

Although the package was heavy

While Mr. Galloway waited

When the game was over

After the crowd dispersed

Subordinating conjunctions are connecting words used to start dependent clauses. They include the words *because*, *although*, *while*, *when*, *after*, *before*, *until*, *since*, *as*, *if*, and *once*, among others. Subordinating conjunctions can be used to join two clauses in a way that places emphasis on one of the clauses over the other:

Because its batteries had run low, <u>the alarm clock suddenly stopped working</u>.

In the example above, the underlined clause is an independent clause. It is placed at the end of the sentence, after the dependent clause *Because its batteries had run low*. This combination and ordering of clauses emphasizes the information at the end of the sentence. Here are a few more examples:

Although pizza is high in calories, <u>it's my favorite food</u>.

While the teacher was away, <u>the students talked loudly</u>.

Until it started to snow, <u>the weather had been gorgeous</u>.

Simple Sentences

A **simple sentence** contains one independent clause:

Ezra went to the store.

This sentence is considered simple because it contains only one independent clause and no dependent clauses. The following sentence is longer, but it is also a simple sentence:

Ezra went to the store and bought some milk.

Complex Sentences

Complex sentences contain an independent clause and one or more dependent clauses.

When Ezra went to the store, <u>he bought some milk</u>.

In this example, the underlined clause is an independent clause. The dependent clause is at the beginning of the sentence: *When Ezra went to the store*.

The following examples are all complex sentences, too:

Although pizza is high in calories, <u>it's my favorite food</u>.

While the teacher was away, <u>the students talked loudly</u>.

Until it started to snow, <u>the weather had been gorgeous</u>.

Each of these examples contains an independent clause (underlined) plus a dependent clause with a subordinating conjunction.

Compound Sentences

Compound sentences contain two or more independent clauses. They can be joined by a semicolon or by a comma and a coordinating conjunction.

The professor gave a great lecture today; we thoroughly enjoyed it.

The professor gave a great lecture today, and we thoroughly enjoyed it.

Sentence Fragments

A **sentence fragment** is a group of words that cannot stand on its own as a complete sentence. Sentence fragments often consist of solitary dependent clauses:

After Martin thought it over.	Fragment

This example is a fragment, because the clause *After Martin thought it* over doesn't provide enough information to stand on its own. We can change this fragment into a simple or complex sentence:

Martin thought it over.	Simple sentence
After Martin thought it over, he decided to attend.	Complex sentence

Sentence fragments can also be created if a sentence is missing its subject or its verb:

Thinking it over in the middle of the afternoon.	Fragment
Martin, who spent a lot of time thinking it over.	Fragment

As with the earlier sentence fragment, these examples do not stand as complete sentences on their own. One way to correct these examples would be to add a subject to the first sentence and a main verb to the second:

Martin was thinking it over in the middle of the afternoon.	Simple sentence
Martin, who spent a lot of time thinking it over, eventually decided to attend.	Simple sentence

Review Questions

1. The puppy barked. The puppy rolled over on his back. I realized the puppy wanted attention. I petted the puppy's head.

   To improve sentence fluency, which of the following best states the information above in a single sentence?

   A. When the puppy barked and I petted the puppy's head and realized he wanted attention, he rolled over on his back.
   B. I petted the puppy's head as I realized he wanted attention and rolled over on his back, and the puppy barked.
   C. When the puppy barked and rolled over on his back, I realized the puppy wanted attention, so I petted his head.
   D. I realized the puppy wanted attention, so the puppy rolled over on his back, and I petted the puppy's head, and the puppy barked.

2. Which of the following is a simple sentence?

   A. Jane's vegetable garden.
   B. Receives plentiful sunshine and produces ample tomatoes, cucumbers, and green beans.
   C. Because it receives plentiful sunshine, Jane's vegetable garden produces ample tomatoes, cucumbers, and green beans.
   D. Jane's vegetable garden receives plentiful sunshine and produces ample tomatoes, cucumbers, and green beans.

3. College tuition costs have continued to escalate rapidly. Many more students are applying for financial aid.

   Which of the following uses a conjunction to combine the sentences above so that the focus is more on students applying for financial aid and less on escalating tuition costs?

   A. Since college tuition costs have continued to escalate rapidly, many more students are applying for financial aid.
   B. College tuition costs have continued to escalate rapidly, and many more students are applying for financial aid.
   C. College tuition costs have continued to escalate rapidly; many more students are applying for financial aid.
   D. College tuition costs have continued to escalate rapidly, many more students are applying for financial aid.

4. Which of the following is an example of a simple sentence?

   A. Andrea was confused by the lack of road signs, and she drove 10 miles out of her way.
   B. Andrea was confused by the lack of road signs and drove 10 miles out of her way.
   C. Because she was confused by the lack of road signs, Andrea drove 10 miles out of her way.
   D. Andrea drove 10 miles out of her way because she was confused by the lack of road signs.

5. The barber shop on Main Street _____.

   Which of the following completions for the above sentence results in a simple sentence structure?

   A. decided to relocate since its lease expired at the shopping plaza.
   B. welcomed many new customers after its grand opening last weekend.
   C. is hiring several more employees, and applicants should inquire within.
   D. is a local landmark located in the city's historic district downtown.

6. Which of the following is a simple sentence?

   A. Mary was interested in archaeology before she studied paleontology.
   B. Since Dan and his friends enjoy skiing, they've decided to try snowboarding.
   C. Shingles on Jenna's garage roof are starting to come loose and must be replaced.
   D. Red apple varieties tend to be sweet, and green apples are crisp and tart.

7. Which of the following is an example of a simple sentence?

   A. The girl with the long, blond ponytail and pink jeans played on the elementary school playground after she completed her homework.
   B. The girl with the long, blond ponytail and pink jeans played on the elementary school playground.
   C. The girl with the long, blond ponytail and pink jeans playing on the elementary school playground.
   D. The girl with the long, blond ponytail and pink jeans.

8. Phil prepared for the final exam. He reviewed his lecture notes. He read chapters in his textbook. He attended a study session.

   Which of the following choices best uses grammar for style and clarity to combine the sentences above?

   A. Phil prepared for the final exam though he reviewed his lecture notes and read chapters in his textbook; he attended a study session.
   B. After Phil prepared for the final exam, he reviewed his lecture notes and read chapters in his textbook when he attended a study session.
   C. To prepare for the final exam, Phil reviewed his lecture notes, read chapters in his textbook, and attended a study session.
   D. Once Phil prepared for the final exam and he reviewed his lecture notes, then he read chapters in his textbook or attended a study session.

9. Which of the following is an example of a complex sentence?

   A. Before Ken may ride the bicycle he purchased from the yard sale, he must put air in the tires and fix the broken kickstand.
   B. Ken may ride the bicycle he purchased from the yard sale.
   C. Ken must put air in the bicycle's tires and fix the broken kickstand.
   D. Ken may ride the bicycle he purchased from the yard sale, but he must put air in the tires and fix the broken kickstand.

10. The man who walks his Labrador retriever by our house _____.

Which of the following allows the above sentence to be completed as a simple sentence?

A. sometimes stops to talk about mutual friends in the neighborhood.
B. sometimes stops to talk, and he likes to discuss mutual friends.
C. sometimes stops to talk although he only discusses mutual friends.
D. sometimes stops to talk when he wants to discuss mutual friends.

11. Which of the following sentences is most clear and correct?

A. The twins were adopted when they were two years old by Larry.
B. Larry adopted his twin sons when they were two years old.
C. Larry adopted his twin sons at the age of two years.
D. Two years old, Larry adopted his twin sons.

12. Samantha forgot to set her alarm clock. Her mother had to drive her to school.

Which of the following uses a conjunction to combine the sentences above so that the focus is more on Samantha's mother driving her to school and less on Samantha forgetting to set her alarm clock?

A. Because Samantha forgot to set her alarm clock, her mother had to drive her to school.
B. Samantha forgot to set her alarm clock, and her mother had to drive her to school.
C. Samantha forgot to set her alarm clock; her mother had to drive her to school.
D. Samantha forgot to set her alarm clock since her mother had to drive her to school.

13. Which of the following is a compound sentence?

A. My neighbor's porch light shines brightly at night and often keeps me awake.
B. Because my neighbor's porch light shines brightly at night, it often keeps me awake.
C. My neighbor's porch light shines brightly at night, and it often keeps me awake.
D. When my neighbor's porch light shines brightly at night, it often keeps me awake.

14. In the Northern Hemisphere, the winter solstice occurs _____.

Which of the following allows the above sentence to be completed as a simple sentence?

A. in late December, and it is the shortest day of the year.
B. in late December; it is the shortest day of the year.
C. in late December; furthermore, it is the shortest day of the year.
D. in late December and is the shortest day of the year.

15. Which of the following is an example of a complex sentence?

   A. Jamie enjoys socializing with friends, but he also appreciates quiet time alone.

   B. Although Jamie enjoys socializing with friends, he also appreciates quiet time alone.

   C. Jamie enjoys socializing with friends; conversely, he also appreciates quiet time alone.

   D. Jamie enjoys socializing with friends and also appreciates quiet time alone.

Answer Key

1. C		**9.** A	
2. D		**10.** A	
3. A		**11.** B	
4. B		**12.** A	
5. D		**13.** C	
6. C		**14.** D	
7. B		**15.** B	
8. C			

Answers and Explanations

1. **(C)** Choice C retains the intent of the original group of sentences by using dependent clauses and transitional words to subordinate the puppy's actions to the subject's response. The other choices muddle the meaning of the original sentences and place them in nonlinear sequences.

2. **(D)** Choice D is an example of a simple sentence containing one subject, *garden*, and one verb, *receives*. Since it contains a dependent clause, Choice C is a complex sentence. Choices A and B do not contain both a subject and a verb and are not complete sentences.

3. **(A)** Through the use of the subordinating conjunction *Since*, choice A positions the dependent clause pertaining to college tuition as secondary to the independent clause addressing students applying for financial aid.

4. **(B)** Choice B is an example of a simple sentence containing one subject, *Andrea*, and one compound verb, *was confused* and *drove*. Choice A is a compound sentence linking two independent clauses with the conjunction *and*, and choices C and D contain dependent clauses, making them complex sentences.

5. **(D)** Choice D provides an example of a simple sentence completion since it connects one verb, *is*, to one subject, *shop*. Choices A and B are complex sentences containing subordinating conjunctions, and choice C is a compound sentence.

6. **(C)** Even though this sentence contains a compound verb, it is composed of one independent clause and is therefore a simple sentence. Choices A and B are complex sentences with dependent clauses, and choice D is a compound sentence.

7. (B) Choice B presents a simple sentence containing one subject, *girl*, and one verb, *played*. Choice A contains a dependent clause and is therefore a complex sentence, and choices C and D are sentence fragments lacking a verb.

8. (C) Choice C retains the intent of the original group of sentences by using a dependent clause to introduce the purposeful sequence of actions performed by the subject, Phil. The other choices distort the meaning of the original sentences through inappropriate subordinate conjunctions.

9. (A) Choice A consists of a dependent clause followed by an independent clause, making it a complex sentence. Choices B and C are examples of a simple sentences, and choice D is a compound sentence.

10. (A) Choice A provides an example of a simple sentence completion since it connects one verb, *stops*, to one subject, *man*. Choice B is a compound sentence, and Choices C and D are complex sentences containing dependent clauses.

11. (B) Choice B clearly and correctly relates the writer's intent, connecting the plural pronoun *they* to the plural antecedent, *twins*. Choice A is less succinct, and choices C and D distort the writer's meaning through confusing word order.

12. (A) Through the use of the subordinating conjunction *Because*, choice A positions the dependent clause pertaining to Samantha's forgetting to set her alarm clock as secondary to the independent clause about her mother driving her to school. The use of the subordinating conjunction *since* in choice D changes the sentences' original intent.

13. (C) Choice C is a compound sentence. It contains two independent clauses joined by a comma and the coordinating conjunction *and*. The first independent clause is *My neighbor's porch light shines brightly at night*. The second independent clause is *it often keeps me awake*. Both of these clauses can stand as complete sentences on their own.

14. (D) Choice D provides an example of a simple sentence completion since it contains one subject, *solstice*, and one compound verb, *occurs* and *is*. The other choices are compound sentences connecting two independent clauses.

15. (B) Choice B consists of a dependent clause followed by an independent clause, making it a complex sentence. Choices A and C are examples of compound sentences, and choice D is a simple sentence.

CHAPTER 46

Points of View

Points of View questions address whether a text is written in the first person, second person, or third person. Questions also distinguish between third-person omniscient and third-person limited narration.

Texts written in the **first-person** point of view are written from the perspective of the narrator. They use first-person singular pronouns, such as *I*, *me*, *my*, and *mine*. They may also use first-person plural pronouns: *we*, *us*, *our*, and *ours*:

> I came home exhausted from the day's events. I wasn't looking forward to cooking dinner. But my family needed a good meal that night—we hadn't had a home-prepared meal in three or four days.

This paragraph contains text written in the first person. The narrator describes events from his or her point of view. The first-person pronouns *I* and *we* are used, which signal that the narrator is telling the story personally.

Texts written in the **second-person** point of view are written as though the narrator is talking to the reader directly. Second-person narratives use second-person singular and plural pronouns: *you*, *your*, and *yours*:

> You came home exhausted from the day's events. You weren't looking forward to cooking dinner. But your family needed a good meal that night—you hadn't had a home-prepared meal in three or four days.

Because of the use of second-person narrative, this paragraph seems to be describing events that happened to the reader. The pronouns *you* and *your* are used to depict the reader's experience.

Finally, texts written in the **third person** relay events from the perspective of one or more characters in the story. Third-person narratives use third-person singular pronouns, such as *he*, *she*, *him*, *her*, and *his*, *hers*. They may also use third-person plural pronouns: *they*, *them*, *their*, and *theirs*:

> Cheryl came home exhausted from the day's events. She wasn't looking forward to cooking dinner. But she felt that her family needed a good meal that night—she knew they hadn't had a home-prepared meal in three or four days.

Third-person texts can take one of two forms. **Third-person limited** narratives describe events from the perspective of only one character in the story. Readers are told how events unfold, but events are explained only from one character's viewpoint. Readers aren't given information from the perspective of other characters in the story.

Third-person omniscient narratives also use third-person pronouns, like third-person limited, but they relay events from the perspective of more than one character. With a third-person omniscient narrative, the reader is able to understand not just how the main character views events, but also how other characters perceive the action that is unfolding.

The preceding example is written in third-person limited narration. It gives the perspective of one character in the story, Cheryl. The following example, however, is written in third-person omniscient narration.

Harlan could never understand why each step of the business agreement required so much legal paperwork. He had had to sign paper after paper, and he tired of reading the fine print. Harlan was conservative when it came to business matters, and he liked to do his research. But he was also a practical sort. He wasn't going to spend hours reviewing texts if those hours would delay progress in the negotiation.

Harlan's lawyer couldn't have disagreed with him more. Martin Shaw was a seasoned contract attorney; Harlan had hired Shaw precisely because of his vast experience. Shaw watched Harlan's actions in the business negotiations with increasing concern. He wanted to protect his client's interests, but he couldn't do so if his client wasn't willing to take his advice. "Slow down," Shaw insisted, as he and Harlan spoke during a meeting break. "We don't need to surge through this all at once today."

This example gives the perspective of two characters in the story, Harlan and his lawyer, Martin Shaw. The first paragraph explains Harlan's perspective, while the second paragraph describes Shaw's.

Review Questions

1. Which of the following is an example of the third-person point of view?

   A. As soon as we get home from school, we are leaving for the concert.
   B. Bobby must stay after school today to make up a test he missed last week.
   C. I'm planning to pick Bobby up from school after I go to the store.
   D. Before you pick Bobby up from school, you should get ready for the concert.

2. Joseph did not want to go to his room that night and thought of many ways to delay his bedtime. His mother knew that Joseph was afraid of the dark, and she realized that she needed to help him overcome this fear while also providing comfort. She gently led him into his bedroom, checked under the bed and in the closet to make sure nothing scary was hiding in those places, and turned on his night light. Joseph felt better and understood that he was safe in his room.

From which of the following points of view is the above passage written?

A. First person
B. Second person
C. Third-person omniscient
D. Third-person limited

3. Which of the sentences in the following set of instructions is an example of the third-person point of view?

A. To make a delicious cup of coffee, I recommend using freshly ground coffee beans.
B. Fill the coffee maker with water up to the desired number of cups.
C. Next, you will add the ground coffee beans, about one tablespoon per cup of water.
D. Once the coffee is brewed, one may add cream and sugar to suit his or her tastes.

4. Which of the following is an example of the first-person point of view?

A. Seagulls along the shore competed for sandwich crumbs very aggressively.
B. Seagulls along the shore competed for our sandwich crumbs very aggressively.
C. Seagulls along the shore competed for your sandwich crumbs very aggressively.
D. Seagulls along the shore competed for his sandwich crumbs very aggressively.

5. When I was a college student, it was difficult for me to make a decision about my college major. At first, I considered majoring in fine arts, but my artistic talents did not seem equal to those of my classmates. I thought a business degree might serve me well later in life, but I found the courses didn't hold my interest. Finally, I decided to major in arts administration so that my appreciation of the arts could lead to gainful employment.

From which of the following points of view is the above passage written?

A. First person
B. Second person
C. Third-person omniscient
D. Third-person limited

6. Which of the sentences in the following set of instructions is an example of the second-person point of view?

A. Anyone may select young tomato plants at the nursery and easily transplant them.
B. I like to dig an ample hole in my garden or a large container to accommodate each new plant.
C. Gently remove the young tomato plant from its original container, place it in the hole, and cover the roots with rich soil.
D. Tomato plants will thrive in direct sunlight, and they prefer to grow in moist soil.

7. Which of the following is an example of the third-person point of view?

   A. I was surprised to hear that inactive volcanos may be dormant for thousands of years.
   B. Although you might believe a volcano is extinct, it could be in an extended dormant period.
   C. In my geology class, I learned that volcanos may remain dormant for thousands of years.
   D. Volcanos believed to have been extinct have erupted again following a long period of dormancy.

8. If you would like to apply for a scholarship this year, your first course of action should be a visit to the Student Services Office on campus. Representatives from this office will help you complete the necessary forms and analyze your financial need, and they will also recommend possible sources of scholarship funds. If you are awarded a scholarship, these funds will be applied to your tuition before the start of the fall semester.

   From which of the following points of view is the above passage written?

   A. First person
   B. Second person
   C. Third-person omniscient
   D. Third-person limited

9. Which of the sentences in the following set of instructions is an example of the first-person point of view?

   A. Before you begin painting a room, clean the walls with mild detergent and water.
   B. Although not an absolute requirement, priming the walls ensures a smooth finish.
   C. Prior to rolling on the paint, I use painter's tape to cover all baseboards and windows.
   D. Once the walls are painted, one must remove the painter's tape before the paint dries.

10. Which of the following is an example of the second-person point of view?

    A. Johnny is hoping for several inches of snow tonight so he can go sledding tomorrow.
    B. Johnny asked me if it will snow overnight so he can go sledding tomorrow.
    C. Johnny will be able to go sledding tomorrow if we get enough snow this evening.
    D. Johnny told you that he is hoping to go sledding tomorrow if it snows this evening.

11. As Katie stepped onto the large, inflatable raft, she felt her excitement about their white-water rafting excursion begin to mount. She had been looking forward to this trip for weeks, and now she and Joel were finally ready to set off on their adventure. Katie looked over at Joel, but his face wore its usual passive expression, and she could not tell if he was as enthusiastic as she was about their impending journey through the rapids.

    From which of the following points of view is the above passage written?

    A. First person
    B. Second person
    C. Third-person omniscient
    D. Third-person limited

12. Which of the sentences in the following set of instructions is an example of the first-person point of view?

    A. Taking care of cats has many challenges, such as establishing an ideal feeding schedule.
    B. In my experience, cats appreciate grazing on dry cat chow, so I give it to them twice each day.
    C. However, some cats prefer moist food, so you may offer it in addition to dry cat chow.
    D. A steady diet of high-quality cat food in both dry and moist varieties serves most cats very well.

13. Which of the following is an example of the third-person point of view?

    A. That retailer ensures that you always receive excellent customer service.
    B. When shopping at that retailer, I've noticed its focus on customer service.
    C. Retailers must prioritize customer service in order to remain competitive.
    D. I am more likely to shop at retailers that provide excellent customer service.

14. I've explained many times why I don't enjoy dining at the restaurant. Since the place is chronically understaffed, I always have to wait at least 30 minutes for a table. For me, the quality of the food served is not worth the long wait. I'm usually disappointed with my lukewarm and uninspired dinner once it finally arrives at my table.

    From which of the following points of view is the above passage written?

    A. First person
    B. Second person
    C. Third-person omniscient
    D. Third-person limited

15. Which of the sentences in the following set of instructions is an example of the third-person point of view?

    A. Journaling can be an effective tool for recording one's thoughts and feelings and charting personal growth over time.

    B. Right before bedtime, I find it therapeutic to write down my daily thoughts and experiences and my reactions to them, which gives me greater insight.

    C. You may prefer to write in your journal at other times of the day or on a less regimented schedule, which is fine, as long as you continue to write and reflect.

    D. Looking back over previous journal entries is also very helpful, for I can see how I've resolved certain issues and pinpoint areas still needing my attention.

Answer Key

1. B	**9.** C
2. C	**10.** D
3. D	**11.** D
4. B	**12.** B
5. A	**13.** C
6. C	**14.** A
7. D	**15.** A
8. B	

Answers and Explanations

1. (B) Only choice B provides an example of the third-person point of view. Choices A and C are written in the first person, and choice D is written in the second person.

2. (C) Choice C is an example of a passage written from the third-person omniscient point of view in which the narrator knows the thoughts and feelings of all the characters. The third-person point of view is indicated by words such as *his*, *him*, *he*, and *she*.

3. (D) Choice D is written from the third-person point of view, as signified by the word *one*. Choice A is written in the first person, and choices B and C are written in the second person, with choice B providing an example of "you" understood. The pronoun *you* is not expressly stated in choice B, but it is implied by the phrasing of the sentence.

4. (B) Because choice B uses the possessive pronoun *our*, it is written in the first person. Choices A and D are written from the third-person point of view, and choice C is written from the second-person point of view.

5. (A) Written from the first-person point of view, this passage uses pronouns such as *I*, *my*, and *me* to relate the narrator's experience of choosing a college major.

6. (C) Choice C is written in the second person, using the understood "you" construction common to imperative sentences or those giving a command. Choices A and D are written in the third person, and choice B is written in the first person.

7. (D) Choice D is written in the third person, a style common in academic writing. Choices A and C are written from the first-person point of view, and choice B is written from the second-person point of view.

8. (B) Pronouns such as *you* and *your* indicate that this passage is written in the second person. The second-person point of view is commonly used in writing that provides directions or instructions.

9. (C) Choice C is written in the first person, signified by the use of the pronoun *I*. Choice A is written in the second person, and choices B and D are written in the third person.

10. (D) Choice D is written in the second person, as indicated by the use of the pronoun *you*. Choice A is written from the third-person point of view, and choices B and C are written from the first-person point of view.

11. (D) Choice D is an example of a passage written from the third-person limited point of view in which the narrator knows the thoughts and feelings of just one character. The third-person point of view is indicated by words such as *she*, *her*, *their*, and *his*.

12. (B) Choice B is written in the first person, as indicated by the pronouns *my* and *I*. Choices A and D are written in the third person, and choice C is written in the second person.

13. (C) Choice C is written in the third person. Choice A is written from the second-person point of view, and choices B and D are written from the first-person point of view.

14. (A) Written from the first-person point of view, this passage uses pronouns such as *I*, *my*, and *me* to relate the narrator's comments.

15. (A) Choice A is written in the third person, as indicated by the use of the pronoun *one's*. Choices B and D are written in the first person, and choice C provides an example of the second-person point of view.

CHAPTER 47

Active vs. Passive Voice

Active vs. Passive Voice questions address whether a sentence is written using active verbs or passive verbs. You must distinguish between the two types of expression.

Active verbs are those that express action directly. When you use an active verb, the sentence typically shows the agent performing the action:

Raquel <u>purchased</u> the clock.   Active

In this sentence, *Raquel* is the agent performing the action. *Purchased* is the verb indicating the action. *The clock* is the object that was acted upon.

Sentences that use active verbs are said to be written in the **active voice**. Active voice sentences usually contain sentence components in this order:

Agent + action + object

Because active sentences often show the agent and the action directly, they tend to be straightforward in meaning and easily understood.

Instead of showing an agent acting, like active sentences do, **passive sentences** show an object being acted upon. When you use a passive verb, the sentence emphasizes the object that received the action:

The clock <u>was purchased</u> by Raquel.   Passive

In this example, *the clock* is the object being acted upon, *was purchased* is the verb showing the action, and *Raquel* is the agent performing the action.

Sentences that use passive verbs are written in the **passive voice**. Passive voice sentences typically contain sentence components in this order:

Object + action + agent

Some passive sentences may not even include the agent of the action at all:

The clock <u>was purchased</u> this morning.   Passive

In this sentence, it's not clear who purchased the clock. Because passive sentences tend to deemphasize the agent of the action, they can seem more obscure in meaning than active sentences. Passive sentences can even be used on purpose to obscure meaning:

A decision <u>was made</u> to terminate your employment.   Passive

Passive verbs are also used to convey meaning with constructions such as *it is* or *it was*:

<u>It is</u> anticipated that the ceremony will last for hours.	Passive
<u>It was</u> hoped that someone would come up with new ways of approaching the problem.	Passive

Helping Verbs

To identify passive sentences, look for helping verbs such as the "be" verbs *is*, *are*, *was*, *were*, and *will be*. Sentences in the passive voice will always contain helping verbs.

The piano <u>was tuned</u> by an expert.	Passive
In the story, many neighborhoods <u>are hit</u> by a devastating storm.	Passive
The tree <u>will be cut down</u> next summer.	Passive

To change a passive sentence into an active one, look for the agent of the action. Move the agent of the action to the subject position in the sentence, and eliminate the helping verb. Use an active verb that shows the action directly instead:

An expert <u>tuned</u> the piano.	Active
In the story, a devastating storm <u>hits</u> many neighborhoods.	Active

In these sentences, the active verbs *tuned* and *hits* have been substituted for the passive verbs. The agents of the action are *an expert* (first sentence) and *a devastating storm* (second sentence). These agents now come first in both sentences, before the active verbs.

If the agent of an action is not made clear in a sentence, such as in the third sentence in the passive examples above, an agent may need to be inserted in order to make the sentence active:

Our tree service <u>will cut down</u> the tree next summer.	Active

Here, we have specified that *our tree service* is performing the action of the sentence. This enables the sentence to use a future-tense active verb.

Review Questions

1. Thirty dollars was spent by Karlee at the craft show last weekend.

   Which of the following changes the sentence above so that it is written in the active rather than in the passive voice?

   A. During the weekend craft show, thirty dollars was spent by Karlee.
   B. Karlee spent thirty dollars at the craft show last weekend.
   C. When Karlee shopped at the craft show, thirty dollars was spent.
   D. At the craft show last weekend, thirty dollars was spent by Karlee.

2. Significant damage to the small, seaside town was caused by the recent hurricane.

   Which of the following changes the sentence above so that it is written in the active rather than the passive voice?

   A. Significant damage was caused by the recent hurricane's high winds to the small, seaside town.
   B. As residents have noted, significant damage was caused by the recent hurricane to the small, seaside town.
   C. Significant damage, including beach erosion, was caused by the recent hurricane to the small, seaside town.
   D. The recent hurricane caused significant damage to the small, seaside town.

3. Higher test scores in mathematics were achieved by students following intensive review sessions.

   Which of the following changes the sentence above so that it is written in the active rather than the passive voice?

   A. Students achieved higher test scores in mathematics following intensive review sessions.
   B. Higher test scores showing proficiency in mathematics were achieved by students following intensive review sessions.
   C. Higher test scores in mathematics, a high priority for the district, were achieved by students following intensive review sessions.
   D. To the relief of district administration, higher test scores in mathematics were achieved by students following intensive review sessions.

4. It was anticipated that the price of the company's stock would plummet following the abrupt resignation of its president.

Which of the following changes the sentence above so that it is written in the active rather than the passive voice?

A. It was anticipated by noted analysts that the price of the company's stock would plummet following the abrupt resignation of its president.
B. Following the abrupt resignation of its president, it was anticipated that the price of the company's stock would plummet.
C. Analysts predicted that the price of the company's stock would plummet following the abrupt resignation of its president.
D. It was anticipated that the price of the company's stock would plummet following the abrupt resignation of its president and the perceived lack of skilled leadership.

5. Articles for the local newspaper are often written by several part-time reporters.

Which of the following changes the sentence above so that it is written in the active rather than the passive voice?

A. Increasingly, articles for the local newspaper are written by several part-time reporters.
B. Articles for the local newspaper focusing on city government are often written by several part-time reporters.
C. Articles for the local newspaper are often written by several part-time reporters who also cover the news in other cities.
D. Several part-time reporters often write articles for the local newspaper.

6. The study investigating sleep disorders in children was conducted by Dr. Jean Allen, a noted child psychologist.

Which of the following changes the sentence above so that it is written in the active rather than the passive voice?

A. A noted psychologist, the study investigating sleep disorders in children was conducted by Dr. Jean Allen.
B. Dr. Jean Allen, a noted child psychologist, conducted the study investigating sleep disorders in children.
C. The study investigating sleep disorders in children, including nightmares and frequent waking, was conducted by Dr. Jean Allen, a noted child psychologist.
D. Over the past few months, the study investigating sleep disorders in children was conducted by Dr. Jean Allen, a noted child psychologist.

7. Data showing snow accumulation totals for the past winter were compiled by local meteorologists.

   Which of the following changes the sentence above so that it is written in the active rather than the passive voice?

   A. Data showing above-average snow accumulation totals for the past winter were compiled by local meteorologists.
   B. For the past winter, data showing snow accumulation totals were compiled by local meteorologists.
   C. Data by local meteorologists showing snow accumulation totals were compiled for the past winter.
   D. Local meteorologists compiled data showing snow accumulation totals for the past winter.

8. It was expected that health insurance costs would decrease for the next fiscal year.

   Which of the following changes the sentence above so that it is written in the active rather than the passive voice?

   A. It was expected that health insurance costs, as well as dental insurance costs, would decrease for the next fiscal year.
   B. Following the negotiation, it was expected that health insurance costs would decrease for the next fiscal year.
   C. Employees expected that their health insurance costs would decrease for the next fiscal year.
   D. It was believed by the employees that health insurance costs would decrease for the next fiscal year.

9. The private lives of celebrities are distorted and exploited by tabloid magazines.

   Which of the following changes the sentence above so that it is written in the active rather than the passive voice?

   A. Tabloid magazines distort and exploit the private lives of celebrities.
   B. The private lives of celebrities, from famous actors and actresses to notable sports figures, are distorted and exploited by tabloid magazines.
   C. For many years, the private lives of celebrities have been distorted and exploited by tabloid magazines.
   D. The private lives of celebrities, a constant source of fascination by avid readers, are distorted and exploited by tabloid magazines.

10. A blue ribbon was presented to the first-place swimmer by the head coach after the meet.

   Which of the following changes the sentence above so that it is written in the active rather than the passive voice?

   A. After the meet, a blue ribbon was presented to the first-place swimmer by the head coach.
   B. The head coach presented a blue ribbon to the first-place swimmer after the meet.
   C. In front of the cheering crowd, a blue ribbon was presented to the first-place swimmer by the head coach after the meet.
   D. A blue ribbon was presented to the first-place swimmer, in front of a cheering crowd, by the head coach.

11. Antibiotics were sometimes overprescribed by general practitioners prior to the revised guidelines.

   Which of the following changes the sentence above so that it is written in the active rather than the passive voice?

   A. Prior to the revised guidelines, antibiotics were sometimes overprescribed by general practitioners.
   B. Although common practice at the time, antibiotics were sometimes overprescribed by general practitioners prior to the revised guidelines.
   C. Prior to the revised guidelines, general practitioners sometimes overprescribed antibiotics.
   D. Antibiotics were sometimes overprescribed to patients requesting these medications by general practitioners prior to the revised guidelines.

12. The idea that the Earth's continents were originally one giant land mass called Pangaea has been widely accepted by scientists.

   Which of the following changes the sentence above so that it is written in the active rather than the passive voice?

   A. It has been widely accepted that the Earth's continents were originally one giant land mass called Pangaea by scientists.
   B. Over the past few decades, it has been widely accepted by scientists that the Earth's continents were originally one giant land mass called Pangaea.
   C. It has been widely accepted by scientists, who have reviewed convincing evidence, that the Earth's continents were originally one giant land mass called Pangaea.
   D. Scientists have widely accepted the idea that the Earth's continents were originally one giant land mass called Pangaea.

13. It is predicted that costs for fresh produce will continue to soar following last summer's extended drought.

    Which of the following changes the sentence above so that it is written in the active rather than the passive voice?

    A. Grocers predict that costs for fresh produce will continue to soar following last summer's extended drought.
    B. Following last summer's extended drought, it is predicted that costs for fresh produce will continue to soar.
    C. It is predicted that costs for fresh produce, including apples, oranges, and berries, will continue to soar following last summer's extended drought.
    D. It is predicted by grocers that costs for fresh produce will continue to soar following last summer's extended drought.

14. The letter of recommendation written by Professor Reed was sent to my prospective graduate program last week.

    Which of the following changes the sentence above so that it is written in the active rather than the passive voice?

    A. Last week, the letter of recommendation written by Professor Reed was sent to my prospective graduate program.
    B. Written by Professor Reed, the letter of recommendation was sent to my prospective graduate program last week.
    C. Professor Reed sent the letter of recommendation he wrote to my prospective graduate program last week.
    D. Sent to my prospective graduate program last week, the letter of recommendation was written by Professor Reed.

15. Perhaps the most famous work of art ever created, the *Mona Lisa*, was painted in the early sixteenth century by Leonardo da Vinci.

    Which of the following changes the sentence above so that it is written in the active rather than the passive voice?

    A. Painted in the early sixteenth century by Leonardo da Vinci, the *Mona Lisa* is perhaps the most famous work of art ever created.
    B. Leonardo da Vinci painted the *Mona Lisa*, perhaps the most famous work of art ever created, in the early sixteenth century.
    C. The *Mona Lisa*, perhaps the most famous work of art ever created, was painted in the early sixteenth century by Leonardo da Vinci.
    D. Perhaps the most famous work of art ever created, the *Mona Lisa* was painted in the early sixteenth century by Leonardo da Vinci and is displayed in the Louvre in Paris.

Answer Key

1. B
2. D
3. A
4. C
5. D
6. B
7. D
8. C

9. A
10. B
11. C
12. D
13. A
14. C
15. B

Answers and Explanations

1. **(B)** The original sentence uses the passive construction *thirty dollars was spent*. In choice B, the passive sentence is rewritten in the active voice in which the subject, *Karlee,* performs the action in the sentence, *spent*.

2. **(D)** The sentence given uses the passive construction *damage was caused*. Choice D presents an example of a sentence written in the active voice in which the subject, *hurricane,* performs the action in the sentence, *caused*.

3. **(A)** Choice A is an example of a sentence written in the active voice in which the subject, *Students,* performs the action, *achieved*. All of the other choices are written with passive voice construction.

4. **(C)** The sentence given uses the passive construction *It was anticipated*. Choice C presents an example of a sentence written in the active voice in which the subject, *Analysts,* performs the action in the sentence, *anticipated*.

5. **(D)** The original sentence uses the passive construction *Articles are written*. In choice D, the passive sentence is rewritten in the active voice in which the subject, *reporters,* performs the action in the sentence, indicated by the active verb *write*.

6. **(B)** Choice B is an example of a sentence written in the active voice in which the subject, *Dr. Jean Allen,* performs the action, *conducted*. All of the other choices are written with passive voice construction.

7. **(D)** The original sentence uses the passive construction *Data were compiled*. In choice D, the passive sentence is rewritten in the active voice in which the subject, *meteorologists,* performs the action in the sentence, *compiled*.

8. **(C)** Choice C is an example of a sentence written in the active voice in which the subject, *Employees,* performs the action, *expected*. All of the other choices are written with passive voice construction.

9. **(A)** The original sentence uses the passive construction *lives are distorted and exploited*. In choice A, the passive sentence is rewritten in the active voice in which the subject, *magazines,* performs the action in the sentence, indicated by the active verbs *distort* and *exploit*.

10. **(B)** The sentence given uses the passive construction *a blue ribbon was presented*. Choice B presents an example of a sentence written in the active voice in which the subject, *coach,* performs the action in the sentence, *presented*.

11. (C) Choice C is an example of a sentence written in the active voice in which the subject, *general practitioners*, performs the action, *overprescribed*. All of the other choices are written with passive voice construction.

12. (D) The sentence given uses the passive construction *idea has been accepted*. Choice D presents an example of a sentence written in the active voice in which the subject, *Scientists*, performs the action in the sentence, *have accepted*.

13. (A) The original sentence uses the passive construction *It is predicted*. In choice A, the passive sentence is rewritten in the active voice in which the subject, *Grocers,* performs the action in the sentence, *predict*.

14. (C) Choice C is an example of a sentence written in the active voice in which the subject, *Professor Reed*, performs the action, *sent*. All of the other choices are written with passive voice construction.

15. (B) The original sentence uses the passive construction *Mona Lisa was painted*. In choice B, the passive sentence is rewritten in the active voice in which the subject, *Leonardo da Vinci,* performs the action in the sentence, *painted*.